CARDIAC EMERGENCY CARE

CARDIAC EMERGENCY CARE

Edited by

EDWARD K. CHUNG, M.D.

Professor of Medicine
Jefferson Medical College of
Thomas Jefferson University
and
Director of the Heart Station
Thomas Jefferson University Hospital
Philadelphia

LEA & FEBIGER · *Philadelphia*

Library of Congress Cataloging in Publication Data

Chung, Edward K.
  Cardiac emergency care.

  Includes index.
    1. Heart—Diseases. 2. Medical emergencies.
3. Coronary care units. I. Title. [DNLM: 1. Emer-
gencies—Congresses. 2 Heart diseases—Congresses.
WG205 C559c]
RC682.C55 1975   616.1′2′025   74-26878
ISBN 0-8121-0516-8

Published in Great Britain by Henry Kimpton Publishers, London
Printed in the United States of America

Print number: 4 3 2

To My Wife, Lisa
and
To Linda and Christopher

PREFACE

It is not the purpose of this book to discuss in depth various subjects in medicine or to describe in detail all possible emergency medical events. The primary intention is to describe common cardiac emergencies which are frequently encountered in our daily practice.

The contents are intended to be clinical, concise, and practical. It is hoped that this book will provide all physicians with up-to-date materials that will assist them directly in the daily care of their patients with cardiac emergency problems.

The book will be particularly valuable to house staff, cardiology fellows, practicing internists, cardiologists, family physicians, and emergency room physicians, as well as coronary care unit nurses. In addition, medical students will derive great benefit from reading this book in learning a general approach to various cardiac emergencies.

I am grateful to all authors for their valuable contributions to *Cardiac Emergency Care*. I also wish to thank my personal secretary, Miss Theresa McAnally, for her devoted and cheerful secretarial assistance. She has been most helpful in handling correspondence with the contributors, as well as in typing several chapters of mine for this book. It has been my pleasure to work with the staff of Lea & Febiger Publishers. In particular, I would like to express my thanks to Mr. R. Kenneth Bussy, Executive Editor, for his indispensable assistance.

Philadelphia   EDWARD K. CHUNG, M.D.

CONTRIBUTORS

A. A. J. Adgey, M.B., M.R.C.P.
Physician, Cardiac Department
Royal Victoria Hospital
Belfast, Northern Ireland

Theodore L Biddle, M.D.
Assistant Professor of Medicine
Cardiology Unit
University of Rochester School of Medicine
Rochester, New York

Albert N. Brest, M.D., F.A.C.P., F.A.C.C.
James C. Wilson Professor of Medicine
Director, Division of Cardiology
Thomas Jefferson University
Philadelphia, Pennsylvania

Stanley K. Brockman, M.D., F.A.C.S., F.A.C.C.
Professor of Surgery
Director, Division of Cardiovascular Surgery
Thomas Jefferson University
Philadelphia, Pennsylvania

Agustin Castellanos, M.D., F.A.C.C.
Professor of Medicine
University of Miami School of Medicine
Miami, Florida

Edward K. Chung, M.D., F.A.C.P., F.A.C.C.
Professor of Medicine
Jefferson Medical College of
    Thomas Jefferson University and
Director of the Heart Station
Thomas Jefferson University Hospital
Philadelphia, Pennsylvania

Jay N. Cohn, M.D., F.A.C.P., F.A.C.C.
Professor of Medicine
Head, Cardiovascular Section
University of Minnesota School of Medicine
Minneapolis, Minnesota

William J. Grace, M.D., F.A.C.P., F.A.C.C.
Professor of Clinical Medicine
New York University Bellevue Medical Center
Director, Department of Medicine,
St. Vincent's Hospital
New York, New York

George H. Khoury, M.D., F.A.A.P., F.A.C.C.
Professor of Pediatrics
Director, Division of Pediatric Cardiology
West Virginia University School of Medicine
Morgantown, West Virginia

Albert Klainer, M.D., F.A.C.P.
Professor of Medicine
Director, Division of Infectious Disease
West Virginia University School of Medicine
Morgantown, West Virginia

Louis Lemberg, M.D., F.A.C.P., F.A.C.C.
Clinical Professor of Medicine
University of Miami School of Medicine
Miami, Florida

J. F. Pantridge, M.D., F.R.C.P., F.A.C.C.
Professor of Cardiology
The Queen's University of Belfast
Belfast, Northern Ireland

Leon Resnekov, M.D., F.R.C.P., F.A.C.C.
Professor of Medicine
Joint Director, Division of Cardiology
University of Chicago School of Medicine
Chicago, Illinois

Sol Sherry, M.D., F.A.C.P., F.A.C.C.
Professor and Chairman
Department of Medicine
Temple University School of Medicine
Philadelphia, Pennsylvania

David H. Spodick, M.D., F.A.C.P., F.A.C.C.
Professor of Medicine
Tufts University School of Medicine
Director, Division of Cardiology
Lemuel Shattuck Hospital
Boston, Massachusetts

Paul Walinsky, M.D.
Assistant Professor of Medicine
Director, Intermediate Coronary Care Unit
Thomas Jefferson University
Philadelphia, Pennsylvania

Leslie Wiener, M.D., F.A.C.P., F.A.C.C.
Professor of Medicine
Director, Coronary Care Unit
Thomas Jefferson University
Philadelphia, Pennsylvania

Paul N. Yu, M.D., F.A.C.P., F.A.C.C.
Sarah McCort Ward Professor of Medicine
Director, Division of Cardiology
University of Rochester School of Medicine
Rochester, New York

CONTENTS

Chapter 1

ACUTE PULMONARY EDEMA

THEODORE L. BIDDLE
PAUL N. YU

Acute congestive heart failure is a common medical emergency. Prompt treatment must be instituted in order to correct the condition and lower the mortality. In this chapter, acute pulmonary edema of both cardiac and noncardiac origin will be discussed, with particular emphasis on a practical overview for clinical management.

Four anatomic compartments of the pulmonary circuit have been delineated in an effort to improve our understanding of the pathophysiology of heart failure[1]: The *vascular compartment* consists of the pulmonary arteries, capillaries, and veins that participate in fluid exchange with the interstitial tissue of the lung. The *alveolar compartment* comprises the alveoli, whose walls are made up of epithelial cells with a lipoprotein layer called surfactant. This layer coats the inner alveolar surface and exerts an "anti-atelectasis effect," stabilizing alveoli and preventing their collapse under conditions of low alveolar volume. The *interstitial space* is interposed between the small pulmonary vessels and the alveoli and also contains small lymphatics and conducting airways. The *lymphatic space* denotes the extensive network of pulmonary lymphatics that drain excess fluid from the alveolar and interstitial compartments. Endothelial cells of the pulmonary capillaries, alveoli, and lym-

This work was supported in part by MIRU Contract No. HV 81331, HL 03966 and HL 05500 from the National Heart and Lung Institute, National Institutes of Health, Besthesda, Maryland.

phatics and other cell types have been dealt with extensively elsewhere.[1,3] Their specific functions, while of great importance, will not be described in this review.

Two important cell-mediated responses in pulmonary edema involve the generation of early symptoms and late pathologic change. The J receptors in the interstitial space act as stretch receptors stimulated by increases in interstitial pressure or fluid; this stimulation results in the characteristic tachypnea of acute congestive heart failure. Also, edema fluid promotes the formation of collagen, reticulum, and elastic fibers in the interstitial space. This phenomenon may lead to the interstitial fibrosis common among patients with chronic elevation of pulmonary capillary pressure.

Traditionally, the pathophysiology of pulmonary edema has dealt with (1) increased hydrostatic pressure or (2) increased permeability of the alveolar–capillary "membrane." This approach cannot account for the wide variety of illnesses characterized by pulmonary edema. In general, one or more of four potential factors are responsible for the production of acute pulmonary edema: (1) elevated pulmonary capillary pressure, (2) damage to the pulmonary capillary "membrane," (3) decrease in plasma osmotic pressure, and (4) impaired lymphatic drainage. Our etiologic approach will deal with both cardiac and noncardiac forms of pulmonary

Table 1-1   *Etiology of Acute Pulmonary Edema*

Cardiac
　Left ventricular failure
　　Myocardial infarction
　　Acute decompensation of chronic left ventricular
　　　failure—aortic, hypertensive, or cardiomyopathic
　　Mitral valve disease
　　Volume overload

Noncardiac
　Altered permeability of pulmonary capillary membrane
　　Inhalation of toxic agents
　　Adult respiratory distress syndrome
　　Bacteremic sepsis
　　Uremia
　　Radiation pneumonitis
　　Disseminated intravascular coagulation
　Decreased plasma osmotic pressure—hypoalbuminemia
　Lymphatic obstruction
　Uncertain etiology
　　High-altitude pulmonary edema
　　Heroin overdose
　　Pulmonary embolism
　　Neurogenic
　　Postanesthetic

edema (Table 1-1). The cardiac forms will be discussed extensively in this chapter, but a broad knowledge of the many causes of pulmonary edema is necessary for intelligent management.

The most common cause of acute pulmonary edema is cardiac disease, whether atherosclerotic, valvular, hypertensive, or myopathic in origin. Pericardial disease will be dealt with in Chapters 12 and 13. Acute or chronic myocardial "failure" occurs when the left ventricle is unable to eject the normal stroke volume. Thus diastolic pressure in the left ventricle rises and results in an elevation of left atrial and pulmonary venous pressure. Normally, plasma oncotic pressure prevents a substantial diffusion of fluid across the normal capillary membrane to the interstitial space. With increasing hydrostatic pressure, however, interstitial and intra-alveolar edema may occur. The amount of lung water in patients with acute myocardial infarction complicated by heart failure has been estimated.[4,5] The lung water measured by a double isotope technique increased with increasing severity of pulmonary congestion by both clinical and radiographic criteria (Fig. 1-1 and 1-2). A significant correlation was found between the pulmonary capillary (wedge) pressure and lung water. In all patients with acute pulmonary

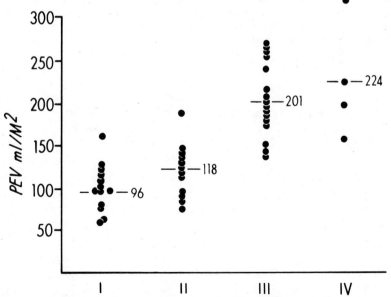

Figure 1-1. Pulmonary extravascular volume (PEV) in patients with acute myocardial infarction, clinical classification. Class I, uncomplicated; class II, S₃ gallop and pulmonary rales; class III, frank pulmonary edema; and class IV, cardiogenic shock. The mean value in each class of patients is represented by a horizontal line. Note progressive increase in PEV from class I to class IV patients.

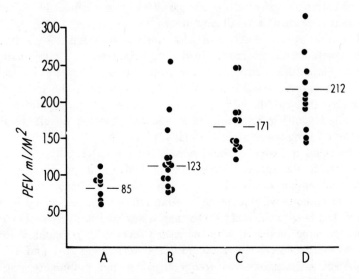

Figure 1-2. Pulmonary extravascular volume (PEV) in patients with acute myo-cardial infarction classified according to changes in the chest x-ray. Class A, normal; class B, pulmonary congestion; class C, interstitial edema; and class D, frank pulmonary edema. The mean value in each class of patients is repre-sented by a horizontal line. A progressive increase in PEV is observed from class A to class D patients.

edema the pulmonary wedge pressure was elevated. With clinical im-provement, both the pulmonary wedge pressure and the lung water de-creased. Increasing arterial hypoxemia has been correlated with more severe pulmonary edema and elevation of lung water.[5]

In patients with left ventricular failure secondary to aortic valve dis-ease, hypertensive cardiovascular disease, or cardiomyopathy, the ele-vated left ventricular end diastolic pressure eventually leads to an in-crease in pulmonary capillary pressure and fluid in interstitial or alveolar compartments of the lungs. Patients with rheumatic mitral stenosis de-velop an elevation of left atrial and, subsequently, pulmonary capillary pressure. The magnitude of mitral valvular obstruction and increase in hydrostatic force largely determine the severity of pulmonary congestion.

Volume overload from excessive intravenous fluid therapy may pre-cipitate acute pulmonary edema but probably only in patients with pre-existing myocardial dysfunction.

Noncardiac types of pulmonary edema are usually related to altera-tions in permeability of the pulmonary capillary membrane.[2] An offending agent may cause damage to the capillary endothelium or alveolar epithelium without deleterious myocardial effects. Pulmonary congestion therefore could occur in the absence of left ventricular dysfunction. Inhalation of smoke or toxic gases such as chlorine, phosgene, hydrogen sulfide, metallic oxides, and nitrogen dioxide may be associated with fulminant pulmonary edema.[6]

The term "adult respiratory distress syndrome" has been used to denote pulmonary parenchymal damage with interstitial edema of several causes. Shock, extracorporeal oxygenation, and mechanical ventilation with high partial pressure of inspired oxygen have all been associated with loss of capillary endothelial integrity. The resultant clinical picture of pulmonary edema with progressive respiratory failure is thought to be secondary to altered permeability, but the exact mechanism of injury has yet to be defined.

Bacteremic sepsis with endotoxemia has resulted in pulmonary edema without an elevated pulmonary capillary pressure. Vasoactive peptides (histamine, serotonin, kinins), as well as local endothelial cell damage, may be responsible for the pulmonary congestion.[7,8] Impaired myocardial function in bacteremic sepsis has been demonstrated in experimental animals.[9,10] This direct myocardial depressant effect may be present in some cases of sepsis in man.[11] Uremia, high doses of radiation, and disseminated intravascular coagulation may also induce pulmonary edema as a result of vascular endothelial injury.

An abrupt fall in plasma protein concentration that results in reduced osmotic pressure may cause pulmonary edema with only moderate volume overload in the absence of left ventricular failure.[2]

Lymphatic obstruction with impaired drainage has produced pulmonary edema experimentally. The clinical counterpart may exist in the pulmonary edema occasionally seen in silicosis and lymphangitic carcinomatosis.[12]

Other syndromes of acute pulmonary edema have been well described clinically, but their precise etiology is unknown. Patients without previous cardiopulmonary disease have manifested pulmonary edema upon sudden exposure to high altitude. The illness is reversed when they descend toward sea level, and other manifestations of heart disease are found to be lacking.[13] Similarly, overdose of intravenous heroin and other narcotics have resulted in florid pulmonary congestion and frequently death in respiratory failure despite normal cardiac function.[14] The pulmonary edema associated with acute pulmonary embolism may occur secondary to changes in vascular permeability or acute pulmonary hypertension[15] (see Chapter 2). In addition, fluid accumulation has been associated with fat embolization. Injuries to the central nervous system and the use of general anesthesia have also been associated with acute pulmonary edema of unexplained etiology.

TREATMENT OF CARDIAC PULMONARY EDEMA

Acute pulmonary edema may be of such rapid onset and of such life-threatening potential that immediate and intelligent management is mandatory. Severe respiratory distress is often accompanied by frothy blood-tinged sputum, cold clammy extremities, and the patient's terrifying fear of drowning in his own secretions.

Pulmonary edema is most commonly secondary to disease of the left side of the heart except for less common noncardiac causes as mentioned in the previous section. Initial management therefore should involve consideration of the exact etiology. The patient may have knowledge of previous heart disease, but acute pulmonary edema is often the first manifestation of cardiac illness. Generally, treatment should follow the history, physical examination, electrocardiogram, and roentgenogram of the chest, but the magnitude of the illness usually demands some emergency therapy while the results of diagnostic tests are being assembled.

The management of acute pulmonary edema will be discussed according to the physiologic approach outlined in Table 1-2.

Improvement in Ventilation

Treatment usually applicable to all cases of acute pulmonary edema, regardless of etiology, includes attention to techniques to optimize venti-

Table 1-2   *Treatment of Acute Pulmonary Edema*

General measures to improve ventilation
Sitting position
Oxygen therapy
Reduction in pulmonary capillary pressure
Decrease in left ventricular filling pressure—rotating tourniquets, morphine, diuretics, phlebotomy
Decrease in impedance to left ventricular ejection—vasodilating agents
Increase in myocardial contractility—digitalis, catecholamines, glucagon
Alteration in capillary permeability
Removal of offending agent
Ventilatory support
Anti-inflammatory agents
Additional measures
Aminophylline
Mechanical ventilation
Bedside cardiac catheterization

latory function. The sitting position is usually the most comfortable and advantageous for several reasons. Venous return to the heart is reduced, thus lowering pulmonary blood volume and congestion. The upright position also decreases the work of breathing and increases vital capacity.[16] The arterial hypoxemia common to acute pulmonary edema warrants oxygen therapy to raise alveolar oxygenation and prevent the metabolic consequences of sustained tissue hypoxia. Pulmonary congestion from left ventricular dysfunction is thought to produce a ventilation–perfusion imbalance responsible for the hypoxemia. In acute myocardial infarction the degree of hypoxemia correlates with the magnitude of heart failure.[17,18]

A mask or nasal catheter is usually adequate for oxygen delivery, and arterial blood gases should be monitored in severe cases of pulmonary congestion. The partial pressure of carbon dioxide is usually normal, but a mild respiratory alkalosis is frequently observed even in lesser degrees of left ventricular dysfunction.[19] Carbon dioxide retention is uncommon in pulmonary edema of cardiac origin unless complicated by coexistent pulmonary disease. If hypercarbia (pCO_2 greater than 50 mm Hg) and severe hypoxemia (pO_2 less than 60 mm Hg) occur despite oxygen therapy and optimum medical treatment, intubation and mechanical ventilation are usually necessary. Care must be exercised, however, for high levels of inspired oxygen (greater than 50%) and prolonged positive pressure ventilation may result in oxygen toxicity or the "adult respiratory distress syndrome."[21] A safe approach would be to increase the inspired oxygen concentration to 30–40% by mask at 4 to 6 liters per minute and measure arterial blood gases if prolonged therapy is necessary. Without intubation, the highest actual level of inspired oxygen delivered even with 100% oxygen flow is about 50–60%.[21] Thus the risk of oxygen toxicity using the standard disposable face mask is low. If the pCO_2 is between 35 and 40 mm Hg, pO_2 is maintained above 80 mm Hg, and the pH is normal, adequate ventilatory support has been provided.

Reduction in Pulmonary Capillary Pressure

A major therapeutic goal in the management of acute pulmonary edema involves the reduction in venous return to the right heart to alleviate further pulmonary congestion. The time-honored use of venous occlusive tourniquets or cuffs on extremities can be safe and efficient if arterial flow is not compromised. This technique can be of only temporary benefit, however, for the major physiologic defect of cardiac decompensation has not been alleviated. Prolonged venous occlusion may result in thrombosis and the threat of embolic phenomenon. Although effective, therefore, rotating tourniquets should be used only in addition to other therapeutic maneuvers.

The therapeutic effectiveness of morphine sulfate is not completely understood, but several beneficial possibilities exist in pulmonary edema of cardiac origin. Vasodilatation probably occurs and decreases venous return and pulmonary capillary hydrostatic pressure.[23,24] Morphine may also alleviate pain or anxiety and provide for a more favorable respiratory pattern. Small doses (4 to 5 mg) may be given intravenously with rapid effectiveness. Subcutaneous or intramuscular routes of injection may result in delayed effectiveness in hypotensive patients with poor peripheral perfusion, but the hazards of drug-induced hypotension or respiratory depression are less than with intravenous use. Our practice has been to administer morphine intravenously in the severe cases of pulmonary edema if the blood pressure is maintained above 100 mm Hg.

Diuretics have been utilized in acute congestive heart failure to promote a reduction in pulmonary capillary pressure by decreasing plasma volume. Furosemide and ethacrynic acid when given intravenously can indeed induce a rapid diuresis; it is questionable however, whether alveolar or interstitial fluid is actually mobilized. A reduction in plasma volume by diuresis would, at least, aid in preventing any further increase in pulmonary capillary pressure. Furosemide appears to have additional beneficial effects in patients with left ventricular failure complicating acute myocardial infarction. A decrease in pulmonary artery pressure occurs 5 to 15 minutes after injection, before any possible diuretic effect, and is probably related to changes in venous capacitance.[25] Thus a decrease in hydrostatic pressure, a reduction in venous return, and the prompt diuretic effect provide a valuable mechanism of treatment.

In severe cases of acute congestive heart failure, phlebotomy may be helpful when other measures are ineffective or for some reason unavailable. Cautious venesection of 300 to 500 ml of blood can be effective in decreasing venous return and, therefore, pulmonary capillary pressure. Plasmapheresis separates red cells from plasma and makes the former available for retransfusion. Severely volume-overloaded patients can be bled 500 ml initially, and, following plasmapheresis, the packed cells can be retransfused during subsequent phlebotomies. This technique provides continued reduction in plasma volume without significant loss of red cells.

A new concept in the treatment of pulmonary congestion involves the reduction in impedance to left ventricular emptying by systemic vasodilatation. If systolic unloading of the ventricle were facilitated, abnormal diastolic volume of the ventricle and hence pulmonary venous pressure would be reduced. Probably some of the therapeutic effects of morphine sulfate involve direct reduction in peripheral resistance by systemic vasodilatation and indirect reduction by the sedative effect. Recent investigation of acute myocardial infarction with agents promoting systemic vasodilatation has further substantiated this new concept of the beneficial effects of reducing blood pressure. Gold and co-workers found that sublingual nitroglycerin reduced pulmonary wedge pressure and arterial pressure in patients with advanced heart failure associated with acute myocardial infarction.[26] The rapid fall in pulmonary wedge pressure was accompanied by an increase in cardiac output. Thus, peripheral blood flow was increased while the hydrostatic force responsible for pulmonary congestion was reduced. These beneficial effects are probably secondary to the peripheral vascular action of nitroglycerin, but they may conceivably be related to changes in the coronary circulation or myocardial contractility. Caution must be exercised in acute myocardial infarction, however, for sublingual nitroglycerin may induce significant hypotension, a reduction in coronary blood flow, and further ischemic damage. The drug may be of benefit in patients with pulmonary congestion who can be closely monitored, ideally with direct measurements of pulmonary wedge pressure and cardiac output.

Reduction in pulmonary capillary pressure by vasodilator therapy can be more safely achieved by intravenous infusions of drugs such as phentolamine or nitroprusside. The same principle of reduction in impedance to left ventricular emptying by peripheral vasodilatation is applicable, but a safer and more predictable drug effect is possible with sustained pump infusion. When treated with nitroprusside, patients with acute myocardial infarction and abnormal elevation of pulmonary wedge pressure undergo a prompt reduction in pulmonary wedge pressure and rise in cardiac output with only a modest decrease in systemic blood pressure.[27,28] Phentolamine and nitroprusside should not be considered first-line drugs in the management of acute pulmonary edema. Like sublingual nitrates, their use may be hazardous if not closely monitored by experienced physicians, with right heart catheterization and precise measurement of pulmonary wedge pressure and cardiac output readily available.

The authors have found nitroprusside to be beneficial in the management of protracted left ventricular failure complicating acute myocardial infarction that is resistant to standard medical therapy. Structural defects such as acute papillary muscle dysfunction and ventricular septal rupture are usually amenable to treatment with nitroprusside. In the former, a reduction in systemic peripheral resistance with nitroprusside facilitates left ventricular emptying and decreases regurgitant flow through the incompetent mitral valve. Acute ventricular septal rupture in myocardial infarction grossly increases pulmonary blood flow and congestion because of the left-to-right shunt. In our laboratory, we have demonstrated a reduction in both left-to-right shunt flow and pulmonary congestion in acute septal rupture treated with intravenous nitroprusside. The initial studies with these new agents are promising, and further investigation is warranted.

Increase in Myocardial Contractility

Another major therapeutic approach in the management of acute pulmonary edema has involved the use of inotropic drugs. True left ventricular failure implies a decrease in myocardial contractility. An increase in stroke volume would theoretically be beneficial both by lowering the elevated pulmonary venous pressure and by increasing renal blood flow to induce diuresis and reduce plasma volume. Agents utilized for this purpose include digitalis, catecholamines, and glucagon.

Digitalis. Digitalis is recommended in acute congestive heart failure as adjunctive therapy to oxygen, rotating tourniquets, morphine sulfate, and diuretics. Many patients can be successfully treated without digitalis, and use of the drug may have serious consequences; patients with acute myocardial infarction appear to be more sensitive to the drug, and toxic rhythm disturbances may result.[30] In addition, the hemodynamic response to digitalis in acute myocardial infarction is unpredictable.[30,31] With an increase in myocardial contractility, oxygen consumption must also increase, and concern is often expressed that the use of digitalis in acute myocardial infarction may actually extend the area of necrosis. If cardiomegaly exists in congestive heart failure, however, an increase in myocardial oxygen consumption by digitalis administered to increase contractility will be offset by a decrease in oxygen requirement produced by the reduction in left ventricular size and wall tension.[29] The problem is unsolved, but it is recommended that digitalis not be used in mild left ventricular failure that can be managed with diuretics alone.

When the severity of acute congestive heart failure warrants digitalis therapy, the intravenous route is advisable. Many patients have nausea and vomiting, and gastrointestinal absorption of an oral dose may be uncertain. The intermediate preparation digoxin can be given in initial doses of 0.5 to 0.75 mg intravenously, with additional 0.25 mg doses in 2 to 4 hours if necessary, depending upon the patient's response. Factors of body size, electrolyte imbalance, and other drug therapy must be considered. It is important to remember that a significant inotropic response can be achieved with doses less than those considered to represent full digitalization.[30]

Digitalis can be of benefit in pulmonary edema due to mitral stenosis only in control of rapid atrial fibrillation. A decrease in the ventricular rate can allow for improved left ventricular filling and a reduction in pulmonary venous pressure. Patients with obstructive cardiomyopathy are made worse by agents that increase contractility. Digitalis would increase the obstruction to left ventricular outflow and is therefore contraindicated in this condition. Digitalization is described in detail in Chapter 7.

Catecholamines. Catecholamines (isoproterenol, epinephrine, dopamine) increase myocardial contractility and hence cardiac output, but their use should be reserved for patients with severe "pump failure" resistant to all other forms of medical therapy. These agents also increase myocardial oxygen demand and are frequently responsible for ventricular arrhythmias if not used cautiously.

Glucagon. Glucagon is rarely effective in patients unresponsive to more standard medical therapy. The drug should be considered, however, in cases of left ventricular failure precipitated by the β-blocking effects of propranolol therapy. Glucagon acts via cyclic AMP and not cardiac β receptors as with catecholamines. Glucagon and not catecholamines, therefore, could be effective in increasing myocardial contractility in the presence of β-blockade.

Other Therapeutic Measures

Aminophylline. Aminophylline is known to have cardiovascular, renal, and pulmonary properties. The drug can increase heart rate and myocardial contractility yet decrease peripheral vascular resistance by smooth muscle relaxation. The net result is usually an increase in blood pressure because of the increased cardiac output despite the peripheral vasodilatation. The diuretic property of aminophylline is due to a direct effect on the renal tubule independent of an increase in renal plasma flow from a rise in cardiac output.[23] Bronchodilatation is a result of smooth muscle relaxation; this property provides a specific use for aminophylline in acute pulmonary edema complicated by bronchospasm. If intense pulmonary congestion or wheezing suggestive of bronchospasm is resistant to treatment previously mentioned, 500 mg of aminophylline may be given by slow intravenous drip. Caution must be exercised because rapid administration may precipitate tachyarrhythmias. It would be wise, if possible, to avoid the drug altogether in acute myocardial infarction because of the risk of potentially fatal ventricular arrhythmias and the increase in myocardial oxygen requirement which could enlarge the area of infarction. Aminophylline should not be given for its cardiac or diuretic properties alone, since safer and more effective drugs are available for these purposes.

Mechanical Ventilation.   Occasionally acute pulmonary edema is of such severity that respiratory failure occurs despite optimum management. Profound hypoxemia (pO_2 less than 60 mm Hg) with increasing hypercarbia (pCO_2 greater than 50 mm Hg) usually indicate that intubation and mechanical ventilation are necessary. Heavy sedation may be required to totally control respiration, but better ventilation and gas exchange should result. Positive end-expiratory pressure (PEEP) of 5 to 20 cm applied with the respirator has additional advantages in refractory hypoxemia. PEEP will increase functional residual capacity of the lungs, which serves to increase airway and alveolar diameter. Alveolar collapse will thus be reduced, and an improvement in distribution of ventilation will decrease physiologic shunting and hypoxemia. The increase in end-expiratory pressure may also decrease venous return. To a degree, this would be beneficial in reducing hydrostatic pressure and pulmonary congestion, but it is also potentially harmful if the reduction in venous return is of such magnitude that left ventricular filling is impaired and cardiac output decreases. Usually, judicious use of PEEP is beneficial in improving ventilation–perfusion abnormalities and is a recommended practice.[32]

Bedside Cardiac Catheterization.   The development of flow-directed balloon-tip cardiac catheters has made right heart catheterization available at the bedside.[33] While not a specific therapeutic agent, this technique can be of help in the measurement of pulmonary artery and wedge pressures as a guide to the most appropriate therapy.[34,35] Cardiac catheterization can aid in the diagnosis of ventricular septal rupture or papillary muscle dysfunction complicating acute myocardial infarction. Generally, cardiac catheterization is indicated in patients with refractory left ventricular failure.

NONCARDIAC PULMONARY EDEMA

Pulmonary edema of noncardiac origin is so frequent and so similar to congestive heart failure that some description is warranted here. As previously stated, alteration in pulmonary capillary membrane permeability is probably the most common cause of noncardiac pulmonary edema. The three basic features of management regardless of etiology include (1) removal of the offending agent, (2) ventilatory support, and (3) consideration of therapy with anti-inflammatory agents. Generally, pulmonary edema is a secondary feature of the illness, and treatment differs from that of the pulmonary congestion of cardiac decompensation.

Industrial exposure to caustic chemicals may produce alveolar or capillary damage sufficient to induce a chemical pneumonia, edema, and hypoxemia.[6] Oxygen therapy is of utmost importance, but digitalis, morphine, and diuretics are usually of little benefit. Corticosteriods are recommended to reduce the intense inflammatory reaction. The prognosis is good if the extent of hypoxemia and need for mechanical ventilatory support are not great.

The "adult respiratory distress syndrome" comprises severe respiratory dysfunction and hemorrhagic pulmonary edema as an end result of many respiratory and cardiovascular insults. Again, pulmonary edema occurs as a result of extensive pulmonary vascular or parenchymal damage and is not secondary to left ventricular dysfunction with pulmonary venous congestion. Appropriate therapy involves treatment of the primary illness and ventilatory support with oxygen, mechanical ventilation, positive end-expiratory pressure, and tracheostomy, if necessary. This topic has been the subject of extensive reviews elsewhere and will not be discussed further here.[20-22,32,36]

Increased membrane permeability and myocardial depression of uncertain cause contribute to the pulmonary edema occasionally present in bacteremic sepsis. Adequate ventilation, corticosteroids, and often inotropic drugs to enhance myocardial contractility are important in managing the cardiovascular manifestations of sepsis.[7,8,11] Disseminated intravascular coagulation, uremia, and radiation therapy may all induce alveolar and capillary damage sufficient to increase membrane permeability. The clinical picture of acute pulmonary edema must not be misdiagnosed as cardiac decompensation, for therapy should not involve the techniques of reducing pulmonary capillary pressure or increasing myocardial contractility previously discussed.

Hypoalbuminemia and lymphatic obstruction are potential sources of pulmonary congestion but are clinically quite rare.

Other syndromes of acute pulmonary congestion are of uncertain or mixed etiology. High-altitude pulmonary edema usually occurs upon rapid ascent to extreme heights. The syndrome is most common in the young, with onset frequently at night following a strenuous day. Oxygen therapy is of supportive value, and morphine or diuretics are of some benefit, but the optimal and most effective treatment—return toward sea level—should not be delayed.[13]

Acute pulmonary edema secondary to the use of intravenous heroin has become a frequent occurrence in major cities. Other narcotics, including oral preparations, have also resulted in this syndrome, but less commonly. Heroin coma with miotic pupils is followed 12 to 24 hours later by tachypnea, severe pulmonary congestion, and profound hypoxemia. Treatment of the overdose itself should include a narcotic antagonist. Oxygen therapy, tracheal suction, and, frequently, mechanical ventilation are necessary for treatment of the pulmonary edema.[14]

Acute pulmonary embolism may result in severe pulmonary edema despite pre-existing normal cardiac function. It has been postulated that acute pulmonary hypertension is responsible for the transudation of fluid, but an exact explanation for the hypertension is lacking.[15] Mechanical obstruction from the thromboembolism and reflex pulmonary vasoconstriction from hypoxia or vasoactive agents (serotonin, histamine) have been suggested. Generally, treatment should include oxygen and anticoagulation with mechanical ventilatory support; angiography and embolectomy should be considered only in cases of shock or severe respiratory failure.

Injuries to the central nervous system and general anesthesia have also been associated with otherwise unexplained pulmonary edema.[2] Therapy, as in other cases of uncertain etiology, should be supportive.

SUMMARY

Acute pulmonary edema is a common medical emergency with many possible causes. Treatment must be administered promptly and specifically according to the cause. Pulmonary edema of cardiac origin occurs when an abnormal increase in pulmonary capillary pressure promotes transudation of fluid from the vascular compartment to the interstitial space. The increase in pulmonary capillary pressure as a consequence of left ventricular failure may be secondary to valvular, ischemic, hypertensive, or myopathic heart disease. Pulmonary edema of mitral stenosis is secondary to mitral valve obstruction and is not truly myocardial failure.

The treatment of acute pulmonary edema of cardiac origin should have three goals: (1) improvement in ventilation by the upright position and oxygen therapy; (2) reduction in pulmonary capillary pressure either by decreasing left ventricular filling pressure with rotating tourniquets, morphine sulfate, diuretics, or phlebotomy, or by decreasing impedance to left ventricular ejection by vasodilating drugs; and (3) increase in myocardial performance with agents such as digitalis. (Digitalization is described in detail in Chapter 7.)

Acute pulmonary edema of noncardiac origin often is the result of altered permeability of the pulmonary capillary membrane; hypoalbuminemia and lymphatic obstruction are uncommon causes. Altered permeability results in interstitial edema due to an "injury" to the pulmonary capillary membrane in the absence of myocardial failure. Treatment should include removal of the offending agent, ventilatory support, and consideration of anti-inflammatory drugs.

Occasional cases of acute pulmonary edema are of mixed or uncertain etiology. This classification includes pulmonary edema secondary to heroin use and to exposure to high altitude.

REFERENCES

1. Robin, E. D., Cross, C. E., and Zelis, R.: Pulmonary edema. (First of two parts.) N. Engl. J. Med. 288:239, 1973.
2. Robin, E. D., Cross, C. E., and Zelis, R.: Pulmonary edema. (Second of two parts.) N. Engl. J. Med. 288:292, 1973.
3. Szidon, J. P., Pietra, G. G., and Fishman, A. P.; The alveolar-capillary membrane and pulmonary edema. N. Engl. J. Med. 286:1200, 1972.
4. Biddle, T. L., Khanna, P. K., Yu, P. N., Hodges, M., and Shah, P. M.: Lung water in patients with acute myocardial infarction. Circulation 49: 115, 1974.
5. Biddle, T. L., Hodges, M., Yu, P. N., Chance, J. R., Kronenberg, M. W., and Roberts, D. L.: Lung water and hypoxemia in acute myocardial infarction. Circulation 50:III 151, 1974.
6. Cordasco, E. M., and Stone, F. D.: Pulmonary edema of environmental origin. Chest 64:182, 1973.
7. Christy, J. H.: Pathophysiology of gram-negative shock. Am. Heart J. 81:694, 1971.
8. Christy, J. H.: Treatment of gram-negative shock. Am. J. Med. 50:77, 1971.
9. Siegal, H. H.: Modifying myocardial response to endotoxin. Clin. Res. 13:220, 1965.
10. Solis, R. J., and Downing, S. E.: Effects of E. coli endotoxin on ventricular performance. Am. J. Physiol. 211:307, 1966.
11. Winslow, E. J., Loeb, H. S., Rahimtoola, S. H., Kamath, S., and Gunnar, R. M.: Hemodynamic studies and results of therapy in 50 patients with bacteremic shock. Am. J. Med. 54:421, 1973.
12. Rusznyak, I., Foldi, M., and Szabo, G.: Physiology and pathology. In L. Youlten (ed.), Lymphatics and Lymph Circulation, 2nd ed. Oxford, Pergamon Press, 1967.
13. Wilson, R.: Acute high-altitude illness in mountaineers and problems of rescue. Ann. Intern. Med. 78:421, 1973.
14. Addington, W. W., Cugell, D. W., Bazley, E. S., Westerhoff, T. R., Shapiro, B., and Smith, R. T.: The pulmonary edema of heroin toxicity—An example of the stiff lung syndrome. Chest 62:199, 1972.
15. Sasahara, A. A.: Pulmonary vascular responses to thromboembolism. Mod. Concepts Cardiovasc. Dis. 36:55, 1967.
16. Ramirez, A., and Abelmann, W. H.: Cardiac decompensation. N. Engl. J. Med. 290:499, 1974.
17. Valencia, A., and Burgess, J. H.: Arterial hypoxemia following acute myocardial infarction. Circulation 40:641, 1969.
18. Fillmore, S. J., Shapiro, M., and Killip, T.: Arterial oxygen tension in acute myocardial infarction. Serial analysis of clinical state and blood gas changes. Am. Heart J. 79:620, 1970.
19. Ramo, B. W., Myers, N., Wallace, A. G., Starmer, F., Clarke, D. O., and Whalen, R. E.: Hemodynamic findings in 123 patients with acute myocardial infarction on admission. Circulation 42:567, 1970.

20. Pontoppidan, H., Geffin, B., and Lowenstein, E.: Acute respiratory failure in the adult. (First of three parts.) N. Engl. J. Med. 287:690, 1972.
21. Pontoppidan, H., Geffin, B., and Lowenstein, E.: Acute respiratory failure in the adult. (Second of three parts.) N. Engl. J. Med. 287:743, 1972.
22. Pontoppidan, H., Geffin, B., and Lowenstein, E.: Acute respiratory failure in the adult. (Third of three parts.) New Engl. J. Med. 287:799, 1972.
23. Goodman, L. S., and Gilman, A. (ed.): The Pharmacological Basis of Therapeutics. 4th ed. New York, Maxmillian, 1970.
24. Zelis, R. F., Mason, D. T., Spann, J. F., and Amsterdam, E. A.: The effects of morphine on the venous bed in man. Demonstration of a biphasic response. Am. J. Cardiol. 25:136, 1970.
25. Dikshit, K., Vyden, J. K., Forrester, J. S., Chatterjee, K., Prakash, R., and Swan, H. J. C.: Hemodynamic effects of furosemide in cardiac failure. N. Engl. J. Med. 288:1087, 1973.
26. Gold, H. K., Leinbach, R. C., and Sanders, C. A.: Use of sublingual nitroglycerin in congestive failure following acute myocardial infarction. Circulation 46:839, 1972.
27. Chatterjee, K., Parmley, W. W., Ganz, W., Forrester, J., Walinsky, P., Crexells, C., and Swan, H. J. C.: Hemodynamic and metabolic responses to vasodilator therapy in acute myocardial infarction. Circulation 48:1183, 1973.
28. Franciosa, J. A., Limas, C. J., Guiha, N. H., Rodriguera, E., and Cohn, J. N.: Improved left ventricular function during nitroprusside infusion in acute myocardial infarction. Lancet I:650, 1972.
29. Smith, T. W.: Digitalis glycosides. (First of two parts.) N. Engl. J. Med. 288:719, 1973.
30. Smith, T. W.: Digitalis glycosides. (Second of two parts.) N. Engl. J. Med. 288:942, 1973.
31. Hodges, M., Friesinger, G. C., Riggins, R. C. K., and Dagenais, G. R.: Effects of intravenously administered digoxin on mild left ventricular failure in acute myocardial infarction in man. Am. J. Cardiol. 29:749, 1972.
32. Leftwich, E. I., Witorsch, R. J., and Witorsch, P.: Positive end-expiratory pressure in refractory hypoxemia. A critical evaluation. Ann. Intern. Med. 79:187, 1973.
33. Swan, H. J. C., Ganz, W., Forrester, J., Marcus, H., Diamond, G., and Chonette, D.: Catheterization of the heart in man with use of a flow-directed balloon-tipped catheter. N. Engl. J. Med. 283:447, 1970.
34. Forrester, J. S., Diamond, G., McHugh, T. J., and Swan, H. J. C.: Filling pressures in the right and left sides of the heart in acute myocardial infarction. A reappraisal of central-venous-pressure monitoring. N. Engl. J. Med. 285:190, 1971.
35. Russell, R. O. Jr., Rackley, C. E., Pombo, J., Hunt, D., Potanin, C., and Dodge, H. T.: Effects of increasing left ventricular filling pressure in patients with acute myocardial infarction. J. Clin. Invest. 49:1539, 1970.
36. Fishman, A. P.: Shock lung. A distinctive nonentity. Circulation 48:921, 1973.

Chapter 2
PULMONARY EMBOLISM AND INFARCTION

SOL SHERRY

Pulmonary embolism is the impaction in the pulmonary vascular bed of detached thrombi, fat globules, gas bubbles, foreign matter, and the like. Since the first is by far the most important, this chapter will be restricted to a discussion of embolism arising from a detached thrombus. Pulmonary infarction, i.e., the necrosis of lung parenchyma resulting from the interference with blood supply, is a variable and relatively unimportant complication of embolism; it will be referred to in the text when indicated. The reader is urged to consult other reviews, particularly two monographs that have appeared in recent years.[1,2]

Approximately 90% of pulmonary emboli originate from a thrombus in the deep veins of the lower extremity; the remainder arise primarily from the prostatic or pelvic veins, the inferior vena cava and its main tributaries or the right heart. On rare occasions, an embolus may originate in the upper extremities or the superior vena cava and its main tributaries.

Pulmonary embolism with or without infarction is a common disorder and a most important cause of morbidity and mortality. It is frequently misdiagnosed. Next to pneumonia, it is the most common acute pulmonary lesion occurring in hospitalized patients today: 30% of pulmonary emboli are seen in cardiac patients, another 30% in noncardiac cases (particulary among the aged), and most of the remainder occur postoperatively. Immobilization, venous disease, and prior cardiopulmonary disease are the factors most frequently predisposing to pulmonary embolism. The overall incidence of pulmonary embolism in general autopsy series ranges from 5% to 14%, but the incidence is considerably higher (25%) in custodial institutions serving aged patients and is highest (30–45%) among cardiac patients; noteworthy is the observation that the incidence of pulmonary embolism has increased progressively over the past several decades.

Embolism to the major vessels, i.e., the main pulmonary artery or its primary branches, occluding the major portion of the circulation through the lungs, though less frequent than embolism of smaller vessels, is the third commonest cause of sudden death (5%) among hospitalized patients and occurs in about 3% of general autopsy series.

Embolism to medium-sized vessels, i.e., lobar and segmental vessels, is observed approximately three to five times more frequently in autopsy series than is embolism of the major vessels, but, since the former is commonly not fatal and often is recurrent, the actual incidence of such episodes is relatively much greater. Furthermore, in contrast to embolism of the major vessels, the presence of medium-sized emboli at autopsy can be considered as only incidental in two thirds of the cases; in the other third, the clinical features are such as to suggest some relation to death. Pulmonary infarction complicates embolism of medium-sized arteries in less than 25% of cases. In cardiac patients, the incidence of infarction following such embolism is considerably increased.

Embolism to small vessels, i.e., subsegmental arteries and their branches, probably occurs with great frequency, but the incidence is difficult to assess. As an isolated and focal lesion, such embolization has little clinical significance, for it usually is not large enough to produce a macroinfarction, and in autopsies the lesion is likely to be overlooked unless there are associated thrombi in the larger vessels. However, multiple small emboli scattered throughout the lungs are frequently observed in association with thrombotic occlusions of larger vessels; under these circumstances, they contribute significantly to the impairment of pulmonary circulation and associated morbidity. Miliary small vessel occlusion is also the major cause of morbidity when nonthrombotic emboli, such as fat, amniotic fluid, air, or nitrogen, are involved.

Pulmonary emboli may be single or multiple and may vary in size from microscopic particles to large saddle emboli that completely occlude the pulmonary artery and its major branches. In addition, a large embolus may break up during its passage through the heart or upon impaction and not only obstruct a major vessel but further embolize into one or more smaller branches in both lung fields. There is also evidence that after impaction, emboli may shift or further fragment into previously unobstructed pulmonary vessels.

PATHOPHYSIOLOGY

Emboli lodging in the pulmonary arterial tree acutely reduce the circulation distal to the site of obstruction. Potentially, the effects are fourfold: (1) Less blood proceeds through the pulmonary circuit to the left heart and systemic circulation: (2) there is a damming of blood behind the mechanical obstruction: (3) hemorrhagic necrosis of the ischemic area may occur; and (4) pulmonary function is impaired (pulmonary capillary perfusion and diffusion; later, ventilation may be compromised as well).

Except for the occurrence of infarction, which must be considered as a localized or focal disorder, the average person is believed capable of withstanding considerable obstruction of the pulmonary arterial bed without serious consequences to the vascular dynamics[3]; in normal animals, a 60% to 70% obstruction is usually well tolerated. Nevertheless, exceptions occur, both in the congested lung, particularly in the presence of underlying heart disease where less extensive occlusions may elevate pulmonary arterial pressure or significantly reduce pulmonary venous outflow, and where pulmonary circulation has been previously impaired by disease or prior embolization.

With a large occlusion of the main pulmonary artery or its primary branches, the effects are acute and primarily mechanical: rapidly rising pulmonary artery pressure, failure of the right ventricle, cyanosis, venous engorgement, and hepatic congestion. The consequences of impaired pulmonary venous return are sharp reduction in left ventricular filling, diminished cardiac output, reduced coronary and cerebral blood flow, hypoxia (also due to pulmonary blood shunting), dyspnea, pallor, tachycardia, and hypotension, often progressing quickly to shock and death. Sudden dyspnea and retrosternal pain frequently are the most prominent initial complaints: The dyspnea is believed to be due to anoxia, apprehension, and stimulation of Hering-Breuer and other reflexes; the angina is usually attributed to acute coronary insufficiency, but direct stimulation of sensory nerves in the wall of a rapidly distending pulmonary artery may also play a significant role.

The effects of embolization to medium-sized vessels depend on the number, size, and distribution of the emboli and the prior state of the lung and circulation. Several patterns may be observed: (1) There may be no observable effects; a transient episode of dyspnea may be the only clue to its occurrence. (2) The picture may be predominantly one of pulmonary infarction, with hemoptysis, pleuritic chest pain, friction rub, and abnormal roentgenographic shadows. Often, however, some elements of this pattern may be absent, notably hemoptysis or evidence of pleural involvement. (3) There may be an acute picture similar to but frequently not as severe as that seen with embolization of the main pulmonary artery or its primary branches: Here, the primary difficulty is extensive and sudden compromise of the pulmonary arterial circulation, in this case by multiple emboli or recurrent embolization; it may or may not be complicated by infarction. (4) There may be a chronic and insidiously developing syndrome of cor pulmonale from progressive pulmonary hypertension that has evolved slowly following repeated episodes of embolization with or without infarction. This is often superimposed upon and obscured by other underlying chronic disease.

Hemorrhagic necrosis of the lung tissue and the overlying pleural inflammation it incites are responsible for the characteristic clinical features of pulmonary infarction: The former accounts for the hemoptysis, cough, and fever; the latter for the pleural friction rub and pain. Since both lung tissue and the visceral pleura are devoid of sensory nerves, infarcts that do not extend to the outer surface of the lung to involve the parietal pleura do not cause pleural pain. When pain is present, it usually occurs over the ribs in the axillary region, but occasionally it may appear in the abdomen along the costal margin or, when there is involvement of the parietal diaphragmatic pleura, in the shoulder or neck. The mechanism of the pain has usually been attributed to friction over an inflamed pleura, but an alternative explanation that may better account for its features (accentuation only on inspiration) is tension exerted during inspiration on those sensitized nerve ends of the parietal pleura that are attached to the intercostal muscles.

CLINICAL FEATURES AND DIAGNOSIS

The manifestations of massive pulmonary embolism (defined for clinical purposes as occlusion of 50% or more of the pulmonary arterial circulation and representing approximately one third to one half of the suspected cases) may include sudden dyspnea; tachypnea; cyanosis; precordial or substernal oppressive pain, occasionally with radiation to shoulders and neck; evidences of right-sided cardiac dilatation and failure; tachycardia; restlessness; anxiety; syncope, occasionally with convulsions; and hypotension.

With massive embolism, death may be sudden or may occur after several hours. In the latter instance, shock with vascular collapse becomes prominent. In 2–3% of the cases, death may be delayed from one to several days, but, if blood pressure spontaneously returns to normal, recovery is likely (unless the course is complicated by recurrence or an underlying disease). The physical signs noted include pulsation in the second left interspace, accentuation of P_2, a pseudopleuropericardial or pleuropericardial friction rub, systolic or diastolic murmurs in the second left interspace, an interscapular bruit, S_3 or S_4 gallop rhythm, increased cardiac dullness to the right, distended neck veins, increased venous pressure with an hepatojugular reflex, and enlarged liver.

Serial electrocardiographic observation reveals transient changes in most patients (85%), but the pattern is extremely variable. The most frequent initial finding is T-wave inversion (40%). The electrocardiographic manifestations of acute cor pulmonale (S_1–Q_3–T_3 pattern, right bundle branch block, P-pulmonale, or right axis deviation) is present in only 25% of patients; left axis deviation is observed more frequently than right axis deviation. Rhythm disturbances (most commonly, ventricular premature beats) are observed in 10%, as is a pseudoinfarction pattern. Patients with prior cardiopulmonary disease have a greater frequency of arrhythmias, conduction disturbances, and QRS changes; patients with extensive embolization demonstrate more QRS, S–T, and T-wave changes. In general, little change occurs during the first 24 hours, but after 5 to 6 days, the QRS, primary S–T segment, and T-wave abnormalities begin to disappear. Roentgenographically, massive pulmonary embolism may result in the appearance of a large pulmonary arterial shadow that is dilated and terminated abruptly; in some cases, the ischemia may produce an increased radiolucency of portions of the lung field (Westermark's sign).

With submassive embolism, i.e., occlusion of less than 50% of the pulmonary circulation and usually involving the medium-sized or smaller vessels, the clinical manifestations may vary from a transient episode of dyspnea or the sudden or insidious worsening of an underlying pulmonary or cardiac disease to the full-blown picture described for massive embolism (submassive embolism in patients with prior embolism or severe underlying cardiopulmonary disease frequently presents with the findings ordinarily attributable to massive embolism); when pulmonary infarction occurs, its manifestations may also be superimposed.

The manifestations of pulmonary infarction are usually less dramatic. They vary in intensity from silent lesions to those characterized by pleuritic chest pain, hemoptysis, cough, moderate dyspnea, fever, tachycardia, pleural friction rub, areas of dullness or flatness on percussion, and diminished breath sounds, occasionally with tubular breathing and rales. The leukocyte count is usually elevated, the sedimentation rate is accelerated, and, subsequently, the serum bilirubin and serum lactic dehydrogenase levels rise. Roentgenographic examination may show typical humped or wedge-shaped shadows; on occasion, the lesions are rounded or indistinguishable from pneumonic infiltrates. At other times, a pleural effusion may be the only clue to an underlying infarct. The average patient with pulmonary infarction runs a moderately febrile course for a few days, which is followed by clearing of roentgenographic and physical signs in 1 to 3 weeks.

Despite the introduction of such diagnostic aids as pulmonary isotopic and ventilation photoscanning and selective pulmonary angiography, the diagnosis of pulmonary embolism with or without infarction is accurately made in no more than 50% of cases when compared to autopsy findings. Frequently, the diagnosis is overlooked because the disorder appears in the guise of congestive heart failure or pneumonia rather than as a distinctive syndrome; furthermore, the cardinal features do not occur with any great regularity. In half of the patients subsequently proved to have recurrent infarction, no evidence of phlebitis, pleural pain, pleural friction rub, or hemoptysis is present, and in any one episode the incidence of each of these features is less than 20%. Thus in the absence of classic features, the diagnosis must be made on the basis of a high index of suspicion followed by confirmatory laboratory findings.

The possibility of pulmonary embolism should be suspected in the presence of one or more of the following symptoms, signs, or laboratory findings: sudden or increased dyspnea, tachypnea, cough, or cyanosis; substernal or pleuritic chest pain; hemoptysis; phlebitis; acute right-sided failure or sudden worsening of congestive heart failure; shock; pulmonary consolidation; pleural friction rub; roentgenographic evidence of pulmonary infiltration, elevated diaphragm, or large areas of increased radiolucency or pleural effusion; unexplained arrhythmias or electrocardiographic changes, particularly when the latter are indicative of acute right-heart strain or dilatation; pulmonary function studies indicating an increased ventilatory dead space, i.e., a reduction in the mean alveolar carbon dioxide tension in the presence of a normal or nearly normal carbon dioxide tension; and unexplained fever, leukocytosis, or elevated erythrocyte sedimentation rate, serum bilirubin, lactic dehydrogenase, and fibrinogen/fibrin split products (normal levels of fibrinogen/fibrin split products and fibrin monomer are rare in pulmonary embolism).

The most reliable screening procedures for excluding an acute pulmonary embolism are pulmonary isotopic photoscanning with technetium-labeled microspheres or macroaggregates of human serum albumin and an arterial pO_2 determination on room air; a negative four-positional (anterior, posterior, and both laterals) lung scan virtually rules out an acute embolism, and acute embolism is extremely rare in the presence of an arterial pO_2 of 90 mm Hg or above on room air.

Confirmation of the diagnosis often can be achieved through the use of either selective pulmonary angiography or pulmonary isotopic photoscanning; on occasion, both techniques will be necessary. Since selective pulmonary angiography provides for direct visualization of the vascular tree, it is the more definitive of the two procedures and is the choice for establishing the diagnosis of pulmonary embolism. However, there are limitations to its usefulness. It is an expensive procedure and requires a skilled team; catheterization of the pulmonary artery is associated with some morbidity; the technique does not distinguish between new and old emboli; the subsegmental and smaller vessels are not visualized adequately; and there may be errors in interpretation unless the angiographer is experienced and strict criteria are used.

Pulmonary isotopic photoscanning has the advantages of convenience and lack of significant morbidity and allows for repeated observation in following the course of the patient. However, unlike pulmonary arteriography, photoscanning does not visualize the pulmonary arterial tree; rather, it is a measure of the distribution of blood flow or pulmonary capillary perfusion, and the cause of defects in perfusion may be misinterpreted, especially in the presence of any underlying pulmonary lesion, e.g., infiltrates, blebs, cysts, emphysema, an acute asthmatic attack, or alterations in perfusion as a result of previous or associated disease. Since the scan is not specific for pulmonary embolism, perfusion defects should be characterized as to whether they are segmental or not and interpreted only as having a high, medium, or low probability of being due to an embolism. While emphysema also may be responsible for high-probability perfusion defects, the confusion usually can be resolved by a radioactively labeled xenon ventilation scan, which is unaffected by pulmonary embolism, at least for a period of 5 days.

Pulmonary isotopic photoscanning is most useful for demonstrating and quantitating the perfusion defect of a pulmonary embolism when the chest roentgenogram is normal; it may also aid diagnosis by revealing multiple perfusion defects (indicative of multiple pulmonary embolism) when only an isolated infiltrate or lesion is present roentgenographically. Resolution of the perfusion defect following embolism occurs progressively (50% in 2 weeks), and this too may be useful diagnostically. Noteworthy is the fact that patients with underlying cardiac disease have an impaired resolution rate.

TREATMENT

The three major therapeutic objectives are general support, prevention of recurrence, and restoration of the pulmonary circulation and altered hemodynamics.

General Measures

Supportive treatment for the usual acute embolism should include bed rest, an analgesic or narcotic [preferably meperidine hydrochloride (Demerol)] for pain and apprehension, and oxygen as indicated. The administration of antimicrobial drugs to prevent bacterial disease of the lungs is not indicated unless a septic infarct is suspected. All sudden effort should be avoided, especially straining at stool. Stool softeners and colonic lavages may prove useful. Pleural effusions may require aspiration, particularly if dyspnea is progressive. Digitalization is indicated if cardiac failure appears or worsens, but it usually results in little benefit. Intravenous diuretics and various antiarrhythmic agents should be used in the appropriate clinical situation in the usual dosages (see Chapter 7).

In the more severe cases, continuous oxygen therapy should be employed, and positive pressure oxygen may prove particularly useful when pulmonary edema is present. Cardiac arrhythmias, which occur in 10% of cases, should be treated appropriately. If shock occurs, fluids and isoproterenol should be given. Intravenous fluids should be monitored by central venous pressure measurements and should be kept below 150 mm saline to prevent pulmonary edema. For hypotension, isoproterenol, because of its inotropic effect on the heart, is the agent of choice. It should be given intravenously slowly by drip (2–4 mg in 500 ml of 5% dextrose in water) usually at a rate of 2 μg/min, to sustain the systolic blood pressure at about 100 mm Hg (preferably at 120 mm Hg in previously hypertensive patients).[4] If hypotension persists despite isoproterenol, 1-norepinephrine (2–6 ml of 0.2% in 500 ml of 5% dextrose in water) should be administered. Aminophylline, 250 to 500 mg (by suppository, intramuscular, or slow intravenous administration), may prove useful, particularly when dyspnea is prominent or pulmonary edema is present. Venesection may be dangerous, however, because of impaired left ventricular filling. The value of pulmonary vasodilators (e.g., papaverine) and bronchodilators (e.g., atropine) is still highly controversial. Pulmonary edema and cardiogenic shock are discussed in detail in Chapters 1 and 3, respectively.

Prevention of Recurrence

Medical. In the absence of contraindications, heparin therapy should be instituted immediately in all patients with pulmonary embolism to lessen the danger of a recurrent and frequently fatal embolic accident (when heparin allergy is present, anticoagulation should be instituted immediately with coumarin compounds). Hemoptysis from pulmonary infarction is not a contraindication to anticoagulant therapy.

Heparin can be administered intravenously or by the intramuscular and subcutaneous routes. Based on control of antithrombotic effects, the intravenous route is most often recommended, particularly for the first several days of therapy.[5] Because of local pain and frequent hematomas, intramuscular injections are the least desirable. Even with the intravenous route, dosages and regimens vary. Continuous intravenous infusion of heparin, though requiring special care in administration, is becoming the preferred mode of therapy; control of dosage is more easily achieved and, more important, evidence is accumulating that bleeding complications can be reduced significantly. A suggested procedure is to begin therapy with a loading dose of 75 IU per pound of body weight, followed by a sustaining infusion of 10 IU per pound per hour through an indwelling plastic catheter placed above the antecubital fossa. Dosage is subsequently adjusted to maintain the activated partial thromboplastin time at twice normal (range, $1\frac{1}{2}-2\frac{1}{2}$)[6]; with Lee-White clotting times, the range is $2-2\frac{1}{2}$ times normal. If the intermittent injection technique is employed, it is suggested that 60,000 IU be given during the first day (e.g., 10,000 units every 4 hours) and that, beginning on the second day, dosage be regulated by coagulation determinations; 1 hour before the next injection, the activated partial thromboplastin time or Lee-White clotting time should be at the level recommended above for sustaining infusions.

Once the dose requirement has been established, the clotting time may be checked once daily at an appropriate time to exclude a possible increase or decrease in the anticoagulant effect of the drug and to allow for variations in heparin requirement during the course of therapy. Not infrequently, patients in whom thrombosis is occurring require more heparin in the first 24 to 48 hours of treatment than is required several days after the institution of therapy. It is recommended that heparin therapy be continued for 7 to 10 days, after which oral anticoagulation with coumarin drugs alone may be relied upon; this will ensure the most potent antithrombotic state and allow the causative peripheral venous thrombus to become firmly fixed to the vessel wall.

While "burning fingers" and an occasional allergic reaction may be seen with heparin, the primary toxicity of heparin therapy is bleeding; usually the incidence is of the order of 5–8%. Some of this risk can be reduced by better control of the anticoagulant state, elimination of aspirin and aspirin-containing compounds, and avoidance of intramuscularly administered medications and invasive procedures. When significant bleeding occurs, the heparin in the circulation can be immediately neutralized with protamine sulfate; the latter reacts with heparin stoichiometrically and on a milligram per milligram basis. Protamine is administered slowly intravenously after dilution in physiologic saline in an amount equivalent to half the last dose of heparin but not in excess of 100 mg.

Oral anticoagulation with coumarin compounds should be instituted several days before the discontinuation of heparin. It should be continued for 6 weeks to 6 months, unless the embolism has occurred as a consequence of immobilization, in which case the drug is continued until full physical activity is resumed. If thrombi recur when anticoagulants are discontinued, anticoagulants should be resumed, and long-term therapy may be necessary. Patients with known recurrent episodes of pulmonary embolism often require prophylactic anticoagulant therapy for years.

The action of coumarin compounds is indirect, i.e., the induction of a hypocoagulable state, in contrast to the action of heparin as an immediate activator of antithrombin III. At present, the aim of therapy is to reduce the level of the prothrombin complex factors (factors II, VII, IX, and X) to approximately 20% of normal and maintain it there. (Antithrombin III levels are increased during coumarin administration, and this may contribute to the antithrombotic effect.) This is achieved by regulating dosage so as to prolong the one-stage prothrombin time test to one and a half to two times the control time as measured by the Quick test. Levels of two and a half times or greater are associated with an increased incidence of bleeding, and levels of less than one and a half times the control may not be effective.

There is little difference in the onset of effect or smoothness of control among the various coumarin derivatives, and vitamin K_1 is equally effective in counteracting their action. Because Factor VII has the shortest half-life of the various vitamin-K-dependent factors (II, VII, IX and X), it is depressed most quickly by coumarin therapy. However, the rapid depression of Factor VII does not provide good antithrombotic protection, but it does enhance the risk of bleeding. Accordingly, previous regimens involving the use of a loading dose are being employed less frequently.[7] A suggested regimen is to give warfarin 10–15 mg daily until the desired effect on the prothrombin time is achieved; the dose is then adjusted to maintain that level. Individualization of dosage is essential, for a variety of drug interactions, other pharmacologic considerations, and metabolic factors influence the sensitivity and response to the coumarin compounds.[8]

Drugs to be avoided during warfarin therapy include aspirin, phenylbutazone, oxyphenbutazone, and indomethacin, and the following drugs have been shown to potentiate its effect: anabolic steroids, certain antibiotics (particularly chloramphenicol and those that affect the intestinal bacterial flora), chloral hydrate, clofibrate, disulfiram, ethacrynic acid, glucagon mefenamic acid, methylphenidate, quinidine, quinine, and sulfinpyrazone. Those agents that inhibit the prothrombinopenic effect of warfarin include barbiturates, corticosteroids, cholestyramine, ethchlorvynol, glutethimide, griseofulvin, haloperidol, meprobamate, and oral contraceptives. Also, older patients, particularly women, are especially sensitive to warfarin, as are individuals suffering from febrile illnesses, malnutrition, steatorrhea, and liver and pancreatic disease; warfarin sensitivity is also increased during the immediate postoperative state. Increased resistance to warfarin is associated with hyperlipidemia and hyperuricemia.

In patients being switched from heparin to warfarin therapy, a period of overlap is necessary because of the delay in the antithrombotic effect of the coumarin. A suggested procedure is to give warfarin 10–15 mg daily for 2–3 days until the desired therapeutic range for the prothrombin time is achieved; then, while maintenance warfarin therapy is continued, heparin dosage is progressively reduced over another 3–4-day period before discontinuation. Since prothrombin times are influenced by the presence of heparin, assays should be carried out on blood specimens with a normal or near normal activated partial thromboplastin time; for patients on sustaining infusions of heparin, this may require the *in vitro* addition of protamine.

Bleeding is a significant hazard with oral anticoagulation, occurring in 3% or more of patients on long-term therapy; vitamin K_1 in doses of 5 to 10 mg is usually corrective. Long-term therapy should not be undertaken unless a reliable laboratory is available and patient cooperation can be assured. Individuals on such therapy should not engage in contact sports and should avoid aspirin and aspirin-containing compounds; they should be observed carefully after even slight trauma (subdural hematoma in the aged is often an unsuspected complication of coumarin therapy). Invasive procedures, including needle biopsies and spinal taps, are to be avoided unless the prothrombin time is first restored to normal or near normal. Other adverse effects are minimal; probably of most interest is the occasional appearance of skin necrosis and the rare "purple toe syndrome." Contraindications to coumarin therapy are similar to those for heparin, with the addition of pregnancy. Not only has coumarin administration been shown to increase teratogenesis in animals during the first trimester, but, unlike heparin, it crosses the placental barrier and can produce fetal hemorrhage. The use of coumarins should also be avoided, when possible, in patients with severe liver disease or advanced renal insufficiency.

Surgical.   Inferior vena caval ligation, plication, or the insertion of a filter or umbrella should be reserved for those patients in whom anticoagulants are contraindicated or must be discontinued or whose disease for one reason or another cannot be successfully managed with this form of therapy. Since these procedures carry a significant incidence of sequelae, they are not indicated unless there has been massive embolism or there is evidence of recurrent embolization (a minor recurrence is observed in about 10% of patients during the first few days of heparin therapy and should not be considered as a failure of anticoagulant therapy unless the episode is clinically significant or recurrence continues with adequate levels of anticoagulation).

Restoration of Pulmonary Arterial Circulation

Medical. Newer thrombolytic agents, when available, should prove useful as adjuncts in the management of pulmonary embolism, for they provide a medical means for rapidly restoring an obstructed pulmonary arterial circulation. Clinical trials (urokinase pulmonary embolism trial[9] and urokinase–streptokinase pulmonary embolism trial[10]) have demonstrated that urokinase and streptokinase lyse pulmonary emboli extensively, reduce the hemodynamic abnormalities, improve pulmonary capillary perfusion, and increase gas exchange. These effects occur fairly rapidly and are most striking in patients with massive embolism; these agents should significantly reduce the need for surgical embolectomy, particularly when the therapy is combined with temporary cardiac bypass to tide the patient over the most critical period. Whether local perfusion of the agent directly into the pulmonary artery has any advantage over intravenous administration remains to be established. At present, thrombolytic agents are not indicated for the treatment of submassive embolism when vital signs are stable; in the absence of complications, the patient is destined to recover and there is little need to increase the risk of bleeding.

Streptokinase is a secretory product of hemolytic streptococci and can be produced readily in large quantities and relatively inexpensively for therapeutic purposes. Its major disadvantage is its antigenicity; this poses problems in dosage and, more important, in retreatment should thrombosis recur. Urokinase, a normal constituent of human urine, is nonantigenic and simpler to use therapeutically, but it is more expensive. Though originally prepared from urine, it is currently being processed from the culture medium of fetal kidney tissue cells. Both agents are given intravenously: For pulmonary embolism, a suggested procedure for streptokinase is to give 250,000 units as a loading dose over a 20-to-30-minute period, followed by a sustaining infusion of 100,000 units per hour for 48 to 72 hours; with urokinase, 2000 units per pound of body weight is given as a loading dose, followed by a sustaining infusion of the same amount per hour for 24 to 48 hours. Heparin therapy is instituted at the termination of the fibrinolytic therapy so as to prevent rethrombosis. Though both agents, when used in appropriate dosage, are capable of lysing large emboli, the intense fibrinolytic state tends to induce bleeding. However, this can be largely avoided by restricting invasive procedures, cut-downs, and intramuscular injections.

Both urokinase and streptokinase are still under evaluation in the United States and neither is yet commercially available. The only available preparation, human fibrinolysin, is a mixture of streptokinase and human plasmin. At the dosages recommended by the manufacturer, the fibrinolytic activity induced in the patient is extremely variable, and little enthusiasm currently exists for using this material for thrombolytic purposes.

Surgical.   Embolectomy may be lifesaving in critically ill patients. However, this procedure requires cardiac bypass, and because of the condition of the patient, mortality from surgical embolectomy is still very high. At present, the embolectomy is indicated only for those patients with angiographic evidence of massive embolism of the main pulmonary artery (or its primary branches) who have sustained peripheral hypotension despite the use of appropriate supportive measures. Pulmonary embolectomy may also be considered for those patients who have survived a massive embolism but in whom pulmonary hypertension resulting from the presence of an accessible embolus is leading to the development of cor pulmonale (see Chapter 17).

PROGNOSIS

The prognosis of pulmonary embolism is difficult to establish because the clinical diagnosis is frequently obscure. Of those who succumb, approximately 90% die immediately or within the first 2 hours. Another 2–3% die of protracted shock during the next 48 hours. Once stable vital signs are established, subsequent mortality approximates 7% and usually is attributable to recurrent embolism or adverse effects on an underlying cardiopulmonary disease. The likelihood of a fatal episode is increased with succeeding embolic attacks and, most important, in the presence of significant impairment of cardiopulmonary reserve.[11] The greatest hope for the management of this problem is prevention.

PROPHYLAXIS

Stasis should be eliminated whenever possible, particularly in the older patient. This includes the wearing of elastic or supportive hose for varicose veins; avoidance of long periods of cramped sitting and of constricting garments about the abdomen and lower extremities; and the use of appropriate measures during periods of immobilization or illness or following surgery, trauma, or fracture. The value of wearing elastic hose during periods of immobilization is very limited, as are foot and leg exercises, even when carried out frequently and in the elevated position. Of more value are physical devices that ensure repeated calf muscle contraction or intermittent pulsation of the leg veins. Early and active ambulation is to be encouraged following illness, surgery, or trauma.

Prophylactic therapy with anticoagulants is to be considered in high-risk groups, i.e., those most likely to develop pulmonary embolism. Included in this category are patients over the age of 50 who will be bedridden or immobilized for extended periods of time as a result of extensive fractures, particularly of the femur, or other forms of trauma, debilitating disease, cardiac failure, myocardial infarction, or surgery, particularly hip arthroplasty. The pharmacologic basis for the use of anticoagulation in the prevention of pulmonary embolism is sound, and its effectiveness in reducing thromboembolic complications following hip fracture or extensive trauma, during the postoperative state, and after acute myocardial infarction has been established in several series of observations.

When indicated, anticoagulant therapy should be instituted immediately; it can be carried out solely with oral agents (coumarin or indandione compounds), for though these agents take several days to induce an appropriate antithrombotic state, the danger period for pulmonary embolism usually begins somewhat later. Anticoagulation should be continued until full mobilization is completed. Anticoagulation is not a contraindication to surgery or other procedures. Surgery can be performed without much danger either before or shortly after the institution of anticoagulant therapy, since hemostasis is not impaired for several days; later, in the chronically anticoagulated patient, surgery can be undertaken after reduction of the level of anticoagulation and with careful attention to wound hemostasis. Despite its proved value, however, physicians have been reluctant to use such prophylactic anticoagulant therapy except in cases of recurrent thrombophlebitis or pulmonary embolism, citing the hazard of bleeding and the difficulties in maintaining adequate anticoagulation in older patients. Some of these difficulties can be avoided by the elimination of a loading dose and a recognition of the various factors that influence drug responsiveness (see above).

Infusions of Dextran 40 to 75 (500–1000 ml on the day of surgery, 500 ml daily for the next 5 days) also can be used to prevent postoperative thrombophlebitis and the attendant risk of pulmonary embolism. Dextran acts presumably by increasing blood flow and preventing surface interactions. However, while effective, it provides little advantage over anticoagulants since it also enhances the risk of bleeding and is tolerated poorly in individuals with an impaired cardiac reserve.

The most promising development in the prevention of deep vein thrombi in immobilized patients is the administration of small doses of heparin, i.e., 5000 units bid subcutaneously into the abdominal wall during periods of high risk. This regimen maintains circulating heparin blood levels at a fraction of that ordinarily achieved with conventional therapeutic doses used in the treatment of pulmonary embolism (see above) and does not significantly affect the Lee-White clotting time and activated partial thromboplastin time, nor does it enhance the risk of bleeding. However there is sufficient circulating heparin to activate enough heparin co-factor (antithrombin III) to block the action of earlier activated enzymes of the clotting reaction (notably Xa and IXa). In several trials, prophylactic therapy with low-dose heparin has strikingly reduced the incidence of venous thrombosis occurring postoperatively (except after femoral fractures and hip arthroplasty) and following acute myocardial infarction as measured by ^{125}I-labeled fibrinogen scanning.[12] Should trials currently under way also reveal a significant reduction in pulmonary embolism, this mode of prophylaxis is likely to receive widespread acceptance.

The utility of platelet function inhibitors, e.g., aspirin, dipyridamole, and sulfinpyrazone, for the prevention of deep vein thrombosis and pulmonary embolism, remains unclear.

SUMMARY

Pulmonary embolism is a frequent clinical problem, often overlooked or misdiagnosed, and is the third most common medical cause of sudden death. Most pulmonary emboli are not diagnosed because they are unsuspected; even when suspected, a diagnosis on clinical grounds (symptoms, signs, and routine laboratory studies alone) is no better than 50% accurate. Most (90% or so) originate from deep vein thrombi in the lower extremities, and such emboli may or may not be complicated by pulmonary infarction.

Large emboli impact in the main pulmonary artery or its major branches and are the most common cause of massive embolism, i.e., obstruction of 50% or more of the pulmonary arterial circulation. When the latter occurs, it may produce sudden death or be associated with severe and persistent hypotension.

Medium-sized emboli impact in the lobar or segmental arteries; they are more frequent than large emboli and are more likely to be associated with pulmonary infarction. Usually, this form of embolization is unassociated with major hemodynamic alteration or severe tachypnea and dyspnea unless the individual has underlying cardiopulmonary disease or has had recurrent bouts of embolization; in these circumstances, medium-sized emboli can produce a clinical picture similar to that of massive embolism, in which there is the sudden appearance of pulmonary hypertension and acute right-heart strain, along with a reduced cardiac output and peripheral hypotension. Pulmonary infarction, i.e., the necrosis of lung parenchyma, is a complication of embolism and, when it occurs, usually is heralded by the appearance of pleuritic chest pain or hemoptysis.

Small emboli impact in the subsegmental vessels and usually go unrecognized clinically.

Eighty per cent or more of patients with pulmonary embolism will recover, and in most of them pulmonary circulation and capillary perfusion will return to normal spontaneously. Of those that succumb, probably half die immediately; another 3% die within the first few hours with persistent hypotension; and of those who establish stable vital signs, an additional 7% die either because of a recurrent embolism or adverse effects on an underlying cardiopulmonary disease. The presence or absence of underlying cardiopulmonary disease represents the single most important factor other than the size of the embolism influencing prognosis.

When pulmonary embolism is suspected, the laboratory procedures of most value in confirming the diagnosis are the arterial pO_2, pulmonary isotopic perfusion lung scanning, and pulmonary angiography. The arterial pO_2 is useful as a screening procedure; pulmonary embolus is very unlikely when the pO_2 is above 90 mm Hg on room air. Lung scanning is also useful as a screen for excluding the diagnosis of embolism, which is highly unlikely in the presence of a normal scan. When a perfusion defect is present, it should be characterized on the basis of its distribution (e.g., segmental) as having a high, medium, or low probability of being due to embolism. Ventilation scans, when used in combination with perfusion scans, increase the diagnostic capability of scanning procedures. Pulmonary angiography is the most specific of all the tests and should be used to resolve the more difficult diagnostic problems or when the direction of patient management is at issue.

The three major therapeutic objectives are general support, prevention of recurrent embolism, and restoration of the pulmonary circulation and altered hemodynamics.

General support is best provided by bed rest, an analgesic, and oxygen as indicated. For hypotension, fluids and pressors are required; isoproterenol is the pressor of choice.

The prevention of recurrent embolism requires either the use of anti-coagulants (heparin is the agent of choice for the immediate institution of an antithrombotic state, followed after a week or so by coumarin therapy) or inferior vena caval interruption. The latter should be used only when there is a contraindication to anticoagulants or when the problem cannot be controlled with these agents.

Enhanced restoration of the pulmonary circulation is necessary only in those patients with severe hemodynamic alterations and, particularly, when hypotension is maintained despite appropriate supportive measures. Such patients are candidates for pulmonary embolectomy or the use of thrombolytic agents (urokinase or streptokinase) when the latter are available.

REFERENCES

1. Hume, M., Sevitt, S., and Thomas, D. P.: Venous Thrombosis and Pulmonary Embolism. Cambridge, Mass., Harvard University Press, 1970.
2. Stein, M., and Moser, K. M. (ed.): Pulmonary Thromboembolism. Chicago, Year Book Medical Publishers, 1973.
3. McIntyre, K. M., and Sasahara, A. A.: The hemodynamic response to pulmonary embolism in patients without prior cardiopulmonary disease. Am. J. Cardiol. 28:288, 1971.
4. Sasahara, A.: Therapy of pulmonary embolism. JAMA 229:1795, 1974.
5. Genton, E.: Guidelines for heparin therapy. Ann. Intern. Med. 80:77, 1974.
6. Basu, D., Gallus, A., Hirsh, J., and Cade, J.: A prospective study of the value of monitoring heparin treatment with the activated partial thromboplastin time. N. Engl. J. Med. 287:324, 1972.
7. O'Reilly, R. A., and Aggeler, P. M.: Studies on coumarin anticoagulant drugs. Institution of warfarin therapy without a loading dose. Circulation 38:169, 1968.
8. Koch-Weser, J., and Sellers, E. M.: Drug interaction with coumarin anticoagulants. N. Engl. J. Med. 285:547, 1971.
9. The urokinase pulmonary embolism trial. Phase I results. Circulation 47 (Suppl. II):II-5, 1973.
10. Urokinase-streptokinase pulmonary embolism trial. Phase II results. JAMA 229:1606, 1974.
11. Gallus, A. S., Hirsh, J., Tuttle, R. J., et al.: Small subcutaneous doses of heparin in prevention of venous thrombosis. N. Engl. J. Med., 288:545, 1973.
12. Paraskos, J. A., Adelstein, S. J., Smith, R. E. et al.: Late prognosis of acute pulmonary embolism. N. Engl. J. Med., 289:55, 1973.

Chapter 3

CARDIOGENIC SHOCK

JAY N. COHN

Shock is best defined as a state of abnormal circulatory function in which impairment of tissue blood flow has resulted in a disturbance in organ function and has initiated a series of feedback mechanisms that may lead to progressively more severe perfusion abnormality.[1] The diagnosis of shock, therefore, can be made only in the presence of a disturbance in organ function, and once the diagnosis is established, it may be assumed that the syndrome is progressive. In its broader sense, the term "cardiogenic," when applied to shock, implies that an abnormality in cardiac function is an important factor in the development and progression of the shock state. However, it is likely that cardiac function is impaired to a varying degree in all patients with shock, regardless of etiology. Therefore, all shock may be considered at least in part cardiogenic shock. In more restrictive usage, however, cardiogenic is taken to indicate that form of shock precipitated by an acute myocardial infarction. In the following review, we shall consider the physiology of shock in general and then discuss in particular the syndrome of shock associated with acute myocardial infarction.

THE DIAGNOSIS OF SHOCK

The diagnosis of shock must be based on the demonstration of inadequacy of tissue blood flow. The normal cardiac output in the adult of between 5 and 6 liters per minute is distributed to the regional vascular beds on the basis of flow requirements. If cardiac output falls below

35

normal levels, or if peripheral requirements increase out of proportion to the increase in cardiac output, then certain regional beds become less adequately perfused. Mild degrees of inadequate perfusion may be well tolerated without symptoms, and even considerable depressions of cardiac output on a more chronic basis may be surprisingly well tolerated by readjustment of peripheral requirements. Acute reductions of cardiac output are less well tolerated, but even in acute illnesses the degree of reduction in cardiac output that precipitates the syndrome of shock may be variable.[2] Such variability probably relates to the distribution of the reduced cardiac output, the individual's neurohumoral response to this reduction, and the unique requirements of this individual's peripheral tissues. Obviously, the flow deficiency that precipitates shock usually begins some time before the full syndrome is detectable. It is during this early preshock phase, when tissue blood flow may not yet be critically reduced, that therapy may be most effective in reversing the disorder. Possible therapeutic intervention before the diagnosis of shock is established will be considered later in this review. Nonetheless, the diagnosis of shock must be based on clear clinical or laboratory evidence of reduced blood flow.

When renal blood flow falls, renal conservation of sodium and oliguria develops. An hourly urine output of less than 20 ml with a urinary sodium concentration of less than 20 mEq per liter is evidence of critical reduction of renal blood flow. The careful timed measurement of urine output is therefore critical to the early diagnosis of shock, especially because the renal vascular bed may be constricted early in shock and reduction of renal blood flow may therefore occur before any change in arterial pressure is detected. The splanchnic, cutaneous, and skeletal muscle circulations also are under the influence of the sympathetic nervous system. Flow in these beds also may be critically reduced even though arterial pressure is still at normotensive levels. Reduction in cutaneous blood flow can be detected from the color and temperature of the skin. Skeletal muscle and splanchnic flow are vital in the maintenance of normal lactate metabolism. A reduction in these flows leads to a rise in blood lactate levels and the development of metabolic acidosis, which may be detected from arterial blood gases.[3] Early in the course of shock, the arterial blood may reveal an isolated reduction in pCO_2 that is indicative of hyperventilation, but the pH subsequently begins to fall and the patient enters a more rapid downhill phase of tissue underperfusion. The skin and muscle flow in the upper extremities is also critical in the maintenance of arterial pulses in the upper extremities and of an auscultatory blood pressure. The thready radial and brachial pulses and unobtainable auscultatory blood pressure associated with shock are due more often to intense upper extremity vasoconstriction than to hypotension.[4]

The cerebral and coronary beds are less affected by sympathetic nervous system activity and are more under the influence of aortic perfusion pressure. The confusion, restlessness, and somnolence associated with shock is usually due to arterial hypotension, but sometimes inadequate cerebral blood flow may be detected even before the blood pressure falls; thus, the sensorium of the patient is another critical guide to the diagnosis of shock. Coronary arterial flow falls as the blood pressure falls, and in the later stages of shock this arterial hypotension is an important factor in progressive deterioration of cardiac function.[5] Indeed, most of the peripheral vascular reactions that contribute to the regional flow deficiencies in shock represent the body's attempt to prevent hypotension, for once hypotension develops, a rapid deterioration of the cardiovascular system can be expected and survival may be very short.

THE HEART IN SHOCK

Regardless of the cause of shock, the heart plays a pivotal role in its progression. In pure hemorrhagic shock, for instance, the reduction of venous return precipitates a fall in cardiac output, which induces the peripheral vascular reactions that are clinically detected as the shock syndrome. If the circulating blood volume is quickly restored to normal levels, no change in cardiac function may be detected. However, if there is some delay in the restoration of this inadequate blood volume and hypotension persists for any length of time, cardiac function begins to deteriorate.[6] Because of the sympathetic discharge that accompanies the low cardiac output, contractility of the myocardium is increased. If this increase in contractility cannot be reflected in an increase in arterial pressure because of a low circulating blood volume, coronary blood flow may be inadequate to provide the oxygen required to maintain enhanced cardiac contractility.[7] Therefore, myocardial function may begin to deteriorate, and left ventricular end-diastolic pressure may begin to rise. This increase in left ventricular diastolic pressure is a further impediment to coronary blood flow, since the effective coronary perfusion pressure is the aortic diastolic pressure minus the left ventricular diastolic pressure.[8] Progressive subendocardial ischemia may develop, because it is the subendocardium that is most vulnerable to reductions in effective perfusion pressure. The resultant failure of the left ventricle may then contribute to the peripheral flow deficiency, and a cardiogenic factor comes to play a role in what was initially pure hypovolemic shock. This same chain of events may influence performance of the heart in all kinds of shock, even those that are initiated by acute myocardial infarction.

The balance between myocardial oxygen supply and oxygen delivery is thus a critical factor in the progression of shock,[9] and this balance takes on even more significance in the patient with coronary disease, as will be discussed later.

The simplest bedside means of evaluating cardiac function is to relate the cardiac output or the stroke volume to the ventricular filling pressure (Fig. 3-1).[10] In the right ventricle the filling pressure represents the central venous pressure or the mean right atrial pressure. In the left ventricle the filling pressure can be assessed either from a measurement of left ventricular end-diastolic pressure or the pulmonary wedge pressure. With the increasing popularity of invasive methods for bedside evaluation of cardiac function, it is now relatively simple to assess both right and left ventricular function in patients with shock. The cardiac output need not be measured directly but can be assessed qualitatively from an evaluation of the adequacy of regional perfusion. Thus, thready

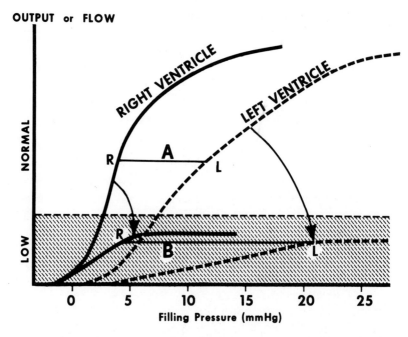

Figure 3-1. The effect of acute myocardial infarction on right and left ventricular function curves. Both curves are depressed downward and to the right (arrows), but the depression of the left ventricle curve usually is greater than that of the right so that the difference between the left and right ventricular filling pressures (line B) is greater after myocardial infarction than in the normal heart (line A). In true "pump failure," output remains in the low (shaded) zone even at very high filling pressures.

pulses, cool skin, low urine output, and metabolic acidosis all may be used as signs of a low cardiac output. Right and/or left ventricular filling pressure must be measured directly with catheters advanced blindly at the bedside by well-established techniques. The right ventricular filling pressure often can be assessed by a careful evaluation of the deep jugular venous pulse as the patient is carefully positioned in bed. Nonetheless, direct measurement of this pressure is usually more satisfactory. In patients with cardiac dysfunction developing as a result of sepsis or of prolonged shock regardless of etiology, right and left ventricular function appear to be relatively equally impaired. Therefore, both the right and left ventricular function curves are shifted to the right, and central venous pressure and left ventricular filling pressure bear a normal relationship to each other, with the pulmonary wedge pressure averaging between 5 and 10 mm Hg higher than the right atrial pressure.[11] In patients with acute cor pulmonale, right ventricular filling pressure is inordinately elevated and often rises to levels higher than the left ventricular filling pressure. In contrast, patients with acute myocardial infarction usually manifest a left ventricular filling pressure considerably higher than the right ventricular filling pressure. Therefore, the central venous pressure will not serve as a reliable guide to the adequacy of myocardial function in the patient with acute myocardial infarction (Fig. 3-1).

VOLUME CHALLENGE

The relative importance of cardiac dysfunction and inadequate venous return in the genesis of the low cardiac output of shock is difficult to evaluate when the ventricular filling pressure is not greatly elevated. The degree of cardiac impairment can best be assessed by sharply augmenting venous return while the ventricular filling pressures and the signs of peripheral blood flow adequacy are monitored.[12] This acute challenge of plasma volume expansion serves two vital purposes in the patient with shock: It provides therapy for the patient whose low cardiac output is due at least in part to inadequate venous return, and it helps to distinguish hypovolemic shock from that due to right or left ventricular dysfunction. A favorable clinical response without much rise in ventricular filling pressure indicates hypovolemia. In contrast, a rise in filling pressure without improvement in the blood flow deficiency indicates cardiac dysfunction, and the ventricle whose filling pressure rises more rapidly is the one that is predominately involved.

In general, patients with a left ventricular filling pressure over 25 mm Hg should not be subjected to volume expansion, because little rise in cardiac output would be expected and there is danger of inducing pulmonary edema.[13] If the left ventricular filling pressure is less than 20 mm Hg, or if the central venous pressure is less than 10 mm Hg and the patient exhibits no signs of left ventricular failure, a cautious trial of volume expansion is indicated. This should be accomplished by administering albumin, dextran, or some other colloidal solution in 50-ml boluses and measuring the ventricular filling pressure after each bolus. As long as the left-side pressure remains below 20–25 mm Hg, or the central venous pressure rises by less than 3 mm Hg per bolus, the challenge should be continued until either the flow deficiency has been corrected or the ventricular pressure rises to these levels. Cessation of the infusion before one of these events has occurred represents an inadequate therapeutic trial.

It is vital that the challenge be carried out rapidly. Thus, a 500-ml expansion should take no longer than 20 minutes to complete. Only by such rapid infusion can one be certain that the vascular compartment is expanded and that venous return will be acutely augmented. Since volume-responsive shock is the only form of shock that can be treated with complete success, it is imperative not to miss a case by circumventing an indicated volume challenge.

HEMODYNAMICS OF ACUTE MYOCARDIAL INFARCTION

Myocardial infarction is characterized by a rise in left ventricular end-diastolic pressure and a fall in stroke volume.[14] This left ventricular failure is an almost invariable accompaniment of myocardial infarction involving the left ventricle, even when symptoms of heart failure are not detectable at the bedside. More rarely, myocardial infarction involves the right ventricle and leads to predominant right ventricular dysfunction.

Although myocardial infarction has traditionally been viewed as a finite process in which the insult has occurred prior to the patient's hospitalization, recent evidence suggests that the area of ischemia and infarction may enlarge significantly during the first few days of hospitalization.[15] The balance between myocardial oxygen consumption and oxygen supply, therefore, must be viewed as a dynamic process that may be influenced by hemodynamic events that characterize the early phase of convalescence. Thus, the elevated end-diastolic pressure, which seems to bear a direct relationship to the severity of the myocardial infarction, may impede subendocardial blood flow and enlarge the area of infarction. Similarly, a reduction in aortic diastolic pressure as a result of a falling cardiac output may also lead to a critical reduction in coronary blood flow. Structural changes also may influence the hemodynamics. Changes in stiffness of the infarcted area may determine whether this area resists stretch or whether it bulges during ejection and whether it can dilate adequately during diastole. Changes in function of the mitral valve apparatus because of ischemic insult to the papillary muscle may lead to valvular regurgitation.

MECHANISMS OF SHOCK AFTER ACUTE MYOCARDIAL INFARCTION

When peripheral blood flow becomes critically reduced after acute myocardial infarction, the prognosis is grave. A mortality rate of between 80% and 95% despite intensive medical therapy has been described from a number of institutions. Autopsy studies of patients dying of myocardial infarction shock usually have revealed extensive damage to the left ventricle with more than 40% of its mass infarcted.[16] These findings have suggested to some that the appearance of shock indicates that the infarction is so extensive that medical therapy is doomed to failure. Nonetheless, the fact that most shock after myocardial infarction develops in the hospital some hours after the onset of clinical signs suggests that the initial insult was indeed compatible with life and that some subsequent changes in the heart or in the peripheral circulation contributed to the further reduction of peripheral blood flow. This concept allows one to postulate that the large infarcts observed at the time of autopsy are made up of an original central zone of infarction and a surrounding infarcted area that may have become progressively larger during the course of hospitalization. If this thesis is correct, a strong plea could be made for instituting aggressive therapy early in the course of myocardial infarction before progressive myocardial damage reduces ventricular function so much that survival is impossible. Such an approach would, of course, depend upon the availability of an effective form of therapy.

The syndrome of shock after acute myocardial infarction must be viewed as a multifactorial event. Some factors are preventable, some are treatable, and some may be beyond help with current therapy.

Initial Central Zone of Infarction

This central infarction usually represents the pathologic equivalent of the episode for which the patient sought medical advice. Since the muscle in this central infarcted zone probably is destroyed within minutes after the initial episode, no therapy to preserve this myocardium is likely to be successful. Depending on the area of this infarction, varying degrees of left ventricular dysfunction will ensue. If this central infarction represents more than 40% of the mass of the left ventricle, or if old and new infarctions render more than half of the left ventricle noncontractile, it is unlikely that the patient will survive the acute episode. Indeed, under these circumstances it is probably unlikely that the patient will even survive long enough to reach the hospital. Therefore, a patient who has reached the hospital some minutes or hours after his acute episode should be viewed as having a central infarcted zone not large enough to be incompatible with survival.

Peri-infarction Ischemic Zone

Around the central zone of necrosis is an ischemic area in which the balance between myocardial oxygen consumption and oxygen supply is tenuous but in which infarction has not yet occurred. Contraction in this ischemic zone may be severly depressed or absent. Thus the ventricle may function as if the infarction is larger than it really is. If events occur that increase the oxygen consumption of this ischemic zone or reduce the delivery of oxygen to this ischemic zone, this area may progress from reversible to irreversible infarction.

Hypovolemia

Circulating plasma volume may be reduced after acute myocardial infarction because of release of catecholamines, sweating, reduced fluid intake, or administration of diuretics.[17] When myocardial function is impaired, the left ventricle requires a higher than normal end-diastolic volume or end-diastolic pressure in order to maintain an adequate cardiac output. If venous return is impaired because of this hypovolemia, the left ventricular filling may fall below its optimal level, and cardiac output may be correspondingly reduced. Hypovolemia is rarely the major factor in development of shock after acute myocardial infarction, but it may be a significant factor often enough that it must be kept in mind and evaluated by the use of a measurement of left ventricular filling pressure.

Peripheral Vasoconstriction

When the cardiac output falls, reflex activation of the sympathetic nervous system ensues. The myocardium is thus stimulated by adrenergic mechanisms to increase its contractility, and the peripheral vascular bed is constricted in order to support arterial pressure despite the reduction in cardiac output. Such a mechanism to maintain arterial pressure is critical to the maintenance of life, for severe hypotension is incompatible with survival. However, the sympathetic nervous system reaction often is inappropriately intense, and arterial pressure may rise to a level above that required to maintain tissue perfusion. Pressure work and oxygen consumption of the left ventricle is thus inordinately increased, and an imbalance between oxygen consumption and oxygen delivery may lead to a further deterioration of left ventricular function.

Inadequate Vasoconstriction

Some patients, particularly elderly individuals or patients with a chronic debilitating disease such as diabetes, may exhibit impairment of the peripheral vasoconstrictor response to a falling cardiac output.[2] In these individuals, blood pressure falls with cardiac output, and reduced aortic pressure may lead to further impairment of myocardial oxygen delivery and progressive enlargement of the area of infarction. Thus, while too much vasoconstriction may be deleterious, so also may too little vasoconstriction.

Arrhythmias

Disturbances in cardiac rhythm may play an important role in the falling cardiac output of shock. Bradyarrhythmias, tachyarrhythmias, and frequent ventricular premature beats may all contribute to the inadequacy of a heart that might otherwise be functioning at a sufficient level to maintain peripheral perfusion. Heart rates below 70 may be deleterious when stroke volume is limited, and even isolated ventricular premature beats may be dangerous in patients with severe ischemia, for the premature beat may consume oxygen without doing any useful work. Rapid heart rates greatly increase myocardial oxygen consumption and may set up a vicious cycle of progressive ischemia and progressive deterioration of cardiac function.

Drugs

The administration of agents that depress myocardial contractility may play an important role in the development of the shock syndrome. Drugs that may be given safely to patients with more normal myocardial function may be hazardous to the patient whose function is at a critical level. Antiarrhythmic drugs such as lidocaine, quinidine, procaine amide, and particularly propranolol all may be culprits. Great caution, therefore, should be exercised in the use of these drugs in patients with mild arrhythmias, particularly when the arrhythmias are a manifestation of left ventricular failure. It is also important to recognize that the cardiac dysfunction that may result from the pharmacologic action of these drugs may long outlast the biologic life of the drug, since positive feedback mechanisms initiated during the period of cardiac dysfunction may continue and progress even though the direct myocardial action of the drug is no longer operating.

Hypoxemia and Acidosis

A reduction in oxygen saturation of arterial blood and lactic acidosis, both of which commonly complicate the course of myocardial infarction shock, may further depress myocardial function, and this may play a role in the progression of the shock syndrome.[18]

PUMP FAILURE AFTER ACUTE MYOCARDIAL INFARCTION

The phrase "pump failure" is diagnostically less restrictive than "shock" because the former does not necessarily require the documentation of hypotension and organ perfusion failure. Indeed, no clear-cut diagnostic criteria for "pump failure" exist. This diagnosis is reserved for the patient with acute myocardial infarction who has severe left ventricular dysfunction but not necessarily "shock." A left ventricular filling pressure over 25 mm Hg with a depressed stroke volume would, in some investigators' view, fulfill the criteria.

What is most critical in this diagnostic category is that the mortality rate in this group of patients is very high. While it does not reach the 85% level reported in shock, the 21-day mortality rate does range from about 30% to 60%. The high risk in this subgroup of patients with acute myocardial infarction may well justify aggressive intervention to attempt to restore peripheral perfusion and, if possible, to reduce myocardial ischemia. Although data on the response of this "pump failure" group to therapy are not available, it is likely that the prognosis would be more easily improved by therapy in this group than in the patients who develop the full-blown shock syndrome.

We shall therefore consider in the following sections therapy to combat left ventricular failure and flow deficiency after myocardial infarction, regardless of whether the stringent criteria for shock are met.

MONITORING THE PATIENT WITH PUMP FAILURE

The patient with pump failure complicating acute myocardial infarction cannot be treated adequately without the following bedside measurements:

Arterial Pressure

Cuff pressure is an unreliable guide to arterial pressure in the patient with pump failure. An indwelling cannula in the brachial, radial, or femoral artery attached to a strain-gauge transducer and a display oscilloscope or recorder is a necessity.

Left Ventricular Filling Pressure

The central venous pressure is a crude and unreliable guide to left ventricular function in acute myocardial infarction. A balloon-tipped catheter in the pulmonary artery or an arterial catheter advanced retrograde from the femoral artery into the left ventricle provide a measurement of left ventricular filling pressure that is vital in selecting therapy and following the patient's course.[19,20]

Urine Output

An indwelling bladder catheter is necessary to assess the adequacy of renal perfusion, which serves as a guide to the course of shock.

Blood Gases

Arterial blood gases should be obtained at frequent intervals to assure that oxygenation is adequate and acidosis has been corrected.

MANAGEMENT OF PUMP FAILURE

General Considerations

The most important early goal of the physician is to correct those contributory factors that may yield to relatively simple therapy. Rhythm and rate must be controlled at most effective levels. Acidosis and hypoxia must be treated. Antiarrhythmic drugs (see Chapter 7) that may depress myocardial function should be stopped, or at least the dosage should be reduced to minimally effective therapeutic levels. An attempt should be made to adjust ventricular filling pressure to optimal levels by the use of plasma volume expanders if the pressure is low or by the application of tourniquets or phlebotomy if the pressure is very high.

Corticosteriods have been recommended as appropriate therapy for all kinds of shock and low flow states. Their use in cardiogenic shock is not based on controlled observations, but evidence does exist that pharmacologic doses of steroids (methylprednisolone 30 mg/kg in a single dose) may prolong the "reversibility" of shock by stabilizing lysosomal membranes. Therefore, steriods might well be administered along with other more specific therapy in the patient with severe shock that is not likely to yield promptly to conventional treatment.

Vasodilator Drugs

When peripheral blood flow is reduced and arterial pressure still is supported at normotensive levels (pump failure, "preshock"), vasodilator drugs have proved to be an effective pharmacologic approach to therapy.[21] Most experience has been gained with the use of sodium nitroprusside (Nipride) given in a continuous intravenous infusion of from 30 to 150 μg/min. Similar responses have been observed to nitroglycerin and the long-acting nitrates, but dosage titration with these latter drugs is more difficult. Phentolamine (Regitine) and trimethaphan (Arfonad) have also been used for their vasodilating properties.

These drugs improve left ventricular performance by lowering the impedance against which the left ventricle must eject blood. Since arterial pressure is reduced and cardiac contractility little altered, the oxygen consumption of the heart is lowered at the same time that its output is increased. The goal of therapy with vasodilators is to reduce left ventricular filling pressure and increase cardiac output without inordinately reducing arterial pressure. The drug dose should be adjusted to attain this goal, and great care must be exercised to avoid hypotension, which can be hazardous in the patient with acute myocardial infarction.

Isoproterenol is also used as a vasodilator agent, but its prominent inotropic and chronotropic properties make it more appropriate to consider this drug in the next section.

Inotropic Drugs

The use of inotropic agents to treat pump failure would appear to be rational, but recent evidence has suggested that such therapy may be harmful in patients with acute myocardial infarction.[15] All inotropic agents augment myocardial oxygen consumption by virtue of their effect on contractility, and further oxygen wasting may result from induced increases in heart rate and arterial pressure.[7] Thus these drugs may aggravate the intramyocardial imbalance between myocardial oxygen consumption and oxygen delivery. Enlargement of the area of infarction or ischemia could result.

Digitalis.   The cardiac glycosides increase cardiac contractility but do not produce much increase in cardiac output in patients with cardiogenic shock.[22] They possess peripheral vasoconstrictor properties that may be deleterious, and arrhythmias may be precipitated, especially in hypotensive patients. These drugs therefore have little place in the acute management of the pump failure of myocardial infarction, although they may still be useful in the treatment of supraventricular arrhythmias (see Chapter 7).

Isoproterenol.   This potent inotropic agent dilates the peripheral vascular bed, especially skeletal muscle, but it also increases heart rate and automaticity. Although it has proved to be a very effective agent in treating low output states not due to ischemic heart disease, its use in myocardial infarction is hazardous because of the marked rise in myocardial oxygen consumption induced by the drug. Its only rational use is in the patient with normal intra-arterial pressure and marked peripheral vasoconstriction in whom low doses may be effective in restoring blood flow without much increase in heart rate.

Norepinephrine and Metaraminol.   These drugs produce both inotropism and peripheral vasoconstriction. When they are administered to a hypotensive patient, the induced increase in myocardial oxygen consumption usually is counterbalanced by a rise in coronary blood flow because of the restoration of aortic diastolic pressure. Thus, these drugs may be tolerated by the ischemic ventricle for short periods.[23] However, regional blood flow often is reduced and the shock state usually is not reversed.

Dopamine and Dobutamine. These sympathomimetic amines have a more selective inotropic effect than either norepinephrine or isoproterenol. Dopamine exerts peripheral vasoconstriction at higher doses but has a renal vasodilator effect at lower doses.[24] Dobutamine has only modest peripheral vasodilator effect at higher doses.[25] Both drugs produce a dose-related increase in cardiac output with little change in heart rate. Although the potency and consistency of their inotropic effect in patients with shock is not well established, the circulatory actions of these drugs may render them the ideal sympathomimetic agents for treating low-output syndromes. Dopamine (Intropin) is already marketed, but dobutamine, which may be more potent and more selective in its action, is still under investigation.

Glucagon. This drug produces an unreliable inotropic effect, but since it is well tolerated and easily administered, a 5-mg intravenous dose as a test for responsiveness may be worthwhile. If a beneficial effect is observed, a continuous infusion of the drug may be administered; however, little experience is available with prolonged infusions of the drug.

Esproquin. This is an inotropic drug that apparently acts by causing selective release of catecholamines in the heart. In preliminary studies it has been demonstrated to exert prolonged cardiac stimulation without much increase in heart rate.[26] It is still under investigation.

Vasoconstrictor Drugs

The only indication for administering a vasoconstrictor drug to the patient with pump failure after acute myocardial infarction is the presence of hypotension. Rapid restoration of arterial pressure is critical to the patient's survival in this situation, and a vasoconstrictor drug counteracts hypotension most rapidly. However, peripheral vasoconstriction increases the work load on the left ventricle and may both increase myocardial oxygen consumption and reduce cardiac output. Norepinephrine, which also possesses inotropic properties, is the drug of choice. It should not be administered, however, unless hypotension is documented by intra-arterial pressure measurement or signs of cerebral underperfusion exist. Angiotensin and methoxamine, which are relatively devoid of direct cardiac effects, probably have no place in the management of pump failure complicating myocardial infarction.

Mechanical Cardiac Assistance

When pump failure persists after correction of those factors that can be specifically treated, after adjustment of the left ventricular filling pressure to above 20 mm Hg, and after a short trial of pharmacologic therapy with vasodilator, inotropic, or vasoconstrictor drugs, then consideration should be given to mechanical cardiac assistance.

Intra-aortic balloon counterpulsation has proved to be an effective means of improving the circulatory status in patients with cardiogenic shock.[27] However, long-term survival has been less common, probably because of the extensiveness of the cardiac damage at the time balloon pumping has been instituted. Many experts feel that early intervention with a mechanical assistance device is preferable to waiting until the patient's condition has deteriorated during ineffective medical therapy.

At present, it is probably advisable for mechanical assistance to be utilized only in institutions with well-trained medical and cardiac surgical teams. Patients probably should not be subjected to mechanical assistance if they have a history of chronic heart failure with considerable cardiomegaly.

Cardiac Surgery

Emergency surgery for the patient with pump failure has been advocated by some institutions. Revascularization of an ischemic zone and excision of dyskinetic areas of the left ventricle have in some cases led to survival that otherwise seemed unlikely. Cardiac surgery is the only hope for patients who respond initially to intra-aortic balloon pumping but cannot sustain their circulation when the pump is turned off. The surgical therapeutic approach is discussed in detail in Chapter 17.

SUMMARY

Shock represents a syndrome of inadequate peripheral blood flow in which insufficient cardiac output is precipitated by inadequate venous return or impairment of cardiac function, or a combination of the two. The diagnosis of shock can be made only when a deficiency of perfusion results in demonstrable abnormalities in organ function, but subtle reductions in perfusion usually precede the appearance of clinical shock, and therapy introduced in this preshock phase may be most effective.

In acute myocardial infarction, an impairment of left ventricular function is an important factor in the genesis of shock, but reduction in venous return, abnormalities in peripheral vascular regulation, disturbances in rhythm, adverse effects of antiarrhythmic drugs, and abnormalities in oxygenation and acid–base balance all may contribute to the circulatory failure. When a state of low peripheral blood flow persists after these nonmyocardial factors have been corrected, the diagnosis of pump failure can be made.

Managing the patient with pump failure requires the monitoring of directly measured arterial pressure, left ventricular filling pressure (pulmonary wedge pressure), hourly urine output, and blood gases. Pharmacologic management includes the use of vasodilator drugs if intra-arterial pressure is adequate and the cautious use of inotropic or inotropic–vasoconstrictor drugs if arterial pressure is low. New inotropic drugs provide some choice in the selection of therapy, but the risks of an increase in myocardial oxygen consumption always must be considered when these drugs are employed.

Mechanical cardiac assistance and emergency cardiac surgery have been the only rational approaches to the patient whose circulation continues to deteriorate despite appropriate pharmacologic therapy. Intra-aortic balloon pumping has been widely employed, but no controlled studies are available to document long-term benefit of the procedure. Earlier intervention with aggressive invasive management may eventually prove to be effective, but careful prospective studies must be carried out.

REFERENCES

1. Thal, A. P., and Kinney, J. M.: On the definition and classification of shock. Prog. Cardiovasc. Dis. 9:527, 1967.
2. Cohn, J. N., and Luria, M.: Studies in clinical shock and hypotension. IV. Variations in reflex vasoconstriction and cardiac stimulation. Circulation 34:823, 1966.
3. Shubin, H., Afifi, A., Rand, W., and Weil, M.: Objective index of hemodynamic status for quantitation of severity and prognosis of shock complicating myocardial infarction. Cardiovasc. Res. 2:329, 1968.
4. Cohn, J. N.: Blood pressure measurement in shock. Mechanisms of inaccuracy in auscultatory and palpatory methods. JAMA 199:972, 1967.
5. Berne, R. M.: Regulation of coronary blood flow. Physiol. Rev. 44:1, 1964.
6. Guyton, A. C., and Crowell, J. W.: Cardiac deterioration in shock. I. Its progressive nature. Int. Anesthesiol. Clin. 2:159, 1964.
7. Sonnenblick, E. H., and Skelton, C. L.: Myocardial energetics: Basic principles and clinical implications. N. Engl. J. Med. 285:668, 1971.
8. Salisbury, P. F., Cross, C. E., and Rieben, P. A.: Acute ischemia of inner layers of ventricular wall. Am. Heart J. 66:650, 1963.
9. Haddy, F. J.: Physiology and pharmacology of the coronary circulation and myocardium, particularly in relation to coronary artery disease. Am. J. Med. 47:274, 1969.
10. Sarnoff, S. J., and Berglund, E.: Ventricular function. I. Starling's law of the heart studied by means of simultaneous right and left ventricular function curves in the dog. Circulation 9:706, 1954.
11. Cohn, J. N., and Tristani, F. E.: Studies in clinical shock and hypotension. VI. Relationship between left and right ventricular function. J. Clin. Invest. 48:2008, 1969.

12. Cohn, J. N., Luria, M. H., Daddario, R. C., and Tristani, F.: Studies in clinical shock and hypotension. V. Hemodynamic effects of dextran. Circulation 35:316, 1967.
13. Russell, R. O., Jr., Rackley, C. E., Pombo, J., Hunt, D., Potanin, C., and Dodge, H. T.: Effects of increasing left ventricular filling pressure in patients with acute myocardial infarction. J. Clin. Invest. 49:1539, 1970.
14. Hamosh, P., and Cohn, J. N.: Left ventricular function in acute myocardial infarction. J. Clin. Invest. 50:523, 1971.
15. Maroko, P. R., Kjekshus, J. K., Sobel, B. E., Watanabe, T., Covell, J. W., Ross, J., Jr., and Braunwald, E.: Factors influencing infarct size following experimental coronary artery occlusion. Circulation 43:67, 1971.
16. Page, D. L., Caulfield, J. B., Kastor, J. A., DeSanctis, R. W., and Saunders, C. A.: Myocardial changes associated with cardiogenic shock. N. Engl. J. Med. 285:133, 1971.
17. Agress, C. M., Rosenburg, M., Binder, M. J., Schneiderman, M., and Clark, W.: Blood volume changes in protracted shock resulting from experimental myocardial infarction. Am. J. Physiol. 166:603, 1951.
18. Wildenthal, K., Mierzwiak, D. S., Myers, R. W., and Mitchell, J. H.: Effects of acute lactic acidosis on left ventricular performance. Am. J. Physiol. 214:1352, 1968.
19. Swan, H., Ganz, W., Forrester, J., et al.: Catheterization of the heart in man with the use of a flow-directed balloon tipped catheter. N. Engl. J. Med. 283:447, 1970.
20. Cohn, J. N., Khatri, I. M., and Hamosh, P.: Bedside catheterization of the left ventricle. Am. J. Cardiol. 25:66, 1970.
21. Cohn, J. N.: Vasodilator therapy for heart failure: The influence of impedance on left ventricular performance. (Editorial.) Circulation 48:5, 1973.
22. Cohn, J. N., Tristani, F. E., and Khatri, I. M.: Cardiac and peripheral vascular effects of digitalis in cardiogenic shock. Am. Heart J. 78:318, 1969.
23. Mueller, H., Ayers, S. M., Giannelli, S., Conklin, E. F., Mazzara, J. T., and Grace, W. J.: Effect of isoproterenol, 1-norepinephrine, and intraaortic counterpulsation on hemodynamics and myocardial metabolism in shock following acute myocardial infarction. Circulation 45:335, 1972.
24. Goldberg, L. I.: Cardiovascular and renal actions of dopamine: Potential clinical applications. Pharmacol. Rev. 24:1, 1972.
25. Akhtar, N., Chaudhry, M. H., and Cohn, J. N.: Dobutamine: Selective inotropic action in patients with heart failure. Circulation 48(Suppl. 4): 538, 1973.
26. Sriussadaporn, S., and Cohn, J. N.: Inotropic properties of an isoquinoline derivative (NC 7197) in man. Am. Heart J. 85:374, 1973.
27. Kuhn, L. A.: Current status of diastolic augmentation for circulatory support. Am. Heart J. 81:281, 1971.

Chapter 4
PREHOSPITAL MANAGEMENT OF ACUTE MYOCARDIAL INFARCTION

J. F. PANTRIDGE
A. A. J. ADGEY

It is, unfortunately, true that more than two thirds of premature deaths from acute myocardial infarction occur before the patient reaches the hospital. Sixty three per cent of the deaths among males aged 50 or less occur within 1 hour,[6] and among patients of both sexes under 65 years with an initial coronary attack, 61% of the deaths occur within the hour.[23] It is clear that hospital coronary care units cannot significantly affect the community mortality from acute myocardial infarction, which is of the order of 40%,[20] since the median time between the onset and hospital admission may be more than 8 hours.[42,44]

Ninety-two per cent of early deaths result from ventricular fibrillation.[1,58] Among those in whom ventricular fibrillation is prevented or corrected, death from shock, pump failure, or rupture need not occur in more than 10%.[2,59]

Since the major problem is outside the hospital, various prehospital schemes have been evolved. These include mobile coronary care units (MCCU's) staffed by (a) medical personnel or (b) trained paramedical personnel and static prehospital coronary care units (life support stations).

MOBILE CORONARY CARE UNITS

An MCCU is defined as "a facility which enables personnel trained in coronary care to reach patients at the site of the heart attack (at home or elsewhere) as soon as possible, to start emergency treatment immediately, and to continue observation and treatment during transport to hospital."[77]

Unfortunately, acceptance of the concept of mobile coronary care has been influenced adversely by the erroneous assumption that large, special, expensive vehicles equipped with highly sophisticated electronic devices are necessary.[74]

Mobile Coronary Care Units Staffed by Medical Personnel

The prototype MCCU was developed at the Royal Victoria Hospital, Belfast, in 1966.[54,55] Family doctors in Belfast were made aware of the problem of coronary deaths outside hospitals and given a special telephone number that allows a rapid response from the coronary care unit. A team, comprised of an intern and a nurse, both trained in coronary care, is able to reach more than 50% of patients within 10 minutes of the receipt of a call from the family doctor or lay individual (Fig. 4-1). The family doctor may activate the mobile unit if a message he has received from a patient, or from the individual with him, suggests

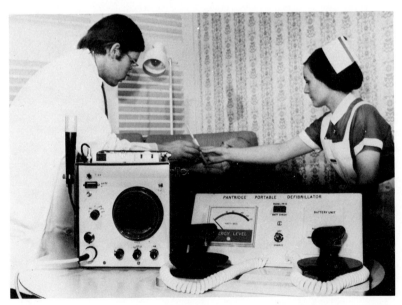

Figure 4-1. Mobile coronary care team in patient's home.

the likelihood of acute infarction. Emergency calls from patients or their relatives are received by the hospital coronary care unit and assessed by a junior doctor. The ambulance depot for the city of Belfast is on the grounds of the Royal Victoria Hospital. No special ambulance is used but two of the 36 ambulances in the ambulance depot have been slightly modified (Fig. 4-2).

A different scheme is in operation for that part of the Belfast population located east of the Lagan River.[7,73] Here, a minivehicle containing the necessary equipment, drugs, and intravenous solutions, is on standby near the Coronary Care Unit of the Community Hospital. A team from the Coronary Care Unit travels in this minivehicle. If the patient is found to have a myocardial infarction, one member of the team will accompany him to the hospital in an ordinary ambulance, monitoring him on the way; the other will drive the minivehicle back to base. This scheme also minimizes the number of ambulance drivers required.

In both schemes, mobile coronary care duty is added to the other duties of the coronary care unit personnel. No individual is unemployed between calls. An important feature of the operation of the Belfast units is that patients are admitted directly to the coronary care unit (Fig. 4-3), thus avoiding the emergency room, which is the most dangerous place in most hospitals for the patient with acute myocardial infarction. It has been reported that those who die in the emergency room or arrive dead account for 60% of deaths in the Middlesex Hospital, London.[56]

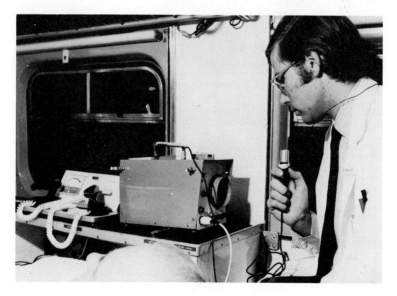

Figure 4-2. Mobile coronary care unit.

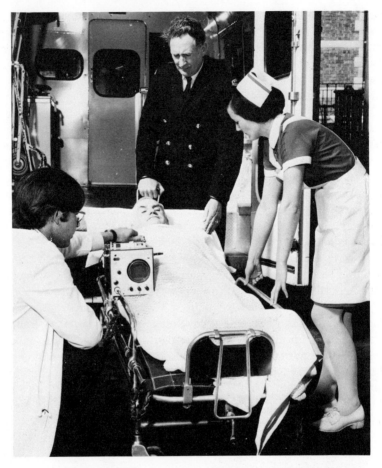

Figure 4-3. Direct transfer of patient to hospital coronary care unit.

The data from the Belfast units indicate that

1. It is possible to get a significant proportion of patients with acute myocardial infarction under intensive care early. Twenty-seven per cent may obtain intensive care within one hour.[2]
2. Patients seen early are at greatest risk of ventricular fibrillation,[59] and correction of ventricular fibrillation outside hospital is a practical proposition.[1,55]
3. Deaths during transport may be eliminated.[58] In the absence of mobile coronary care, transport deaths account for a varying proportion of coronary deaths, depending on transport time and dis-

tance. The percentage of deaths occurring during transport is quoted as 2%,[5] 10.9%,[44] 13%,[50] and 15%.[27]

4. The early initiation of intensive care and the correction and prevention of arrhythmias and autonomic disturbances may limit the size of the area of infarction.[57] Thus, a low incidence of shock, pump failure, and hospital mortality has been recorded among those seen early.[2,56,57,59] The hospital mortality of less than 10% among patients seen within 1 hour and managed by the mobile coronary care team is to be contrasted with a mortality of 25.6% among those patients in the Bristol study who contacted their doctors within 1 hour but who presumably received no therapy in that time.[41] A hospital mortality of 6% has been recorded among patients who received intensive care within 1 hour; this contrasts with a hospital mortality of 20% among those seen later.[25] Patients managed by the Belfast MCCU within 3 hours of the onset of acute myocardial infarction had a significantly lower hospital mortality and incidence of cardiogenic shock than those seen later.[2]

That the magnitude of the area of infarction may be influenced by hemodynamic disturbance and pharmacologic intervention has been experimentally confirmed.[39,40] Braunwald's group found that following coronary ligation in the dog the severity and extent of the ischemic injury was increased by hypotension, by tachycardia, and by the administration of positive inotropic agents—isoproterenol and ouabain. The administration of a beta-blocking agent (propranolol) diminished the severity and extent of ischemic injury.

MCCU's staffed by medical personnel have been developed in the United States, in Australia, in Japan, and in many parts of Europe (Table 4-1). In the Soviet Union, dialing the number 03 will summon emergency care. The emergency care network in the Soviet Union comprises more than 2,500 stations in which some 12,000 doctors work. For each 10,000 of the urban population there is one "normal" ambulance staffed by a doctor, a feldsher, and an orderly.[12] In 1960 special ambulances were put into commission in Moscow for which specialist teams of doctors were appointed by the Moscow City Health Department.[46] The staff of the specialist team consisted of one medical specialist and two or three feldshers. In 1970 there were twelve specialist cardiologist teams in Moscow, eight in Leningrad, and four in Kiev.[12] The special team and special ambulance are summoned by the doctor in the "first strike" or "normal" ambulance. There was no evidence in 1970 that the "normal" ambulance was equipped to provide intensive care for patients with acute myocardial infarction. Cardiac arrest in the prehospital

Table 4-1   *Mobile Coronary Care Units*

Location	Staffing[a]
Great Britain	
Ballymena[30]	M
Barnsley[65]	M
Belfast[55,7]	M
Brighton[76]	P
Dudley[32]	M
Edinburgh	M
Manchester (Salford)[14]	M
Newcastle upon Tyne[17]	M
Eire	
Dublin[21]	P
Switzerland	
Basle[70]	M
Zurich[70]	M
Norway	
Oslo[37]	M
Holland	
Amsterdam[19]	M
Utrecht[69]	M
Australia	
Sydney[52,53]	M
Perth[61]	M
Japan	
Tokyo[45]	M
United States	
New York City[24,62]	M
Columbus, Ohio[36]	P
Charlottesville,[15,16]	M
Los Angeles[34]	P
Pittsburgh[64]	P
Philadelphia[8,9]	M
Seattle[13]	P
Portland, Ore.[63]	P
Miami[49]	P
Oklahoma[28]	N
Chicago[29]	M
Nassau County, N.Y.[33]	P
New Jersey[67]	M

[a] M = Staffed by medical personnel; N = staffed by nursing personnel; P = staffed by paramedical personnel.

phase was managed by the specialist team with a success rate of 30% to 45% in Moscow, Leningrad, Kiev, and Kaunas.[12] In the Soviet Union attention is given to early hospitalization and intensive care during transport. It was reported that in one of the Moscow districts "the mortality rate among hospitalized patients was 2.5 times less in comparison with those treated at home."[11] Chazov records that "in Moscow of 4,000 patients transported to hospital only four died during transport and in Sverdlovsk not a single one of 6,000 patients died during transport."[11]

Since it is difficult to obtain medical personnel to staff MCCU's in some areas, the use of paramedical personnel has been suggested.

Mobile Coronary Care Units Staffed by Paramedical Personnel

These have been developed in many areas in the United States (Table 4-1). In Los Angeles County, for instance, there are 28 such units.[35] Most of the paramedical units concentrate on the correction of ventricular fibrillation, and some have had remarkable success. In Seattle the system devised by Cobb operates through the fire department.[13] An aid car, of which there are 10 strategically placed in Seattle (population 575,000), and an MCCU are dispatched simultaneously when an emergency call reporting a "coronary episode" or "collapse" reaches the fire department. Resuscitation measures are initiated by the personnel in the aid car and completed by the personnel in the MCCU. Originally, the personnel of the MCCU were physicians, but these units are now staffed by highly trained paramedical individuals. These "Emergency Medical Technicians"[3] have had 1,022 hours of instruction and are trained to "near physician level." Attention was also directed toward training some members of the public in resuscitation techniques.[4]

Among the patients resuscitated in the first 2 years of the operation of the Seattle paramedical scheme there were 57 long-term survivors, and in the last year 64 long-term survivors were reported. Cobb's experience in Seattle leads him to believe that telemetering of the cardiogram to the base hospital is not necessary.[13] Rose, in Portland (Oregon),[63] and Nagel, in Miami,[49] on the other hand, consider this facility important. Nagel's data concerning the surroundings in which ventricular fibrillation occurred and the activity immediately preceding its onset are of interest: Among 340 patients who had ventricular fibrillation outside the hospital, he reports that 55% had ventricular fibrillation while at work or in a public place and less than 17% developed it during sleep (Table 4-2). This contrasts with the view that sudden death is usually unwitnessed.[43]

Equipment of Mobile Coronary Care Units

1. The drugs and intravenous solutions normally available in a coronary care unit, including beta-blocking agents.
2. A *battery-operated* monitoring oscilloscope.
3. A *battery-operated* permanent recording facility (cardiograph or tape recorder).

Table 4-2   *Location of Occurrence of 340 Cases of Acute Ventricular Fibrillation and Nature of Activity Preceding Onset in Miami, Florida*[a]

Location of occurrence	
Home	45%
Work	12%
Public place	43%
Activity preceding onset	
Rest or sleep	17%
Mild or moderate	65%
Strenuous	17%

[a] Data from City of Miami Fire Department, reported by Nagel.[49]

4. A *battery-operated* DC defibrillator.
5. Oxygen supply, Ambu bags, endotracheal tubes, suction apparatus.

The hardware should be sturdy and, as far as possible, foolproof. Since the apparatus may have to be carried some distance, occasionally up several flights of stairs, monitoring equipment and defibrillators must be light and compact. While the defibrillators most commonly used are clumsy, expensive, and heavy, small defibrillators are available.

STATIC PREHOSPITAL CORONARY CARE UNITS (LIFE SUPPORT STATIONS)

Static prehospital coronary care units have been established in New York in skyscraper buildings where one or more physicians practice (Table 4-3). Such units also exist in some industrial complexes. These units include monitoring equipment and defibrillators. Units also operate in several stadiums in the United States, and spectators have been suc-

Table 4-3   *Static Prehospital Coronary Care Systems (Life Support Stations)*

City	Location
Rochester, N.Y.	Kodak[22]
New York City	Bankers Trust Buildings[51]
	Consolidated Edison
	New York Life Insurance Company
	New York Giants stadium
New Orleans	Saints football stadium
Lincoln, Neb.	University of Nebraska athletic stadium[10]

cessfully resuscitated from ventricular fibrillation. It has been estimated that if all football stadiums were equipped, "from 60–100 lives could be saved each fall."[10]

COMBINED STATIC AND MOBILE
PREHOSPITAL CORONARY CARE

Schemes have been proposed and one in large part implemented in New York.[26]

MANAGEMENT
Pain Relief

Immediate pain relief is regarded as particularly important in the management of acute myocardial infarction. The autonomic disturbances so frequent at the onset may respond only to pain relief.[75] The catechol release may be diminished by the immediate control of pain. Morphine is the drug most frequently administered; however, adverse effects have been documented.[68,71] Profound hypotension and bradycardia may follow the injection of morphine, particularly when the patient is moved. Adverse hemodynamic effects also occur following the administration of pethidine to patients with acute myocardial infarction.[47] Heroin is the most satisfactory of the narcotic drugs in the control of pain, particularly severe pain. Given in a standard intravenous dose of 5 mg, "it causes little effect on the cardiovascular system."[38] It has a more rapid action and less emetic effect than morphine.[18] (Heroin is not available for clinical use in some countries.)

There is evidence that nitrous oxide may offer an alternative to the use of narcotic drugs in the acute phase of myocardial infarction.[31,72] Since the use of narcotic drugs by paramedical personnel is a serious problem, there is need for detailed investigation of the value of nitrous oxide.

Correction of Autonomic Disturbance and Cardiac Arrhythmias

This subject may have received inadequate attention. Bradycardia within the first 2 hours occurs in 37.5% of patients who come under intensive care within the first hour.[59] Ventricular ectopic beats occur in the first 2 hours in 85% of patients and ventricular fibrillation occurs in 14% of these patients who are treated within the first hour.[59]

Among patients seen within 30 minutes, only 17% will have a normal heart rate and normal blood pressure. Thirty-five per cent will show evidence of sympathetic overactivity, and 48% will show evidence of vagal overactivity.[59]

Antiarrhythmic agents are less effective when the heart rate is outside the normal range. There is evidence that lidocaine is less effective when heart rate is over 90.[59]

It should be noted here that there are dangers inherent in the administration of antiarrhythmic agents in the presence of severe acidosis.

Changes During Transport

Alterations of the heart rate and hemodynamic changes during transport have been inadequately documented. An inappropriately rapid heart rate (≥ 110) that is likely to affect adversely the magnitude of the infarct occurs during movement in one third of patients.[48] Pain relief before transport does not significantly reduce the incidence of a rapid heart rate. The prophylactic administration of practolol is of limited value, but the more potent negative chronotropic beta-blocking agent sotalol (MJ 1999) usually prevents tachycardia (this drug is not available for clinical use in the United States, where propanolol is the only β-blocking agent available).[48] The beta-blocking agent does not give rise to significant bradycardia when administered along with atropine.[48]

SUMMARY

In the consideration of the problem of coronary artery disease, most emphasis is placed on preventive measures. The logic of primary prevention is irrefutable. However, since the etiology is multifactorial, it appears unlikely that much progress will be made in this direction in the immediate future. The coronary care unit was an important advance, but the hospital coronary care unit must be supported by some form of prehospital coronary care scheme to enable the patient to get intensive care quickly and at the time when the risk of death is greatest.

The logistics of prehospital coronary care will depend on the local situation. Staffing of MCCU's by medical personnel may be difficult in many areas, and it has been shown in many parts of the United States that paramedical personnel are capable of resuscitating patients from ventricular fibrillation. Doubt, however, exists about whether they are able to manage the arrhythmias and the autonomic disturbance so frequently present in the acute phase of myocardial infarction. There is, at present, no standardized approach to the correction of these difficulties. Careful titration of the dose of the necessary drugs is required. Since the arrhythmias and the autonomic disturbance influence the magnitude of the infarct and, therefore, the incidence of shock, pump failure, and the long-term prognosis, there will continue to be a place for the operation of MCCU's staffed by physicians. This will be particularly true if the physicians are oriented toward further elucidating the problems of acute myocardial infarction and developing a simplified therapeutic regime for stabilization of the rhythm and the hemodynamic state and correction of the autonomic difficulty. If such a regime should evolve, it might be initiated not only by paramedical personnel but also in some situations by the patient himself.[66] Highly efficient automatic spring injectors exist; the drugs to be carried in such syringes and the dosage are problems to be solved.

Any consideration of prehospital coronary care would be incomplete without reference to public education directed toward reducing the delay between the onset of symptoms and request for medical help. The American Heart Association is involved in publicity programs with this purpose.[79]

The advice frequently given to a stricken individual to proceed immediately to the emergency room of the nearest hospital[60,79] is far from prudent, since 22% of patients seen within 30 minutes of the onset of chest pain will have a systolic blood pressure of not over 80 mm Hg.[59] It would appear more appropriate to advise the victim to lie down immediately and to request someone else to summon medical help immediately.

The involvement of the family doctor in coronary care is also important. If paramedical individuals are able to deal with ventricular fibrillation, then the family doctor should also be able to do so. In rural areas, family doctors, after adequate training, might staff MCCU's.

Early initiation of coronary care will not only result in more patients surviving to reach a hospital but will also limit the size of the infarct in many patients, allowing these patients to be discharged from the hospital sooner.[78]

The coronary care unit and intermediate coronary care unit are discussed in detail in Chapters 5 and 6.

REFERENCES

1. Adgey, A. A. J., Nelson, P. G., Scott, M. E., Geddes, J. S., Allen, J. D., Zaidi, S. A., and Pantridge, J. F.: Management of ventricular fibrillation outside hospital. Lancet i:1169, 1969.
2. Adgey, A. A. J., Allen, J. D., Geddes, J. S., James, R. G. G., Webb, S. W., Zaidi, S. A., and Pantridge, J. F.: Acute phase of myocardial infarction. Lancet ii:501, 1971.
3. Alvarez, H., III, Miller, R. H., and Cobb, L. A.: Medic 1: The Seattle advanced paramedic training program. In National Conference on Emergency Cardiac Care. Washington, D.C., National Academy of Sciences, 1973.
4. Alvarez, H., III, and Cobb, L. A.: Experiences with CPR training of the general public. In National Conference on Emergency Cardiac Care. Washington, D.C., National Academy of Sciences, 1973.
5. Armstrong, A., Duncan, B., Oliver, M. F., Julian, D. G., Donald, K. W., Fulton, M., Lutz, W., and Morrison, S. L.: Natural history of acute coronary heart attacks: A community study. Br. Heart J. 34:67, 1972.

6. Bainton, C. R., and Peterson, D. R.: Deaths from coronary heart disease in persons fifty years of age and younger. N. Engl. J. Med. 268:569, 1963.
7. Barber, J. M., Boyle, D. McC., Chaturvedi, N. C., Gamble, J., Groves, D. H. M., Millar, D. S., Shivalingappa, G., Walsh, M. J., and Wilson, H. K.: Mobile coronary care. Lancet ii:133, 1970.
8. Binnion, P. F., Makous, N., and Keller, W. W.: Cost of a mobile coronary care unit. Am. Heart J. 83:723, 1972.
9. Binnion, P. F., Mandal, S., and Makous, N.: The mobile coronary care unit. JAMA 223:923, 1973.
10. Carveth, S. W.: Cardiac resuscitation program at the Nebraska football stadium. Dis. Chest 53:8, 1968.
11. Chazov, E. I.: First aid in myocardial infarction, p. 313. In D. G. Julian and M. F. Olwer (ed.), Acute Myocardial Infarction: Proceedings of a Symposium. Edinburgh, Livingstone, 1968.
12. Chazov, E. I.: The Role of Mobile Coronary Care Units, Moscow. Copenhagen, WHO Regional Office for Europe, 1970.
13. Cobb, L. A., and Alvarez, H., III: Medic 1: The Seattle system for management of out-of-hospital emergencies. In National Conference on Emergency Cardiac Care. Washington, D.C., National Academy of Sciences, 1973.
14. Cohen, L: Personal communication, 1973.
15. Crampton, R. S., Stillerman, R., Gascho, J. A., Aldrich, R. F., Hunter, F. P., Jr., Harris, R. H., Jr., and McCormack, R. C.: Prehospital coronary care in Charlottesville and Albemarle County. V. Med. Mon. 99:1191, 1972.
16. Crampton, R. S., Aldrich, R. F., Stillerman, R., Gascho, J. A., and Miles, J. R., Jr.: Reduction of community mortality from coronary artery disease after initiation of prehospital cardiopulmonary resuscitation and emergency cardiac care. In National Conference on Emergency Cardiac Care. Washington, D.C., National Academy of Sciences, 1973.
17. Dewar, H. A., McCollum, J. P. K., and Floyd, M.: A year's experience with a mobile coronary resuscitation unit. Br. Med. J. iv:226, 1969.
18. Dundee, J. W., Clarke, R. S. J., and Loan, W. B.: Comparative toxicity of diamorphine, morphine, and methadone. Lancet ii:211, 1967.
19. Dunning, A. J.: Personal communication, 1973.
20. Fulton, M., Julian, D. G., and Oliver, M. F.: Sudden death and myocardial infarction. Circulation 40 (Suppl. 4):182, 1969.
21. Gearty, G. F., Hickey, N., Bourke, G. J., and Mulcahy, R.: Pre-hospital coronary care service. Br. Med. J. iii:33, 1971.
22. Goldstein, S., Moss, A. J., and Greene, W.: Sudden death in acute myocardial infarction. Arch. Intern Med. 129:720, 1972.
23. Gordon, T., and Kannel, W. B.: Premature mortality from coronary heart disease. The Framingham study. JAMA 215:1617, 1971.
24. Grace, W. J., and Chadbourn, J. A.: The mobile coronary care unit. Dis. Chest 55:452, 1969.
25. Grace, W. J., and Chadbourn, J. A.: The first hour in acute myocardial infarction (AMI): Observations on 50 patients. Circulation (Suppl 3) 41:160, 1970.
26. Grace, W. J.: Coronary care: Pre-hospital care of acute myocardial infarction. Report to American Heart Association, 1973.
27. Haigh, M. H.: The Role of Mobile Coronary Care Units, Moscow. Copenhagen, WHO Regional Office for Europe, 1970.
28. Honick, G. L., Nagel, T., and Daniels, A.: A nurse staffed mobile coronary care unit. Okla. State Med. Assoc. J. 63:565, 1970.
29. Jarvis, D., and Kushnir, S.: Mobile coronary-care team's efforts save patients from premature death. Hosp. Top. 49:49, 1971.
30. Kernohan, R. J., and McGucken, R. B.: Mobile intensive care in myocardial infarction. Br. Med. J. iii:178, 1968.
31. Kerr, F., Ewing, D. J., Irving, J. B., and Kirby, B. J.: Nitrous-oxide analgesia in myocardial infarction. Lancet i:63, 1972.

32. Kubik, M. M., Bhowmick, B. K., Stokes, T., and Joshi, M.: Mobile cardiac unit. Experience from a West Midland town. Br. Heart J. 36:238, 1974.
33. Lambrew, C. T., Schuchman, W. L., and Cannon, T. H.: Emergency medical transport systems: Use of ECG telemetry. Chest 63:477, 1973.
34. Lewis, A. J., Ailshie, G., and Criley, J. M.: Pre-hospital cardiac care in a paramedical mobile intensive care unit. Calif. Med. 117:1, 1972.
35. Lewis, A. J.: Personal communication, 1973.
36. Lewis, R. P., Frazier, J. T., and Warren, J. V.: Mobile coronary care: An approach to the early mortality of myocardial infarction. (Abstr.) Am. J. Cardiol. 26:644, 1970.
37. Lund, I.: Resuscitation of cardiac arrest by doctor-manned ambulance services in Oslo. In National Conference on Emergency Cardiac Care. Washington, D.C., National Academy of Sciences, 1973.
38. MacDonald, H. R., Rees, H. A., Muir, A. L., Lawrie, D. M., Burton, J. L., and Donald, K. W.: Circulatory effects of heroin in patients with myocardial infarction. Lancet i:1070, 1967.
39. Maroko, P. R., Kjekshus, J. K., Sobel, B. E., Watanabe, T., Covell, J. W., Ross, J., Jr., and Braunwald, E.: Factors influencing infarct size following experimental coronary artery occlusions. Circulation 43:67, 1971.
40. Maroko, P. R., Libby, P., Covell, J. W., Sobel, B. E., Ross, J., Jr., and Braunwald, E.: Precordial S-T segment elevation mapping: An atraumatic method for assessing alterations in the extent of myocardial ischemic injury. Am. J. Cardiol. 29:223, 1972.
41. Mather, H. G., Pearson, N. G., Read, K. L. G., Shaw, D. B., Steed, G. R., Thorne, M. G., Jones, S., Guerrier, C. J., Eraut, C. D., McHugh, P. M., Chowdhury, N. R., Jafary, M. H., and Wallace, T. J.: Acute myocardial infarction: Home and hospital treatment. Br. Med. J. iii:334, 1971.
42. McDonald, T. L.: The London Hospital, p. 29. In D. G. Julian and M. F. Oliver (ed.), Acute Myocardial Infarction: Proceedings of a Symposium. Edinburgh, Livingstone, 1968.
43. McDonald, E. L.: Personal communication, 1971.
44. McNeilly, R. H., and Pemberton, J.: Duration of last attack in 998 fatal cases of coronary artery disease and its relation to possible cardiac resuscitation. Br. Med. J. iii:139, 1968.
45. Miura, I.: Mobile coronary care unit, p. 5. In Proceedings V Asian-Pacific Congress of Cardiology, Singapore, 1972.
46. Moiseev, S. G.: The experience of rendering first aid to myocardial infarction patients in Moscow. Sov. Med. 25:30, 1962.
47. Muir, A. L.: The circulatory effects of analgesics in myocardial infarction, p. 285. In D. G. Julian and M. F. Oliver (ed.), Acute Myocardial Infarction: Proceedings of A Symposium. Edinburgh, Livingstone, 1968.
48. Mulholland, H. C., and Pantridge, J. F.: Heart rate changes during movement of patients with acute myocardial infarction. Lancet i:1244, 1974.
49. Nagel, E. L., Hirschman, J. C., Nussenfeld, S. R., Rankin, D., and Lundblad, E.: Telemetry-medical command in coronary and other mobile emergency care systems. JAMA 214:332, 1970.
50. Nixon, P. G. F.: Flying squad services, p. 318. In D. G. Julian and M. F. Oliver (ed.), Acute Myocardial Infarction. Proceedings of a Symposium. Edinburgh, Livingstone, 1968.
51. Nolte, C. T.: Delivery of early coronary care. Ind. Med. 42:26, 1973.
52. O'Rourke, M.: Modified coronary ambulances (Abstr.), p. 51. In Proceedings of V Asian-Pacific Congress of Cardiology, Singapore, 1972.
53. O'Rourke, M.: Modified coronary ambulances. Med. J. Aust. 1:875, 1972.
54. Pantridge, J. F., and Geddes, J. S.: Cardiac arrest after myocardial infarction. Lancet i:807, 1966.
55. Pantridge, J. F., and Geddes, J. S.: A mobile intensive-care unit in the management of myocardial infarction. Lancet ii:271, 1967.

56. Pantridge, J. F.: The Role of Mobile Coronary Care Units, Moscow. Copenhagen, WHO Regional Office for Europe, 1970.
57. Pantridge, J. F.: The effect of early therapy on the hospital mortality from acute myocardial infarction. Quart. J. Med. 39:621, 1970.
58. Pantridge, J. F.: Mobile coronary care. Chest 58:229, 1970.
59. Pantridge, J. F., Webb, S. W., Adgey, A. A. J., and Geddes, J. S.: The first hour after the onset of acute myocardial infarction, p. 173. P. N. Yu and J. F. Goodwin (ed.), Progress in Cardiology. Vol. 3. Philadelphia, Lea & Febiger, 1974.
60. Paul, O.: Prehospital management of acute myocardial infarction. Med. Clin. N. Am. 57:119, 1973.
61. Robinson, J. S., and McLean, A. C. J.: Mobile coronary care. Med. J. Aust. 2:439, 1970.
62. Risati, M. C., Granatelli, A., Lustig, G. J., McGinn, T. G., and Arluck, S. B.: Community hospital mobile coronary care unit. N.Y. State J. Med. 70:2462, 1970.
63. Rose, L. B., and Press, E.: Cardiac defibrillation by ambulance attendants. JAMA 219:63, 1972.
64. Safar, P., Esposito, G., and Benson, D. M.: Ambulance design and equipment for mobile intensive care. Arch. Surg. 102:163, 1971.
65. Sandler, G., and Pistevos, A.: Mobile coronary care: The coronary ambulance. Br. Heart J. 34:1283, 1972.
66. Sarnoff, S. J.: A plan for reducing the prehospital mortality due to acute myocardial infarction. Carl J. Wiggers Award Lecture, Circulation Group, American Physiological Society, 1970.
67. Schwartz, M. L.: Early Coronary Care Systems: The Greatest Medical Problem. New York, Act Foundation, 1971, p. 8.
68. Shillingford, J. P.:, p. 292. In D. G. Julian and M. F. Oliver, (ed.), Acute Myocardial Infarction: Proceedings of a Symposium. Edinburgh, Livingstone, 1968.
69. Stad Utrecht gaat als eerste in Nederland twee cardulances in gebruik nemen (Introduction in Utrecht of the first two "cardulances" used in the Netherlands). Technische Gids voor Ziekenhuis en Instelling (Amsterdam) 39 (940): p. 207, 1970.
70. Steinbrunn, W.: Personal communication, 1973.
71. Thomas, M., Malmcrona, R., Fillmore, S., and Shillingford, J.: Haemodynamic effects of morphine in patients with acute myocardial infarction. Br. Heart J. 27:863, 1965.
72. Thornton, J. A., Fleming, J. S., Goldberg, A. D., and Baird, D.: Cardiovascular effects of 50% nitrous oxide and 50% oxygen mixture. Anaesthesia 28:484, 1973.
73. Walsh, M. J., Shivalingappa, G., Scaria, K., Morrison, C., Kumar, B., Farnan, C., Chaturvedi, N. C., Boyle, D. McC., and Barber, J. M.: Mobile coronary care. Br. Heart J. 34:701, 1972.
74. Warren, J. V.: Early Coronary Care Systems: The Greatest Medical Problem. New York, Act Foundation, 1971, p. 7.
75. Webb, S. W., Adgey, A. A. J., and Pantridge, J. F.: Autonomic disturbance at onset of acute myocardial infarction. Br. Med. J. iii:89, 1972.
76. White, N. M., Parker, W. S., Binning, R. A., Kimber, E. R., Ead, H. W., and Chamberlain, D. A.: Mobile coronary care provided by ambulance personnel. Br. Med. J. iii:618, 1973.
77. World Health Organization: The Role of Mobile Coronary Care Units, Moscow. Copenhagen, WHO Regional Office for Europe, 1970.
78. Wilson, C., and Pantridge, J. F.: ST segment displacement and early hospital discharge in acute myocardial infarction. Lancet ii:1284, 1973.
79. Yu, P. N.: Prehospital care of acute myocardial infarction. Circulation 45:189, 1972.

Chapter 5
CORONARY CARE UNIT

LESLIE WIENER

With few exceptions,[1,2] intensive coronary care has been accepted as an integral part of customary hospital practice. It has been more than a decade since the opening of the first coronary care unit. During this time, the coronary care unit has changed in concept from a place where high-risk patients were grouped to ensure prompt cardiopulmonary resuscitation to a more intricate treatment center where arrhythmias that lead to cardiac arrest and early pump failure are more effectively treated.

This chapter reviews many aspects of the development of the coronary care unit concept. It will provide a description of the operations of the unit, including a classification of the arrhythmias that are commonly encountered in acute myocardial infarction as well as a discussion of some of the current methods of treatment of these arrhythmias. Emphasis will also be given to the development of new methods for managing the still unsolved problem of pump failure. Consideration will be given to iatrogenic hazards of the CCU technique, including errors in the interpretation of the oscilloscope and electrical leakage. Finally, the present and future value of the coronary care unit will be examined.

PERSONNEL

At present there is a wide disparity in the implementation of the concept of intensive coronary care. The variation is seen not merely in differences in physical design of facilities or type of hospital but instead in

65

method of operation. The success of the coronary care unit has, to a large extent, been dependent on a team approach. Lack of a plan that allocates to each member specific functions and responsibilities results in increased morbidity and mortality. An ideal coronary care unit team consists of a director, specially trained nursing personnel, paramedical assistants, attending physicians, and house staff.

Much of the form and direction of the coronary care unit stems from the personality and professional competence of the unit director. The responsibilities of the director are diverse and should consist of functioning as a liason between all members of the team; organizing and participating in the training of nurses, paramedics, and house staff; providing specialized technical expertise in coronary care as a consultant to the attending physician; assuming responsibility for initiating emergency measures when necessary; establishing the protocols for treatment and assigning specific duties to various members of the team; contributing to decisions regarding administrative policies of the unit; selecting monitoring and supportive equipment to be used in the unit; introducing new methods for coronary care. The delegation of these responsibilities to a unit director has now become common practice in most coronary care units. Nonetheless, many of these responsibilities can be shared with a committee of physicians.

Considerable effort must be made to train nurses specialized in the principles and practices of intensive coronary care. As part of the team approach, the nurse has emerged as the key to successful coronary care. The initiation of prophylactic emergency medical treatment is often predicated upon the nurse's observations. It is fundamental then that the nurse be empowered to act according to the training she has received. This training should prepare the nurse to recognize premonitory, potentially lethal, cardiac arrhythmias as well as early signs and symptoms of circulatory failure. He or she must be able to evaluate the effectiveness of all therapy on an ongoing basis. The nurse must act to initiate defibrillation or cardiopulmonary resuscitation when necessary and, of course, decide when a physician is to be notified.

A typical system of training for coronary care nurses involves a comprehensive indoctrination program consisting of didactic lectures at a nurse-to-nurse level, supplemented by physician-to-nurse lectures, team conferences, programmed texts, and audiovisual aids. It is recommended that the initial training course be 4 to 6 weeks long and include a review of cardiopulmonary physiology, with special emphasis on coronary heart disease. Additional training is necessary in the technological aspects of coronary care unit care; this training includes instruction in interpreting electrocardiograms and utilizing electronic monitoring devices. The nurse must also achieve proficiency in the cardiopulmonary resuscitation procedure and must fully understand the concepts of electrical pacing, defibrillation, and synchronized countershock. Once the nurse has been judged competent, she can be assigned to a regular rotation in the unit. Optimal, effective coronary care requires a nurse-to-patient ratio of approximately 3 to 1. A training program without continuing education is clearly insufficient.

The use of an increasingly complex technology for patient monitoring for diagnosis and treatment has given rise to the need for cardiology technicians, electronics technicians, and biomedical engineers.

Cardiology technicians contribute to the team effort by setting up and maintaining more elaborate items of monitoring equipment. Their assistance is invaluable in charting the course of those patients who require invasive cardiac catheterization monitoring. In this context, they may assist in the actual catheterization procedure by preparing sterile set-ups of special trays, balancing and calibrating equipment for pressure recordings and cardiac output. They ensure steady and continuous operation of these devices by periodic observation at regular intervals. Working in conjunction with the nursing staff, they have extended cardiac electronic surveillance to include early recognition and management of circulatory failure. Highly motivated nurses and other paramedical personnel familiar with patient care problems are selected for training in this technical specialty. The cardiology technician should be included in the comprehensive indoctrination and continuing education program developed by the unit director.

In larger hospitals and university centers, a biomedical engineer is responsible for planning and supervising new construction, maintenance, surveillance, and repair of equipment. In addition, his or her services can be extended to the important role of educating all staff members who work with life-support equipment, regardless of professional station or job title. The first step in any education program is to acquaint personnel with principles of electrical safety. Hospital workers operating electrical equipment should have a general appreciation of their purpose and operation, as well as their limitations. Thus, standards can be set for all medical personnel working with expensive electrical equipment. In each case the biomedical engineer should focus attention on those principles that relate to specific duties of personnel at different levels. Staff members should be observed periodically in the performance of their duties when electrical instruments, both line-powered and battery-operated, are used. Such surveillance guards against lowering of standards that may result in unsafe practices.

The biomedical engineer's services also include the development and testing of new items of electronic equipment. His or her advice should be sought whenever purchase of additional medical equipment is considered. Together with electronics technicians, the biomedical engineer can be called upon to establish a program of regular, periodic inspections and testing of equipment for safety features and standards of performance. A permanent record or log should indicate the date, condition of apparatus, and tests made. Each device tested should be tagged as approved. At the least, trained maintenance personnel should measure leakage currents and inspect controls, connections, lines, plugs, fuses, and grounds. Equipment occasionally brought into critical care areas, e.g., portable x-ray units, must be checked as rigorously as life-support equipment. When necessary, repair or modification of electrical equipment can often be performed in house at considerable financial savings to the hospital.

In small hospitals, an interested member of the professional staff or the unit director might be encouraged to develop expertise in physics and medical electronics. An outside biomedical engineering service may then be engaged in to run the unit's electrical safety and maintenance program.

An attempt must be made to balance the responsibility of the physician for his own patient against the probability that his busy schedule will permit him to be in the unit for only a brief period on any given day. Accordingly, the attending physician must be willing to delegate some of his normal responsibility to a centralized medical authority, e.g., the director of the CCU who in turns directs members of the team who are always present in the unit. The presence of the attending physician at CCU committee meetings and conferences is desirable and strengthens the group approach. The attending physician should provide those general and specific recommendations pertinent to his patient's needs, but the team should be empowered to act on their own in emergencies to initiate the established protocol for treatment.

In many small hospitals, a resident house staff may not be available and many of their responsibilities must be assumed by the attending staff and unit director through the participation of highly trained nursing personnel. However, in large hospitals with adequate house staffs, the coronary care unit provides a unique experience in physician training. A significant amount of responsibility for patient care may be assumed by the well-trained house officer. Thus, when the coronary care unit nurse detects a significant change in a patient's course, he or she can instantly call upon the house officer or attending physician. The house officer may then make decisions that eliminate delays in treatment due to communication problems. As a consequence, the training program for house staff in coronary care should include a complete review of cardiac arrhythmias, practical experience with the use of specialized coronary care equipment, a refresher course in the recognition and treatment of the complications of myocardial infarction, and a review of the pharmacology of antiarrhythmic and other cardiac drugs. The role of the house staff physician as a member of the team must be anticipated by prior orientation and explanation in order to assure treatment that provides each patient with the benefit of expert care.

ADMISSION AND DISCHARGE POLICY

It has been clearly demonstrated that death following acute myocardial infarction occurs early in the clinical course. Approximately 70% of the total mortality occurs in the first 5 days after admission or earlier.[4] The remaining deaths occur during the subsequent weeks of hospitalization. There is evidence that these late deaths are due to circulatory failure and concomitant secondary arrhythmias.[5] Accordingly, aggressive prophylactic management of arrhythmias could not be expected to significantly influence the outcome in this group of patients. In view of the clinical importance of the period immediately following the onset of symptoms, it is crucial that the unit policy encourage the earliest possible admission of suspected myocardial infarction patients.[6] Since there is a striking decrease in mortality after the first 2 days of myocardial infarction, it appears less crucial to admit patients when symptoms indicate that onset was more than 2 days before.[7]

Because of the considerable pressure for admission of patients with proven or suspected myocardial infarction, the discharge policy of the unit is important in determining the number that can be accommodated. In general, patients with proven transmural myocardial infarction should be monitored for at least 72 hours or until 2 days have passed since the successful suppression of the last life-threatening arrhythmia.

DIAGNOSIS OF ACUTE MYOCARDIAL INFARCTION

In a significant percentage of patients (38%) the correct identification of acute myocardial infarction presents a problem. Killip and Kimball[8] have established criteria for the diagnosis of acute myocardial infarction in three separate categories:

A. Acute transmural infarction—pain, Q waves, changing ECG, enzyme rise
B. Acute infarction (probably subendocardial)—pain, ST–T abnormalities, changing ECG, enzyme rise
C. Possible infarction—pain, abnormal ECG, enzymes nonspecific

In group A and B the hospital mortality rate was 30%, while in group C the mortality was only 3%. Thus the mortality statistics upon which the efficacy of coronary care units may be judged will depend upon the accuracy of a diagnosis of myocardial infarction.

CARDIAC ARRHYTHMIAS

The principal contribution of the coronary care unit to the successful management of acute myocardial infarction derives from the early recognition and prompt control of cardiac arrhythmias leading to cardiac arrest.

Typically, cardiac arrhythmias can be classified according to their site of origin, such as atrial, atrioventricular junctional, and ventricular. Conduction disturbances can be described according to the anatomy involved and the degree of block manifested (i.e., bundle branch block; first, second, and third degree AV block).

Tachyarrhythmias

Ventricular ectopic beats are observed in about 80% of patients with acute myocardial infarction.[9] The potential for degeneration into ventricular tachycardia or fibrillation is present when ventricular ectopic beats occur with a frequency of more than five per minute, when they are grouped, when there is a changing QRS configuration (multifocal beats), and when they fall in close proximity to the preceding T wave ("vulnerable period"). Under these circumstances immediate antiarrhythmic therapy is advised in order to prevent the ventricular fibrillation. In most cases, successful suppression can be achieved by an intravenous lidocaine bolus (50–100 mg in up to three successive doses, if necessary). When control has been accomplished, an intravenous drip diluted in 5% dextrose solution at from 1 to 4 mg per minute can be expected to maintain control. When the arrhythmia persists following attempts at weaning lidocaine, Pronestyl or quinidine should be added. In 80% of cases lidocaine successfully suppressed the arrhythmia, while 10% required additional antiarrhythmic therapy.[10] In the remaining 10%, who are refractory to all drugs, "overriding" by artificial cardiac pacing may be successful (see Chapters 7 and 10).

Persisting sinus tachycardia and atrial tachyarrhythmias (fibrillation or flutter) are often present in conjuction with developing left ventricular failure.[9] Accordingly, digitalization is often required. The use of digitalis glycosides does not preclude the need for other antiarrhythmic agents (see Chapter 7). Quinidine given by mouth may be effective in converting and suppressing most atrial tachyarrhythmias. If atrial tachyarrhythmia persists, it should be converted with direct current synchronized countershock (see Chapter 9).

Bradyarrhythmias

During myocardial infarction, sinus bradycardia and AV junctional rhythm may evolve as a consequence of increased vagal tone. Initially, intravenous atropine in 0.3-mg increments up to a total of 2 mg is given, with subsequent doses as needed every 2–4 hours. If the sinus bradycardia or AV junctional arrhythmia is caused by a falling cardiac output, then an intravenous Isuprel drip (1 mg in 500 ml dextrose in water administered at 1 to 2 ml per minute) is preferable to atropine.

While a critical rate-dependent reduction in cardiac output, indicated by decreased systemic blood pressure, mental confusion, congestive heart failure, and Adams-Stokes syndrome, represents an urgent indication for artificial pacing, other justifications for insertion of pacemaker catheters remain uncertain. A strong case for prophylactic insertion of pacing electrodes can be made by examining the high mortality of myocardial infarction associated with second- and third-degree AV block.[11] Control of the electrical activity of the heart by pacing has an advantage over drug therapy in that it is more reliable and predictable and that unlike drugs, its action is instant and can be terminated at will. On the other hand, Lown and co-workers[12] found that AV block in acute myocardial infarction evolves gradually and that there is time to employ medical measures first. According to this group, the critical factor in determining need for drug therapy is the ventricular rate. Atropine is used first, and if the ventricular rate does not increase, then isoproterenol is chosen. This more conservative approach is supported by the observation that the risk of ventricular fibrillation in acute AV block is greatest during pacemaker insertion.[13,14] Moreover, ventricular fibrillation is a major complication associated with artificial pacing, occurring in 5–21% of cases. Contrasted with Lown's considerations, a recent study of patients under continuous electrocardiographic monitoring has demonstrated that some patients develop complete AV block abruptly, from one beat to the next.[15] In this group, the precipitous onset of complete AV block did not allow time for the initiation of pacing. Those patients prone to sudden onset of complete AV block were identified as having anteroseptal myocardial infarctions resulting in a bundle branch block. Hence, a more aggressive approach (pacemaker insertion) in the presence of any phase of AV block complicated by anteroseptal myocardial infarction seems warranted. Scott and associates[16] recently reported that 18% of their patients with complete AV block following acute myocardial infarction developed ventricular fibrillation unrelated to any form of therapy. This arrhythmia is observed to evolve from frequent or critically timed premature ventricular contractions, coincident with bradycardia.

Based on these observations, the following criteria for pacemaker insertion are suggested (see also Chapter 10):

Mobitz type II second-degree AV block resulting from anterior myocardial infarction or bilateral bundle branch block

Symptomatic Wenckebach (Mobitz type I) AV block in which drug therapy fails to maintain the ventricular rate satisfactorily (between 60 and 80 beats per minute); or if drug therapy becomes compromised by increasing coronary insufficiency and myocardial irritability

Symptomatic complete AV block in acute diaphragmatic myocardial infarction

All acute anterior myocardial infarctions complicated by complete AV block

Acute left or right bundle branch block (may or may not be associated with hemiblocks) in acute anterior myocardial infarction (prophylactic pacing)

Frequent premature ventricular contractions (more than 5 or 6 per minute) in the presence of second-degree or complete AV block (bradytachycardia syndrome)

HEMODYNAMIC MONITORING FOR CIRCULATORY FAILURE

Pulmonary Artery and Pulmonary Wedge Pressure

The development of a flow-directed, balloon-tipped catheter that can easily be introduced at the bedside into the pulmonary artery without fluoroscopic monitoring may achieve for hemodynamic monitoring what the electrocardiogram has accomplished for bedside detection of cardiac arrhythmias. In acute myocardial infarction, knowledge of left ventricular filling pressure is essential for reliable quantification of myocardial performance. On-line measurement of this pressure will provide a quantitative means for anticipation of pulmonary edema. It also allows optimum volume support in low-flow, low-pressure states and continuous assessment of the hemodynamic effects of complex therapeutic interventions (pharmacologic, electrical, and surgical).

Before the advent of a simple means for bedside monitoring of pulmonary artery pressure, central venous pressure had been widely employed as a guide to fluid therapy. In particular, it was assumed that pulmonary edema could be recognized from elevations in right heart filling pressure.

However, the use of central venous pressure monitoring for this purpose assumes that right ventricle function reflects changes in the left ventricular function. Forrester and co-workers[17] have presented clear evidence that central venous pressure correlates poorly with pulmonary artery wedge pressure after myocardial infarction. Furthermore, it is not infrequent for even directional changes in central venous pressure to be misleading.

Although the balloon-tipped, flow-directed catheter may be advanced into the pulmonary artery simply and with reasonable safety, this invasive approach is not entirely without hazard.[18] Accordingly, application of this method for monitoring patients with myocardial infarction is not likely to be as widespread as noninvasive electrocardiographic monitoring. At present, our patient selection criteria for specialized invasive hemodynamic monitoring in acute myocardial infarction include patients manifesting left ventricular failure and/or cardiogenic shock; patients requiring rapid infusion of intravenous fluids, including blood replacement; patients requiring pharmacologic therapies known to have potent depressant effects on myocardial contractility; and patients with risk factors predisposing to left ventricular failure and cardiogenic shock (for instance, massive infarction, ventricular arrhythmias, and previous infarction). It is essential that this last group be identified and their cardiac function characterized if the concept of aggressive management by prophylaxis, so successful in the management of cardiac arrhythmias, is to be extended to the management of pump failure.

Patients in whom cardiac pump complications develop tend to be older than those without these complications. The average age of patients with left ventricular failure and/or shock following myocardial infarction is slightly more than 65 years.[19] While shock occurs in any adult age group, it is not commonly seen before the sixth decade. The incidence of previous myocardial infarction as well as hypertension seems to significantly influence the potential for left ventricular failure.[20] Moreover, anterior myocardial infarction and diabetes mellitus are particularly common in cardiogenic shock patients.[21,22] In the absence of electrocardiographic evidence of transmural myocardial infarction and marked elevation in cardiac enzyme levels, left ventricular failure is unlikely.[23] However, subendocardial infarction affecting such vital areas as the papillary muscle may produce severe mitral regurgitation, resulting in congestive heart failure and shock. It has been our policy to anticipate severe left ventricular dysfunction in patients manifesting acute myocardial infarction. Consequently, pulmonary artery pressure monitoring is employed whenever the aforementioned clinical profile of pump failure is found.

The effectiveness and simplicity of the balloon-tipped catheter technique permits serial monitoring of pulmonary artery wedge pressure. In addition to providing an index of left ventricular function, high-quality wedge tracings may disclose acute mitral regurgitation due, for example, to papillary muscle dysfunction. However, central pulmonary artery pressure measurement will suffice for continuous monitoring of left ventricular pressure. The end-diastolic pulmonary artery pressure in most circumstances appears to closely approximate left ventricular end-diastolic pressure (Fig. 5-1). In this more central location, the potential hazard of pulmonary infarction resulting from continuous peripheral pulmonary arterial obstruction (wedged catheter) is avoided.

The catheter insertion technique involves isolation of a suitably sized antecubital vein. Since the wave forms must be recognized, fluid columns cannot be used. Appropriate strain gauges and display systems are necessary since proper guidance requires the recognition of sequential entry into the right atrium, right ventricle, and pulmonary artery. Because the method is invasive, surgical draping and sterile technique are mandatory. The catheter is prepared for monitoring by filling from a pressurized fluid source through a flush system (Fig. 5-2). Physiologic

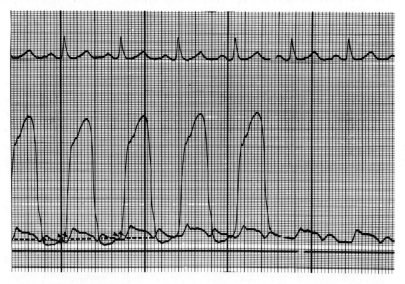

Figure 5-1. Pulmonary artery pressure and left ventricular pressure are recorded simultaneously. Note that the end-diastolic pulmonary artery pressure and end-diastolic left ventricular pressure are located at the same pressure level. In the last third of the tracing, pulmonary artery pressure is recorded simultaneously from both transducers, indicating that the calibration and sensitivity of each transducer were identical.

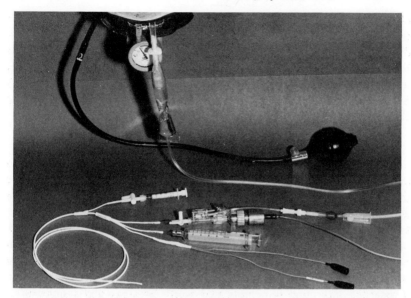

Figure 5-2. Bedside setup for monitoring pulmonary artery pressure and cardiac output. The catheter terminates in four parts (top to bottom): (1) syringe and stopcock connected through a lumen to a distal balloon; (2) transducer connected through a controlled continuous-flush device (limiting flow to 2 to 3 ml/hr.) to a distal-tip catheter opening sampling pulmonary artery pressure; (3) syringe for room-temperature saline injection (thermal dilution cardiac output) connected to a catheter lumen opening 20 cm proximal to the catheter tip; and (4) electric terminals from a distal-tip thermistor connecting to a Wheatstone bridge. (Catheter supplied through the courtesy of American Catheter Corporation, Stokes Road, Medford, N.J. 08055.)

saline with four units of heparin per milliliter is pressurized to 300 mm Hg in an air-free plastic bag. The continuous flow of 2 to 3 ml/hr allowed by the flush system through the catheter prevents clotting and consequent loss of catheter function. A rapid flush valve simplifies filling and flushing the system and permits dynamic response testing of the catheter transducer system.

The principal complications attendant upon use of this catheter system include cardiac arrhythmias, pulmonary emboli and infarction, and infection. Because of the nature of its construction, cardiac arrhythmias are less frequent with the use of this device than with other types of catheters. During insertion, the balloon-tipped surface tends to cushion the impact as the catheter is manipulated through the sensitive endocardial surfaces along the right ventricular outflow tract. Premature ventricular contractions are only occasionally encountered during passage of the catheter (11%).[18] Pulmonary emboli and infarction can be avoided with low-dose heparin, a continuous flush system, and withdrawal of the catheter from the pulmonary artery wedge position after balloon inflation or during spontaneous advancement. The risk of serious infection can be reduced by topical antibiotic ointment (Neosporin) applied at the site of incision, sterile dressings, and removal of the catheter as soon as the clinical condition warrants.

Cardiac Output Determination

Cardiac output determination provides an additional vital insight into the management of critically ill patients. The simultaneous measurement of cardiac output and left ventricular filling pressure provides objective assessment of left ventricular function in the Frank Starling framework. In myocardial infarction, the relationship of left ventricular stroke work to left ventricular end-diastolic pressure invariably shows the most pronounced depression of left ventricular function in patients experiencing cardiogenic shock. Similar but less profound changes are noted when myocardial infarction is complicated solely by signs and symptoms of heart failure. Manipulation of preload by rapid infusion of volume expanders in patients with normal or mildly elevated left ventricular filling pressures or application of potent rapid diuretics when left ventricular filling pressure is markedly elevated (>20 mm Hg) can establish an optimal left ventricular pressure on an individualized basis. Thus, cardiac function may be measured in order to achieve optimal cardiac output in a manner appropriate to the metabolic requirements of the body. Occasionally in cardiogenic shock the infarcted ventricle does not fully utilize its reserve capacity. In these cases, further increase in end-diastolic pressure can augment stroke work and avert irreversible changes.

Cardiac output may be measured by central venous injection of Cardiogreen followed by densitometric determination made via blood sampled from a peripheral artery (dye dilution curve). However, this technique requires considerable equipment and technical expertise. An adequate and simple index of cardiac output may be obtained by sampling from the pulmonary artery. Close correlation between mixed venous oxygen saturation and cardiac output measured by the dye dilution method has been demonstrated (Fig. 5-3). Recently, the flow-directed, balloon-tipped catheter has been modified to permit rapid and accurate measurement of cardiac output by the thermal dilution technique. A thermistor system is balanced against a Wheatstone bridge at the patient's body temperature. A 10-cc volume of physiologic saline or 5% dextrose in water at room temperature is injected rapidly into the right atrium by means of the proximal lumen of a specially designed balloon-

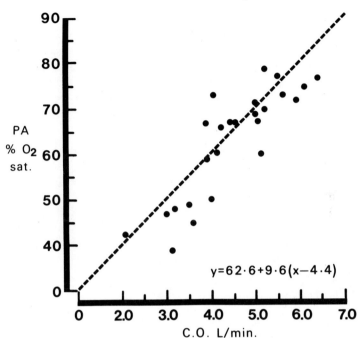

Figure 5-3. Pulmonary artery (*PA*) oxygen saturation correlated with cardiac output (*CO*).

tipped catheter. The off-balanced output from the Wheatstone bridge caused by the change in pulmonary artery blood temperature is amplified and recorded. The area under the temperature–time curve may be determined by planimetry, calculated from the Stewart-Hamilton indicator dilution equation, or computed immediately with an analogue computer.

HAZARDS OF THE CORONARY CARE UNIT

The coronary care unit as a mode of therapy for acute myocardial infarction has distinct advantages, but it has certain limitations and even dangers.

The electrocardiogram as displayed on the oscilloscope is often difficult to interpret because of rapid sweep, baseline instability, 60-cycle interference, patient movement, and pacemaker artifacts.[24] The use of electronic filtering circuits, while minimizing these difficulties, often distorts the basic nature of the ECG wave forms. It is important for the personnel staffing the unit to be familiar with these aberrations so that the electrocardiogram will not be misinterpreted.

Leakage of electrical currents can result in ventricular fibrillation.[25]

The moist skin under monitoring electrodes may provide a low-resistance pathway for current. Intravascular catheters and, in particular, cardiac pacing catheters form a direct electrical pathway to the heart. Since the ischemic heart can be fibrillated by currents as low as 150 micro-amperes, extreme care must be taken to protect patients from extraneous current leakage. For safe operation within the unit, the following guide-lines should be observed:

1. Defibrillation equipment should be readily available whenever electrical devices are applied to the patient.
2. Electrical equipment should be checked before and after being applied to the patient in order to prevent current leakage.
3. Equipment should be adequately grounded to avoid the vast majority of hazards.
4. Ground circuits should be tested periodically to see that they lead to a common ground.
5. New equipment and wiring within the CCU should have properly isolated circuits.

ACCOMPLISHMENTS OF CORONARY CARE UNITS

It is quite clear, from statistics from coronary care units throughout the world, that the original plan in intensive coronary care has already reached a point of maximal effectiveness. No further decrease in mortal-ity rate can be expected from aggressive prophylactic management of cardiac arrhythmias. The residual 15–20% mortality rate reflects our inability to combat death from pump failure. In the system of manage-ment outlined here at least 80% of patients with true cardiogenic shock die and once overt congestive heart failure develops, the mortality is approximately 40%.[19,26-28]

It is now widely accepted that pump failure in myocardial infarction is usually the result of very extensive structural damage to the left ven-tricle.[29] Accordingly, pharmacologic management with potent inotropic agents cannot be expected to provide sustained improvement once circu-latory failure becomes fully developed. Recently, the effectiveness of mechanical devices for support of the failing left ventricle has been demonstrated.[30] However, there is little reason to believe that, once cir-culatory failure resulting from extensive progressive myocardial infarc-tion becomes evident, the ultimate outcome will be significantly altered. If a further reduction in mortality is to be achieved, it appears that the concept of aggressive management by prophylaxis must be extended into the area of pump failure. Recent studies have offered some hope that the cause of pump failure can be identified.[31,32] At present, this requires specialized myocardial metabolic studies involving cardiac catheterization. It is to be anticipated that subsequent correlations will permit development of a bedside noninvasive, clinical profile for recognition of these high-risk patients. Once the high- and low-risk categories are separated, therapeutic alternatives chosen from a variety of medical and surgical methods can be applied in a more individualized and rational manner.

SUMMARY

A unified plan to reduce mortality from acute myocardial infarction has been considered. The concepts of monitoring and treatment of cardiac arrhythmias appearing in the coronary care unit are fundamental in reducing mortality. It has been demonstrated that ventricular fibrillation and cardiac standstill are at times reversible and that, with appropriate prophylactic treatment of premonitory arrhythmias, the occurrence of these cardiac catastrophes can often be prevented. The current mortality of 15–20% will not be reduced further until the problem of pump failure can be solved. The next step in the battle against sudden death from myocardial infarction involves an extension of the concept of aggressive management by prophylactic means to include circulatory failure.

Prehospital management of acute myocardial infarction (mobile coronary care) is treated in Chapter 4, and the intermediate coronary care unit is described in detail in Chapter 6.

REFERENCES

1. Bloom, B. S., and Peterson, O. L.: End results, cost and productivity of coronary care units. N. Engl. J. Med. 288:72, 1973.
2. Mather, H. G., Pearson, N. G., and Read, K. L. Q.: Acute myocardial infarction: home and hospital treatment. Br. Med. J. 3:334, 1971.
3. U.S. Department of Health, Education, and Welfare: Coronary Care Units. Public Health Service Publication No. 1250, 1966.
4. Grace, W. J., and Soscia, J. L.: Reducing mortality from acute myocardial infarction: Current ideas. Cardiol. Dig. 4:29, 1969.
5. Lown, B., Vassaux, C., Hood, W. B., Jr., Fakhro, A. M., Kaplinsky, E., and Roberge, G.: Unresolved problems in coronary care. Am. J. Cardiol. 20:494, 1967.
6. The Current Status of Intensive Coronary Care, Symposium. New York, The Charles Press, 1966.
7. Oliver, M. F., Julian, D. G., and Donald, K. W.: Problems in evaluating coronary care units. Am. J. Cardiol. 20:465, 1967.
8. Killip, T., III, and Kimball, J. T.: Treatment of myocardial infarction in a coronary care unit. Am. J. Cardiol. 20:457, 1967.
9. Lown, B., Klein, M. D., and Hershberg, P. I.: Coronary and precoronary care. Am. J. Med. 46:705, 1969.
10. Lown, B., and Vassaux, C.: Lidocaine in acute myocardial infarction. Am. Heart J. 76:568, 1968.

11. Friedberg, C. K., Cohen, H., and Donoso, E.: Advanced heart block as a complication of acute myocardial infarction. Role of pacemaker therapy. Prog. Cardiovasc. Dis. 10:466, 1968.
12. Lown, B., Fakhro, A. M., Hood, W. B., Jr., and Thorn, G. W.: The coronary care unit: New prospectives and directions. JAMA 199:156, 1967.
13. Paulk, E. A., and Hurst, J. W.: Complete heart block in acute myocardial infarction. A clinical evaluation of the intracardiac bipolar catheter pacemaker. Am. J. Cardiol. 17:695, 1966.
14. Parsonnet, V., Zucker, I. R., Gilbert, L., Rothfield, E. L., Brief, D. K., and Albert, J.: Evaluation of transvenous pacemaking of the heart in complete heart block following acute myocardial infarction. Isr. J. Med. Sci. 3:306, 1967.
15. Stock, R. J., and Macken, D. L.: Observations on heart block during continuous electrocardiographic monitoring in myocardial infarction. Circulation 38:993, 1968.
16. Scott, M. E., Geddes, J. S., Patterson, D. Z., Adgey, A. A. J., and Pantridge, J. F.: Management of complete heart block complicating acute myocardial infarction. Lancet ii:1382, 1967.
17. Forrester, J. S., Diamond, G., McHugh, T. J., and Swan, H. J. C.: Filling pressures in the right and left side of the heart in acute myocardial infarction. N. Engl. J. Med. 285:190, 1971.
18. Swan, H. J. C., Ganz, W., Forrester, J., Marcus, H., Diamond, G., Chonette, D.: Catheterization of the heart in man with use of a flow-directed balloon-tipped catheter. N. Engl. J. Med. 283:447, 1970.
19. Scheidt, S., Ascheim, R., and Killip, T., III: Shock after acute myocardial infarction. Am. J. Cardiol. 26:556, 1970.
20. Mintz, S. S., and Katz, L. N.: Recent myocardial infarction: An analysis of five hundred and seventy-two cases. Arch. Intern. Med. 80:205, 1947.
21. Norris, R. M., Brandt, P. W. T., Caughey, D. E., Lee, A. J., and Scott, P. J.: A new coronary progenetic index. Lancet i:274, 1969.
22. Stock, E.: Prognosis of myocardial infarction in a coronary care unit. Med. J. Aust. 2:377, 1967.
23. Wiener, L.: Rational therapeutic approach to cardiogenic shock. Cardiovasc. Clin. In Press.
24. Arbeit, S. R., Rubin, I. L., and Gross, H.: Dangers in interpreting the electrocardiogram from the oscilloscope monitor. JAMA 211:453, 1970.
25. Electrical charges can be dangerous. JAMA 201:27, 1967.
26. Gunnar, R. M., Cruz, A., Boswell, J., et al.: Myocardial infarction with shock: Hemodynamic studies and results of therapy. Circulation 33:753, 1966.
27. Wan, S. H., Thompson, P. L., Dowling, J. T., et al: Cardiogenic shock. A review of one year's experience. Med. J. Aust. 1:1000, 1971.
28. Ratshin, R. A., Rackley, C. E., and Russell, R. O., Jr.: Hemodynamic evaluation of left ventricular function in shock complicating myocardial infarction. Circulation 45:127, 1972.
29. Page, D. L., Caulfield, J. B., Kastor, J. A., DeSanctis, R. W., and Sanders, C. A.: Myocardial changes associated with cardiogenic shock. N. Engl. J. Med. 285:133, 1971.
30. Mueller, H., Ayres, S. M., Giannelli, S., Jr., Conklin, E. F., Mazzara, J. T., and Grace, W. J.: Effect of isoproterenol, I-norepinephrine, and intraaortic counterpulsation on hemodynamics and myocardial metabolism in shock following acute myocardial infarction. Circulation 45:335, 1972.
31. Smullens, S. N., Wiener, L., Kasparian, H., Brest, A. N., Bacharach, B., Noble, P. H., and Templeton, J. Y., III: Evaluation and surgical management of acute evolving myocardial infarction. J. Thorac. Cardiovasc. Surg. 64/4:495, 1972.
32. Wiener, L., Kasparian, H., Brest, A. N., and Templeton, J. Y., III: Surgical management of acute evolving myocardial infarction: A coronary circulatory, metabolic and angiographic profile. Am. J. Cardiol. 29:296, 1972.

Chapter 6
INTERMEDIATE CORONARY CARE UNIT

WILLIAM J. GRACE

For as long as his life is at high risk, the patient with a myocardial infarction should receive treatment with the basic principles of coronary care. These basic principles are as follows:

1. All the patients are in one area.
2. All the patients are on continuous ECG monitoring.
3. The monitor is under constant "eyeball" scrutiny by trained persons.
4. Those in charge of the patients have an aggressive attitude about the control of cardiac arrhythmia.

The period of maximum risk to the hospitalized patient is the first few days of hospitalization. Death, however, may occur at any time during the hospital stay. Data from this hospital (St. Vincent's New York) indicate that although the peak death rate occurs on the first few hospital days, some 30% of the deaths occur after the fifth hospital day. Information obtained from other institutions also indicates that from 20% to 35% of the hospital deaths from acute transmural myocardial infarction occur after discharge from the coronary care unit.[1-7]

For some time it was felt that these deaths were inevitable and that they are due to pump failure (shock state and congestive heart failure).

From our own experience it is apparent that the greatest proportion of these late deaths are sudden and unexpected. Figure 6-1 shows the data from St. Vincent's Hospital indicating that more than 31% of the deaths occur after the fifth day.[8] Figure 6–2, from a series of almost 3000 patients, indicates that at the end of a week of hospitalization only 75% of the deaths have been accounted for.[8] Because of these findings, it is clear that the period of ECG monitoring must be extended beyond the traditional 4 or 5 days in the coronary care unit if we are to derive the maximum benefit for in-hospital patients with acute myocardial infarction. Patients with transmural myocardial infarction continue to be at risk after this time.

The main reason for discharging patients from the traditional coronary care unit at the end of 4 or 5 days has been the belief which dominates coronary care: that time of the maximum risk is now past. A secondary reason for discharging patients from the coronary care unit at this time is the pressure on the staff and the hospital to admit new patients to such high-priority beds. An additional reason for discharge from the coronary care system is the need to begin mobilization and rehabilitation of the patient, which is troublesome and awkward in the environment of the intensive care or coronary care system. Consequently, our traditional practice has been to discharge patients from the

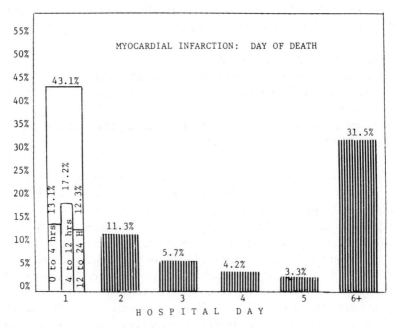

Figure 6–1.

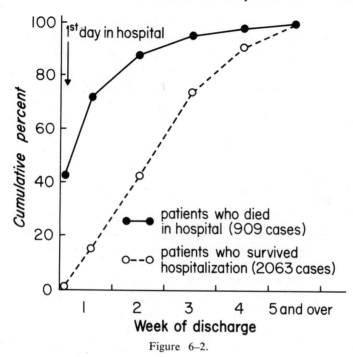

Figure 6–2.

coronary care unit to the general hospital after the fourth or fifth hospital day. As stated above, however, this does not provide maximum security for patients with acute myocardial infarction, and is less than ideal because a significant number of deaths, many of which are sudden and unexpected, are yet to come.

A solution to these problems is to continue monitoring patients with acute myocardial infarction after the fifth hospital day and through the fourteenth hospital day, but in an environment different from the coronary care system. This setting should permit the patient to begin walking and taking care of himself while he is still under the surveillance of continuous electrocardiograph monitoring. Although this can be done with "hard-wire" type of monitoring, use of telemetering equipment is probably simpler and more convenient for the patient.

Some institutions have solved this problem by continuing the monitoring beyond the fifth hospital day and through the fourteenth day, while maintaining the patient in the same place in the hospital. Others, by increasing the size of the coronary care unit, have begun mobilization while the patient is still in the coronary care unit. In some institutions, neither of these solutions has been possible because of space limitations. Our solution to the problem has been to set up a special separate monitoring system, referred to as the Intermediate Coronary Care Unit (ICCU), where our patients have continuous electrocardiographic monitoring via telemetry. The immediate goals of this intermediate coronary care system are to begin early mobilization, to get the patient up and about, and to try to combat the inevitable depressive reaction that occurs. This intermediate type of care tells patients that although they are not truly "out of the woods" and although they still require intensive care, they are doing well, even though some continuous surveillance is necessary.

THE INTERMEDIATE CORONARY CARE UNIT

Our original attempts to monitor beyond the fifth hospital day consisted of interrupted ECG rhythm strip monitoring. At this time there was no electronic telemetry equipment available. We devised equipment so that the patient was continuously attached to ECG leads and an ECG technician or paramedic could visit the bedside of the patient every 6 hours and record a rhythm strip." Although the mechanics and logistics of this system worked out well, we continued to have deaths in our intermediate coronary care system every month. After 8 months, this attempt was given up. We then switched to continuous electrocardiographic monitoring by using a telemetry system.

All patients with transmural myocardial infarction were transferred to this intermediate coronary care system after the seventh hospital day. (Patients with preinfarction angina, persistent chest pain without Q waves in the electrocardiogram, probably should be under intensive cardiac monitoring until all of these indications of impending disaster have subsided. We feel that the patient with persistent chest pain should be kept in the CCU and not the ICCU.) The "hard-wire" monitoring was then removed and telemetry system was attached to the patient. With this equipment, the patient could be up or seated by his bedside in a chair, or he could walk to the bathroom or around the room; his electrocardiogram was continuously transmitted to the master monitor bank. This hospital uses a system of "monitor watchers," and the patient's electrocardiogram is transmitted from the ICCU to the main monitor bank in the coronary care system. The same monitor watchers who scan the oscilloscopes on the coronary care unit also watch the oscilloscopes from the ICCU. A "slave unit" was placed at the nurses' desk, adjacent to the intermediate coronary care unit, for observation by the nurses on that floor. A hot-line telephone was installed from the monitor watchers desk to the nurses' station. A "panic button" was installed, and when it is activated in the ICCU or at the monitor watchers' station, a call for the hospital resuscitation team is made by the telephone operating service, which orders the team to proceed to the intermediate coronary care unit. (The "crash cart" equipment list is presented as appendix A.)

This telemetry system proved satisfactory. Arrhythmias were readily detected and dealt with, and successful cardiac resuscitation was carried out in the ICCU. During the first year of this telemetry system, the anticipated mortality rate of one death per month was greatly diminished. We then had the satisfying experience of operating the system for 18 consecutive months without a death. Since then, there have been only a few unsuccessful attempts at cardiac resuscitation, mainly in patients with "straight line" electrocardiograms. (The regulations now in force for the ICCU are presented as appendix B.)

RECENT EXPERIENCE IN THE ICCU

We have analyzed our last 138 consecutive patients with acute transmural myocardial infarction. There were 36 hospital deaths (26%). Thirty-two of these deaths occurred in the CCU (89%) and two in the general hospital following the discharge from the ICCU. There were two deaths in the ICCU: A 56-year-old man had had an acute anterior infarction and complete heart block; his temporary pacemaker was still in place when he died suddenly and unexpectedly on the tenth hospital day (intractable ventricular fibrillation). The second patient to die in the ICCU had severe valvular heart disease in addition to the acute myocardial infarction; his death was also sudden, unexpected, and associated with arrhythmia. There were two hospital deaths after discharge from the ICCU: an 87-year-old man died suddenly and unexpectedly; and a 61-year-old man also died suddenly during the third week of hospitalization.

In brief, there were 36 deaths from acute transmural myocardial infarction in 138 consecutive patients in 10 months. Four deaths (11%) occurred after discharge from the CCU, two in the ICCU and two following discharge from the ICCU. This recent experience continues to bear out the inference we drew from the original study, namely, that the post-CCU deaths were numerous and that they could be prevented.[13]

A recent analysis of late deaths by Wilson and Adgey supports these findings.[13] For example, they report that more than one third of the episodes of late ventricular fibrillations were sudden and unexpected. Of those patients suffering episodes of late ventricular fibrillation, 57% survived to leave the hospital. The authors conclude that "the data presented here indicates that continued monitoring of those at risk, and the prevention or correction of late ventricular fibrillation may give long term rewards."

Two additional careful reviews of the natural history of acute myocardial infarction in the hospitalized patient have appeared[14,15] very recently. Both of these papers report the high death rate following discharge from the Coronary Care Unit and emphasize that at least one third and probably more of these deaths are sudden and unexpected arrhythmic deaths. The authors of both of these papers indicate that longer monitoring of patients is indicated than has been current practice.

Return of Patients to Coronary Care Units

In an earlier publication,[9] we indicated the main reasons for transferring patients out of the ICCU back to the CCU. The same reasons apply as they did when this unit was first begun. The rates of return are approximately the same. A major reason for returning to the CCU is recurrent chest pain, presumably due to an extension of the infarction, which occurs in approximately 5% of the patients. Approximately 10% of the patients are returned because of the onset of arrhythmias that cannot be controlled by simple oral medication in the ICCU, as our ICCU does not permit adequate nursing service to monitor continuous intravenous medication.

After the fourteenth hospital day, the electronic monitoring system is discontinued and the patient is transferred from this unit to a bed in the general hospital. From there on, an individual decision is made by the patient's own physician as to how much more hospitalization is necessary. In general, another week is spent in the hospital.

Recent Trends

Hospitalization beyond the second week may not be necessary for the patient without complications.[10,11] There is little in our experience that would contradict this. Most physicians with extensive CCU experience have seen isolated episodes of patients dying on the twenty-first to twenty-fifth hospital day, or just as they are about to leave the hospital. Such events are rare, and each hospital will have to ask itself whether the cost-effectiveness of monitoring beyond the fourteenth day is reasonable. At present, it does not seem to be wise to extend monitoring beyond the first 14 days.

Continued experience in this and other CCU's would lead one to believe that there are patients with acute transmural myocardial infarction who at the end of the period of intensive cardiac (CCU) monitoring can be classified as either high-risk or low-risk patients. For example, of 117 patients observed in the ICCU, 17 had to be returned to the

CCU for further management. Nine of these were returned for arrhythmias and six for recurrent chest pain. Of these 17 patients, there were four who had had no complications in the CCU originally and no further complications in the CCU on the second round. They all left the hospital without further event. Patients who had complications during their first time in the CCU had to be referred back to the CCU from the ICCU twice as often as those who had none. Of those patients who had to be referred back to the CCU from ICCU, twice as many had complications within the first few days in the original CCU. Of the patients who went through the initial period on the CCU without complications of recurrent arrhythmia or any evidence of pump failure, none died in the hospital.

Patients with complications in the CCU such as recurrent arrhythmias, unstable blood pressure, congestive heart failure, and bundle branch block were most often the ones who had to be returned to the CCU from the ICCU. Deaths did occur in this group.

Additional information based upon experience in other CCU's indicates that the patient who had bundle branch block or complete AV block during the first few hospital days is a high-risk patient for the remainder of the hospital stay.[6,12] For such patients a more prolonged hospitalization, more than 2 weeks, might be indicated, even without a continuous monitoring system.

A recent publication indicates that precordial mapping for detection of ST vector elevation may be a strong indication of extension of the infarction. This author has no personal experience with this method but would certainly endorse the general concept that recurrent ST elevation or persistent chest pain is a forewarning of disaster and would be an indication for continued monitoring.

THE NURSING RESPONSIBILITY IN INTERMEDIATE CORONARY CARE

A nurse assigned to the ICCU must be as knowledgeable about ischemic heart disease and its complications, and about arrhythmia control, as are the nurses in the emergency room or the ICU or CCU of the hospital. In our own particular instance, these nurses are taught to use the electrical defibrillator and, after they have satisfactorily completed these training sessions, they are given a written statement that they have been taught to use it. After this, they may, and are urged to, defibrillate the pulseless patient in the ICCU setting.[13] The principles of cardiac resuscitation are taught to the entire nursing staff. In addition, they have a responsibility of working with patients through periods of depression and as they face the problems of rehabilitation.

PSYCHOLOGICAL REACTIONS

Although serious behavioral disturbances occur in approximately 1% of the patients in the ICCU, minor degrees of depression are almost universal. We generally refer to this as the "coronary blues." Although it affects everyone to some degree it certainly affects some more than others. We have had our patients interviewed by a psychiatrist, who confirmed this general feeling. He felt that the monitoring system did not promote this depression; indeed, it tended to produce a feeling of security.

SUMMARY

Long-term cardiac ECG monitoring (10–14 days) following admission to the hospital for patients with acute myocardial infarction has been found to be practical and useful. It is practical in the sense that available equipment functions well and that systems can be devised to utilize the equipment. Long-term ECG monitoring in our hands and in hands of others has shown to be useful in saving lives.

Because of logistic and administrative problems, monitoring beyond the fifth hospital day in the coronary care unit may need to be done in a hospital area separate from the CCU. Such a unit is called an intermediate coronary care unit. It provides a bridge between the intensive care of the CCU and the beginning of mobilization and discharge planning for the patient. In the ICCU the patient's ECG is monitored, as in the CCU; here, too, rehabilitation is begun.

Several studies have shown that approximately one third of the deaths from acute myocardial infarction are going to occur following discharge from the CCU, but while the patient is still in the hospital. Most studies indicate that at least half of these deaths are sudden and unpredicted.

Our experience in ICCU monitoring has effected a reduction in the number of deaths following discharge from the CCU through early detection of ventricular premature contractions, prevention of ventricular fibrillation, and early detection of ventricular tachycardia and prompt resuscitation.

APPENDIX A

"Crash Cart" Equipment List

I. *Top of Cart*
    Defibrillator w/jelly
    ECG machine

Intubation tray w/the following:
1) Laryngoscope handle and blade—check to see that bulb works
2) Metal stylet and ET tube #34 or #36
3) Test cuff w/syringe—leave attached w/clamp
4) Xylocaine viscous
5) TR. Benzoin and 1 roll of $\frac{1}{2}''$ adhesive tape
3 CVP catheters and 3 CVP manometers
Ambu Bag
Tourniquet

II. *First Drawer* (working front to back)
Section #1
  Epinephrine and atropine
  Aminophylline
  Bicarbonate
  Calcium chloride and gluconate
  Dextrose
Section #2
  Benadryl and cedilanid
  Digoxin and ephedrin
  Mannitol
  Heparin and inderal
  Neosynephine and regitine
Section #3
  Isuprel and lasix
  Leuphad, pronestyl, and tensilon
  Quinidine and Solu-Cortef
  Valium
  Xylocaine

III. *Second Drawer* (working front to back)
Section #1
  Needles—#18g, #20g
  50-cc syringes
Section #2
  3-cc syringes and medication added labels
  10-cc syringes
Section #3
  Alcohol wipes
  Polycaths—#14g, #18g, Bacitracin ointment
  Butterfly #19, #21
  2 intracardiac needles

IV. *Third Drawer* (working front to back)
Section #1
  ET tubes #30, #32 (2 each)
  Airways #5—2
  Tracheostomy adapter set

Section #2
ET tubes #34, #36 (2 of each)
Extra laryngoscope blades (#3, #4) bulbs, batteries
Section #3
ET tubes #38, #40 (2 of each)
O_2 tubing and O_2 flowmeter
V. *Shelves under Drawers*
1 box—electrode jelly
1 box—ECG paper
1 tube—Cardio Creme
Adhesive tape 1″ and 2″ Paper tape and regular
Suction catheters #14
Levine tubes one #16 and #18
Irrigating set
Sterile gloves—2 pairs each size, 7½ and 8
Arm boards—2 long, one short
Cut-down tray
Tracheostomy tray
VI. *Side Shelves*
   TOP   Lidocaine Bristojects
            Epinephrine Bristojects
            Calcium Chloride Bristojects
            Sodium Bicarbonate Bristojects
   BOTTOM   3 bottles 5% sodium bicarbonate 500 cc
               3 bags 500 D_5W
               1 bottle—germicidal
               2 boxes—4 × 3 (sterile)
               6 boxes microdrip and IV tubing
               4 IV extension tubes
               1 portable suction machine

APPENDIX B

Regulations for ICCU (St. Vincent's Hospital, New York)

The Chief of Medicine or his representative will establish bed priority for all patients on CCU Cronin 9 and ICCU on SJE and Smith 7*. Daily rounds will be made on all floors and records kept of available space by the physician.

The facilities of the ICCU consist of Smith 728—4 male beds and Smith 738—2 female beds; SJE 365—4 male beds. These are to be occupied on first priority by patients with transmural infarcts transferred there from Cronin 9, usually on the seventh day of illness if there have been no complications. Second priority is to be given to patients with non-transmural infarcts. Patients in shock, or in other ways desperately ill, are not acceptable. No

* Smith 7   ICCU—Private Service
  SJE   ICCU—Teaching Service

patients will be admitted directly to the Unit without the expressed approval of the physician-in-charge, i.e., representative of Chief of Medicine. Patients with temporary transvenous pacemakers but without acute myocardial infarction may be accepted at the discretion of the Chief of Medicine. Patients with acute myocardial infarction on leaving Cronin 9 will not be accepted on St. Josephs Hall, except in the ICCU. If no bed is available, the patient will be held on Cronin 9 until such is ready. We hope to apply the same procedure on Smith 7.

Equipment on Hall:

Smith 7—Defibrillator, ECG, Code 99 Cart, Tracheostomy Set, etc.:

The cart may be used for emergencies on the floor and is not to be moved to any other floor. The other equipment is specifically for the ICCU only.

SJE—Defibrillator, ECG, Code Cart, Tracheostomy Set, etc.:

The same regulations apply.

The nurses on both floors have received instruction in defibrillation procedures. The Chief Resident is to be summoned simultaneously when calling a "Code 99." The nurses will institute resuscitation procedures immediately and may defibrillate when necessary.

The authorized nurses may defibrillate (electrically) the pulseless patient if no physician is immediately available.

Monitoring:

ICCU Smith 7: Remote telemetry is being used for four of the patients. Electrodes may be initially attached to the patient on Cronin 9 just prior to transfer. These are connected to a small portable transmitter which is easily carried about by the patient. The signal, via radio waves, is transmitted to the antenna and receiver on Smith 7 and then by special wiring to the monitor console bank on Cronin 9. This console bank is constantly observed by a technician on Cronin 9 who also monitors the ECG's of patients on CCU.

This system will permit continuous monitoring of the ambulatory patient. A special telephone connects the floors involved. The nurses must notify the console bank technician when the patient is being bathed, is in a non-transmitting area, such as bathroom or x-ray Department, or is disconnected from the system when an electrocardiogram is taken. Otherwise, the change in the patient signal would be misinterpreted. It must be emphasized that good communications between the floors is essential for the effective operation of this system.

The electrodes will be changed every 48–72 hours, or more often if necessary, by the nurses. Rhythm strips will be taken by the Cronin 9 technician every hour from the console bank, mounted, and read on Cronin 9, as are the ECG's on the other Cronin 9 patients. Any change in the ECG will be reported to the designated nurse on the ICCU immediately. The rhythm strips will be sent to the floor every eight hours.

In the event that there are more than four patients on Smith 7 ICCU, a decision will have to be made as to which patient to remove from telemetering. This decision will be made by the Chief of Medicine and the private physician or delegate of the Chief of Medicine and the private physician. Daily priority rounds will be made by the Chief of Medicine or his delegate.

ICCU St. Joseph's Hall: Same as on Smith 7.

Patient Privileges in ICCU:

A commode is available. It is anticipated bathroom privileges will be permitted on Smith 7, since bathroom facilities are available. A radio with an ear-plug is permitted, so there will be no interference with the other patients' rest. A television set of the small, personal type with ear-plug may be used. No telephones are permitted.

Transfer off ICCU:

We anticipate a stay of 7–14 days on the ICCU and then transfer to a general hospital bed for the remainder of convalescence. Earlier transfer may be required, depending on pressure of bed requirements on Cronin 9. The situation will be reviewed in daily rounds.

Transfer Back to Cronin 9:

1. Recurrence of severe pain.
2. Recurrent arrhythmia which requires more than occasional oral medication.

Visitors:

Limited to two visitors per patient at one time. Restricted visiting (one visitor a a time) to be explained to the patient by the doctor.

REFERENCES

1. Hoffrendahl, S.: Influence of treatment in a coronary care unit on prognosis in acute myocardial infarction. Acta Med. Scand. Suppl. 519:1, 1971.
2. McGrive, L. B., and Krall, M. S.: Evaluation of cardiac care units and myocardial infarction. Arch. Intern. Med. 130:677, 1972.
3. MacMillan, R. L., et al.: Changing perspectives in coronary care. Am. J. Cardiol. 20:451, 1967.
4. Oliver, M. F., Julian, D. G., and Donald, K. W.: Problems in evaluating coronary care units. Am. J. Cardiol. 20:465, 1967.
5. Meltzer, L. E.: The functional anatomy of the coronary care unit, p. 380. *In* W. Likoff, Arteriosclerosis and Coronary Heart Disease. B. Segal, and W. Insull (ed.), New York, Grune & Stratton, 1972.
6. Weinberg, S. L., and Col, J. J.: The changing coronary care unit: Cardiovascular therapy, p. 79 *in* H. Russek and B. Zohman (ed.), Changing Concept in Cardiovascular Disease. Baltimore, Williams & Wilkins, 1972.

7. Soler, N. G., et al.: Coronary care for myocardial infarction in diabetics. Lancet i:475, 1974.
8. Most, A. S., and Peterson, D. R.: Myocardial infarction surveillance in a meteropolitan community. JAMA 208:2433, 1969.
9. Grace, W. J., and Yarvote, P. M.: Acute myocardial infarction: The course of the illness following discharge from the coronary care unit. Chest 59:15, 1971.
10. Hutter, A. M. Jr., Sidel, V. W., Shine, K. I., and DeSanctis, R. W.: Early hospital discharge after myocardial infarction. N. Engl. J. Med. 288:1141, 1973.
11. Boyle, J. A., Lorimor, A. R., et al.: Early mobilization after uncomplicated myocardial infarction (Medical Division, Royal Infirmary, Glasgow) Lancet ii:346, 1973.
12. Atkins, J. M., Leshin, S. J., Blomquist, G., and Mullins, C. B.: Ventricular conduction blocks and sudden death in acute myocardial infarction. N. Engl. J. Med. 288:281, 1973.
13. Wilson, C., and Adgey, A. A. J.: Survival of patients with late ventricular fibrillation following acute myocardial infarction. Lancet ii:124, 1974.
14. Yanowitz, F., and Fozzard, H. A.: A medical information system for the Coronary Care Unit. Arch. Intern. Med. 134:93, 1974.
15. Bornheimer, J., Haywood, J. L., and deGuzman, M.: Analysis of in-hospital deaths from myocardial infarction after Coronary Care Unit discharge. Arch. Intern. Med. In press.

Chapter 7

TACHYARRHYTHMIAS

Edward K. Chung

With the availability of direct current cardioverters and artificial pacemakers in the past decade, the therapeutic results of the management of various arrhythmias have improved appreciably. For the best therapeutic results, a precise diagnosis of the arrhythmia is necessary, because some drugs are more effective or even almost specific for certain arrhythmias.[1] For instance, digitalis is usually the drug of choice for the treatment of various supraventricular tachyarrhythmias, especially atrial fibrillation with rapid ventricular response. Conversely, digitalis is ineffective or even contraindicated in the treatment of ventricular tachyarrhythmias.[2]

It is essential first to remove the cause of the arrhythmia, if it is apparent. For instance, the first and most important step in the treatment of digitalis-induced arrhythmia is the immediate discontinuance of digitalis.[2] In addition, underlying etiologic factors significantly influence the therapeutic result. For example, ventricular tachycardia associated with acute myocardial infarction is best treated with lidocaine (Xylocaine), whereas digitalis-induced ventricular tachycardia responds best to diphenylhydantoin (Dilantin) or potassium.[1-3] (See Chapter 15.)

Because prevention of recurrence is important in the management of tachyarrhythmias, long-term maintenance therapy with digitalis and other antiarrhythmic drugs is often necessary. In such long-term therapy, quinidine is known to be best for preventing recurrence of atrial fibrillation or flutter,[4] while procaine amide (Pronestyl) is known to be best for the prevention of ventricular tachyarrhythmias.[5] Propanolol (Inderal) has been the most effective agent in the treatment of arrhythmias precipitated by exercise, emotional stress, or excessive sympathetic stimulation and of arrhythmias related to Wolff-Parkinson-White syndrome.[6,7] Bretylium tosylate, though still under investigation, reportedly is very effective in the treatment of refractory ventricular tachyarrhythmias.[8]

Carotid sinus stimulation is probably the simplest way of terminating tachyarrhythmias, particularly supraventricular tachycardia, and it is often effective.[9]

Direct current (DC) shock is an extremely effective measure for terminating various acute tachyarrhythmias, including life-threatening ventricular fibrillation. In addition, DC shock is indispensable in terminating chronic atrial fibrillation or flutter that is refractory to various antiarrhythmic agents.[10]

The primary indication for the insertion of an artificial pacemaker is, needless to say, Adams-Stokes syndrome due to complete AV block.[11] Less commonly, the artificial pacemaker is indicated in treating symptomatic and drug-resistant sinus bradycardia, sinoatrial (SA) block, and sinus arrest. In addition, the artificial pacemaker (overdriving) is often life-saving in the treatment of refractory tachyarrhythmias, particularly ventricular tachycardia.[11,12]

Use of various antiarrhythmic drugs combined with the DC cardioverter and artificial pacemaker is not uncommon in treatment of malignant cardiac arrhythmias.[1]

There are three major clinical categories of cardiac arrhythmias: tachyarrhythmias, bradyarrhythmias, and bradytachyarrhythmias. Bradytachyarrhythmias are a combination of bradyarrhythmias and tachyarrhythmias; they are best treated with an artificial pacemaker with a slightly overdriving pacing rate (80–100 beats per minute).[1]

The therapeutic approaches differ greatly, depending upon the origin, as well as the type, of the tachyarrhythmias.[3] Among the tachyarrhythmias encountered are premature (atrial, AV junctional, or ventricular) contractions (extrasystoles), atrial tachyarrhythmias (atrial tachycardia, flutter and fibrillation), AV nodal (junctional) tachyarrhythmias (paroxysmal and nonparoxysmal form), and ventricular tachyarrhythmias (ventricular tachycardia, flutter and fibrillation).[13]

MANAGEMENT OF VARIOUS TACHYARRHYTHMIAS

Premature Contractions (Extrasystoles)

The first step in management of extrasystoles is to remove any obvious cause of the development of premature contractions, regardless of the origin of the ectopic impulses. For example, as mentioned above, digitalis-induced premature contractions, particularly those that are ventricular in origin, are best treated by discontinuance of digitalis.[2] Sedation is another important method of eliminating premature beats, especially in high-strung or nervous individuals. Premature contractions are often eliminated by stopping heavy smoking or excessive ingestion of coffee.[1]

If the premature contractions are frequent (6 beats or more per minute), particularly in such conditions as acute myocardial infarction, various antiarrhythmic agents (see Table 7-1) may be required.[3] Supraventricular (atrial or AV junctional) premature contractions are best treated with quinidine, but Propranolol (Inderal) is almost equally effective in this situation. Digitalis is particularly effective when premature contractions are associated with heart failure.[2] Lidocaine (Xylocaine) is the drug of choice for the treatment of ventricular premature contractions associated with acute myocardial infarction or occurring during catheterization and cardiac surgery.[14,15]

Treatment of ventricular premature contractions is indicated in the following situations[13] (Figs. 7-1 and 7-2):

Frequent ventricular premature contractions (6 beats or more per minute)

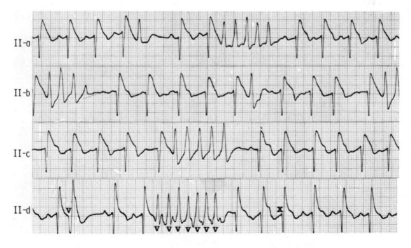

Figure 7-1. Figures 7-1 and 7-2 were obtained from the same patient. In figure 7-1, leads II-a,b,c, and d are continuous. The basic rhythm is sinus with first degree AV block (P–R interval: 0.24 sec). Note frequent ventricular premature beats with short runs of ventricular tachycardia (marked V) initiated by the "R-on-T" phenomenon. Also there are occasional supraventricular premature beats (marked X).

Table 7-1   Common Antitachyarrhythmic Drugs^a

Drug	Full Dosage	Maintenance Dosage	Onset of Action	Maximum Effect	Duration of Action	Indications	Toxicity	
							Dosage-dependent	Dosage-independent
Digoxin (Lanoxin)	0.5–1 mg IV initially, then 0.25–0.5 mg q̄ 2 hr as needed (total: 1–2.5 mg)	0.125–0.75 mg (average: 0.25 mg) daily (PO)	10–30 min	2–3 hr	3–6 days	SV tachyarrhythmias (AF, AFl, AT, AV NT)	Almost all known arrhythmias, aggravation of CHF, anorexia, nausea, vomiting, color vision, blurring vision, headache, dizziness, confusion	Allergic manifestations (urticaria, eosinophilia), idiosyncrasy, thrombocytopenia, GI hemorrhage and necrosis
Deslanoside (Cedilanid-D)	0.8–1.6 mg IV initially, then 0.4 mg q̄ 2 hr as needed (total: 1.2–2 mg)	—	10–30 min	2–3 hr	3–6 days			
Ouabain (G-Strophantin)	0.25–0.5 mg IV initially, then 0.1 mg q̄ ½ hr as needed (total: 0.5–1.2 mg)		3–10 min	½–1 hr	12 hr–3 days			
Lidocaine (Xylocaine)	75–100 mg direct IV q̄ 10–20 min as needed (total: 750 mg) or 200–250 mg IM q̄ 10–20 min as needed	1–5 mg/min IV infusion	At once	At once	Minutes	Primary: V tachyarrhythmias Secondary: SV tachyarrhythmias	Dizziness, drowsiness, confusion, muscle twitching, disorientation, euphoria, cardiac and respiratory depression, convulsion, hypotension, AV & IV block	
Procaine amide (Pronestyl)	1–2 g/200 cc 5% D/W IV drip, 100 mg q 2–4 min (1 g in ½–1 hr) (total: 2 g) or 1 g PO initially, then 0.5 g q̄ 2–3 hr (total: 3.5 g)	0.25–0.5 g q̄ 3–6 hr (PO)	At once / Rapid	Minutes / 1–2 hr	6 hr / 6–8 hr	Primary: V tachyarrhythmias Secondary: SV tachyarrhythmias	AV & IV block, ventricular arrhythmias, LE, nausea, vomiting, lymphadenopathy, hypotension, convulsion	Allergic manifestations (eosinophilia, urticaria) agranulocytosis
Quinidine gluconate	0.8 g/200 cc 5% D/W IV drip, 25 mg/min or 0.4–0.6 g IM initially, then 0.4 g q̄ 2–4 hr (total: 2.6 g)		10–15 min / 10–15 min	Not immediate / 30–90 min	6–8 hr / 6–8 hr	Primary: SV tachyarrhythmias Secondary: V tachyarrhythmias	AV, IV block, nausea, vomiting, photophobia, diplopia, headache, tinnitus, diarrhea, ventricular arrhythmias	Respiratory depression, hypotension, convulsion, rashes (macular or papular), thrombocytopenic purpura, hemolytic anemia
Quinidine sulfate	Oral route (see text p. 41)	0.3–0.4 g q̄ 6 hr (PO)		2–3 hr	6–8 hr			
Diphenylhydantoin (Dilantin)	125–250 mg IV q̄ 10–20 min as needed (total: 750 mg/hr)	100–200 mg q̄ 6 hr (PO)	At once	Minutes	4–8 hr	Primary: Digitalis-induced arrhythmias Secondary: Nondigitalis-induced arrhythmias (ventricular)	Cardiac depression, hypotension AV, SA block, sinus bradycardia, ataxia, tremor, gingival hyperplasia	Allergic manifestations (urticaria, purpura and eosinophilia)
Propranolol (Inderal)	1–3 mg IV initially, then second dose may be repeated after 2 min. Additional medication should not be given less than 4 hr (total: 10 mg)	10–30 mg q̄ 6 hr (PO)	At once	Minutes	3–6 hr	Various tachyarrhythmias	SA, AV block, CHF, nausea, vomiting, diarrhea, asthma, cardiogenic shock	Erythematous rashes, paresthesias of hands and fever

Key to the table: IV: intravenous injection; IM: intramuscular injection; q: every; D/W: dextrose in water; PO: orally; IV block: intraventricular block; LE: lupus erythematosus; CHF: congestive heart failure; GL: gastrointestinal; AF: atrial fibrillation; AFl: atrial flutter; AT: atrial tachycardia; AV NT: AV nodal tachycardia; SV tachyarrhythmias: supraventricular tachyarrhythmias; V tachyarrhythmias: ventricular tachyarrhythmias.
^a Reprinted with minor changes from Chung.[3]

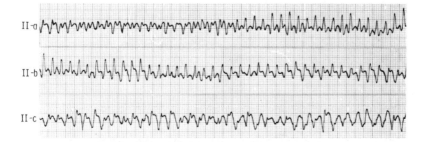

Figure 7-2. Leads II-a,b, and c are continuous. Ventricular fibrillation.

R-on-T phenomenon (ventricular premature contraction superimposed on the top of the T-wave of the preceding beat)

Multifocal ventricular premature contractions

Grouped or paired ventricular premature contractions

Ventricular premature contractions after the termination of ventricular tachycardia or fibrillation

For long-term therapy of the ventricular premature contractions, procaine amide (Pronestyl) is the drug of choice.[5] Dilantin is probably the best agent for the treatment of digitalis-induced premature beats.[16]

Supraventricular Tachyarrhythmias

Again, the first step in management is the elimination of the cause, if apparent. For instance, atrial fibrillation associated with thyrotoxicosis cannot be treated satisfactorily unless the thyroid function returns to euthyroid level.

Carotid sinus stimulation is often effective in terminating paroxysmal atrial or AV nodal (junctional) tachycardia.[9] Of the antiarrhythmic agents, digitalis is usually the drug of choice in the treatment of various supraventricular tachyarrhythmias, especially atrial fibrillation (Figure 7-3). Needless to say, in digitalis-induced supraventricular tachyarrhyth-

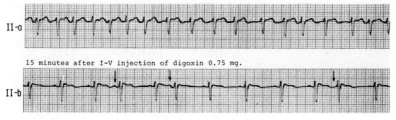

15 minutes after I-V injection of digoxin 0.75 mg.

Figure 7-3. Leads II-a and b are not continuous. Atrial fibrillation (lead II-a) has converted to sinus rhythm (lead II-b) by digitalization. Note occasional atrial premature beats (indicated by arrows).

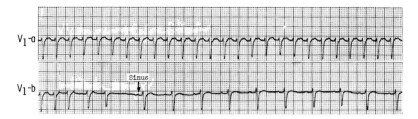

Figure 7-4. Leads V_1-a and b are continuous. Paroxysmal supraventricular (most likely atrial) tachycardia (rate: 187 beats per minute) has been converted to sinus rhythm (indicated by arrow) by intravenous injection of propranolol (Inderal), 1 mg.

mias, digitalis must be discontinued immediately.[2] Diphenylhydantoin (Dilantin) or potassium has been found to be effective in terminating digitalis-induced supraventricular tachyarrhythmias[2,16] (see Chapter 15). Quinidine is the best agent for preventing the recurrence of atrial fibrillation or flutter.[4] Propranolol (Inderal) is the most effective agent in the treatment of arrhythmias precipitated by exercise, emotional distress, or excessive sympathetic stimulation (Figure 7-4), as well as of supraventricular tachyarrhythmias related to the Wolff-Parkinson-White syndrome.[7] Procaine amide (Pronestyl) is less commonly used for the treatment of supraventricular tachyarrhythmias, and lidocaine (Xylocaine) is rarely used in this situation.[14,45]

Direct current shock is often very effective in terminating various acute supraventricular tachyarrhythmias[10] (Figure 7-5). Elective cardioversion is another important therapeutic means of terminating chronic atrial fibrillation or flutter.[10]

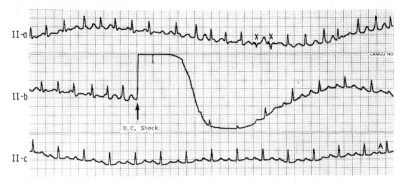

Figure 7-5. Leads II-a,b, and c are continuous. Atrial fibrillation has converted to sinus rhythm by DC shock. Note occasional aberrant ventricular conduction (marked X) and one atrial premature beat (marked A).

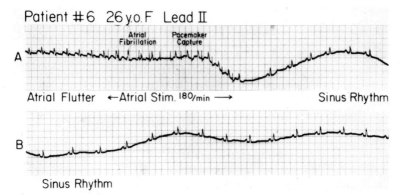

Figure 7-6. The rhythm strips *A* and *B* are not continuous. Atrial flutter is terminated by the atrial stimulation (rate: 180 beats per minute), and the sinus rhythm is restored. (Reprinted with permission from Chung.[3])

Artificial pacemakers (overdriving rate) are occasionally needed in the suppression of various supraventricular tachyarrhythmias (Figure 7-6) that are refractory to various antiarrhythmic agents and DC shock.[11] Direct current shock and artificial pacemakers are discussed in detail elsewhere (see Chapters 9 and 10). Sedation, in conjunction with other therapeutic measures, is often beneficial for the treatment of supraventricular tachyarrhythmias.

Ventricular Tachyarrhythmias

Once again, the first step in treatment is elimination of any apparent cause of ventricular tachyarrhythmias. Digitalis should be stopped immediately when ventricular tachyarrhythmias are due to digitalis toxicity.[2]

Direct current shock is the most effective way of terminating ventricular tachycardia, flutter, and fibrillation[10] (Figure 7-7). Defibrillation, in addition to all necessary cardiopulmonary resuscitation, should be carried out immediately for the treatment of ventricular fibrillation or flutter (Figure 7-8). However, DC shock should be avoided in digitalis-induced ventricular tachycardia,[2] because DC shock often produces new cardiac arrhythmias, particularly ventricular fibrillation, in this situation.

Lidocaine (Xylocaine) is the drug of choice for the treatment of ventricular tachycardia associated with acute myocardial infarction or arising during anesthesia and cardiac catheterization[14,15,17] (Figure 7-9). Procaine amide (Pronestyl) is probably the next most commonly used drug in this situation.[17] Quinidine and propranolol (Inderal) are less effective for the treatment of ventricular tachyarrhythmias. Diphenylhy-

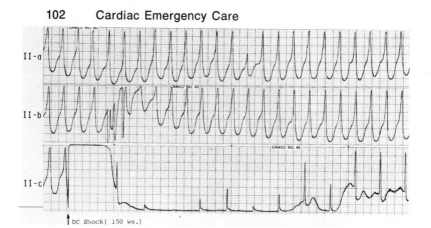

Figure 7-7. Leads II-*a,b,* and *c* are continuous. Ventricular tachycardia (rate: 150 beats per minute) is terminated by DC shock (150 w).

dantoin (Dilantin) is the best drug for the treatment of digitalis-induced ventricular tachycardia.[2,16] Bretylium tosylate, which is still under investigation, has been reported to be very effective in the treatment of refractory ventricular tachycardia.[8]

When ventricular tachyarrhythmias are refractory to antiarrhythmic

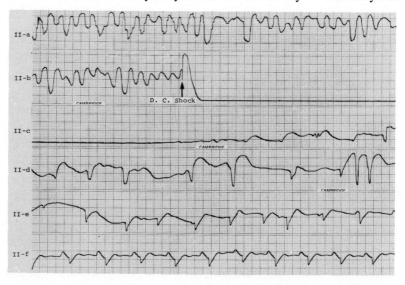

Figure 7-8. Leads II-*a,b,c,d,e,* and *f* are continuous. Ventricular fibrillation is terminated by DC shock, and sinus rhythm is restored. Note that there are ventricular premature contractions and unstable AV junctional escape rhythm in leads II-*d* and *e* before sinus rhythm is established.

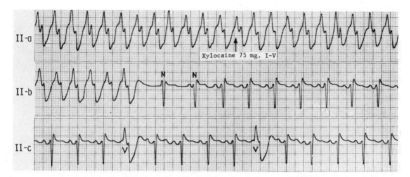

Figure 7-9. Leads II-*a* and *b* are continuous. Ventricular tachycardia is terminated by intravenous injection of Xylocaine, 75 mg. Note occasional AV nodal (junctional) premature beats (marked *N*) and ventricular premature contractions (marked *V*). The configurations of the isolated ventricular premature beat and the tachycardia beats are identical.

agents and DC shock, an artificial pacemaker (overdriving pacing rate: 100–120/min) is often life-saving.[11]

ANTITACHYARRHYTHMIC AGENTS (See Table 7-1)

Digitalis

Guide to Digitalization. Digitalis is one of the oldest and most valuable drugs available for medical practice. However, digitalis intoxication is often unavoidable because the margin between therapeutic and toxic dose is relatively narrow.[2] This narrow margin becomes further reduced in elderly and seriously ill patients with various modifying factors such as renal insufficiency, hypokalemia, and hypoxia. It has been shown that the therapeutic dose is approximately 60% of the toxic dose.[2]

Before a physician attempts to digitalize a patient, the following guidelines must be observed[2]:

• The physician should know whether digitalis is definitely indicated. He should know whether the patient is suffering from congestive heart failure and/or supraventricular tachyarrhythmias. Needless to say, two major indications for digitalis therapy are congestive heart failure and various supraventricular tachyarrhythmias, except, of course, those that are digitalis-induced.

In addition, he should be aware that there is no contraindication to digitalization. The only true contraindication is digitalis toxicity. Another probable contraindication for digitalization is idiopathic hypertrophic subaortic stenosis, since digitalis improves the contractile state of the left ventricular myocardium, which further reduces the left ventricular outflow tract. Deterioration induced by digitalization in this situation usually improves upon withdrawal of digitalis.

• The physician should attempt to obtain precise information about previous digitalization; in particular, full information regarding digitalization within 3 to 4 weeks is important. Not only the duration of digitalization, but also exact information concerning the preparation, dosage, and route of administration is indispensable.

If the clinical symptoms are rather mild and a history of previous digitalization is unclear, I prefer not to give any digitalis until a definite indication for digitalization is established. Serum digitalis determination by radioimmunoassay is extremely valuable when a history of previous digitalization is unclear.

• It is essential to take a control electrocardiogram immediately before digitalization, regardless of the clinical situation, except when the patient is suffering from an unusually acute condition. The most important reason for this is to confirm a fundamental mechanism of the cardiac rhythm, so that any cardiac arrhythmia that develops after digitalization will be clearly evident. Any new cardiac arrhythmia that develops during or after digitalization strongly suggests digitalis intoxication, since almost every known type of rhythm disturbances may be induced by digitalis (see Chapter 15). A control electrocardiogram will also reveal any unexpected abnormalities, such as acute myocardial infarction or hypokalemia, which directly influence the efficacy of digitalis therapy and the probability of digitalis toxicity. In addition to the control electrocardiogram, frequent follow-up electrocardiographic tracings are needed until the patient becomes fully digitalized. The electrocardiogram should be taken as soon as any change in cardiac rhythm is detected by physical examination or if digitalis toxicity is suspected. For the confirmation of the current cardiac mechanism, long strips of leads II and V_1 are adequate.

• Choice of preparation and method of digitalization directly and indirectly influence the efficacy of digitalis and the development of digitalis intoxication. In an emergency, such as acute pulmonary edema, particularly when it is associated with supraventricular tachyarrhythmias, a short-acting preparation such as Cediland-D or digoxin should be given intravenously. If there are any modifying factors, short-acting preparations are always preferable. If the clinical situation is not urgent, oral administration with a slower method is advisable. Every physician should be very familiar with the preparation he has chosen. He should be aware of precise oral and parenteral dosages, as well as the advantages and disadvantages of the particular preparations. Every physician should be fully familiar with at least one preparation for intravenous use in order to obtain very rapid digitalization and one preparation for oral use for slow digitalization.

I believe that digoxin has proven to be the most useful preparation in most clinical situations. There is no point in changing from one preparation to another unless a definite advantage will be obtained or allergy to the original preparation is discovered.

• Modifying factors, such as hypokalemia, and various cardiac as well as noncardiac diseases directly influence the efficacy of the drug and the development of digitalis toxicity.

• In the past 10 years, several methods[18,19] have been developed for determining serum digitalis level in order to establish an optimal therapeutic dosage and to diagnose digitalis toxicity accurately. The clinical importance of serum digitalis determination lies in the fact that there is reasonably close correlation between the digitalis content of blood tissue and that of other tissue, so that the blood levels reflect total body and myocardial concentrations (see Chapter 15).

At present, it is generally agreed that patients with obvious digitalis intoxication have significantly higher serum or plasma levels of digoxin or digitoxin than nonintoxicated patients. Nevertheless, substantial overlap between toxic and nontoxic serum or plasma cardiac glycoside levels exists. This is a problem particularly in patients who suffer from intractable congestive heart failure or various complex cardiac arrhythmias. It is extremely important to remember that the dosage of digitalis varies not only from patient to patient but also from time to time in the same patient. Similarly, toxic and nontoxic serum or plasma digitalis levels may differ from patient to patient, depending largely upon various modifying factors. In general, serum digoxin levels of 2.0 ng/ml or below and serum digitoxin levels of 20 ng/ml or below are considered to be nontoxic, although intoxicated patients may have serum levels within this range.[18,19] Serum digitalis determination by radioimmunoassay method is extremely valuable when the values of serum digitalis levels are interpreted in conjunction with the total clinical picture and electrocardiographic findings.

• Refractory congestive heart failure requires careful evaluation in order to determine whether the patient needs more digitalis or whether digitalis must be discontinued. The presence of any modifying factors and the re-evaluation of the initial diagnosis are additional factors to be considered in treating refractory congestive heart failure. It should be re-emphasized that digitalis intoxication is an important cause of refractory congestive heart failure (see Chapter 15).

• At times, digitalis-induced arrhythmias may be so complex that experienced electrocardiographers disagree about the mechanism of the cardiac rhythm. A given tracing may suggest a variety of mechanisms, and the cardiac rhythm may change form every few seconds or minutes. It may be reasonable to state that disagreement about the mechanism of the cardiac rhythm during digitalization is in itself often sufficient evidence to suspect digitalis intoxication.

Methods of Digitalization[2] **(Table 7-2).** Choice of the proper digitalis preparation and method of digitalization directly influence the therapeutic effect of digitalis and the incidence of digitalis intoxication. There are four methods of digitalization in most clinical situations: very rapid parenteral digitalization (within 12 hours); rapid oral digitalization (within 24–48 hours); moderately rapid oral digitalization (within 2–3 days); and slow oral digitalization (within 5–8 days). The choice depends upon the degree of urgency, the nature of the underlying heart disease, and the presence or absence of cardiac arrhythmias.

Very Rapid Parenteral Digitalization (within 12 Hours). For urgent situations such as acute pulmonary edema due to left ventricular failure and supraventricular tachyarrhythmias, very rapid parenteral digitalization is indicated. Short-acting preparations such as digoxin, deslanoside, or ouabain are commonly used:

Digoxin (Lanoxin): The usual initial dose of digoxin is 0.5 to 1 mg given intravenously; 0.25–0.5 mg may be given thereafter every 2 to 4 hours as needed.

Deslanoside (Cedilanid-D): The initial dose of deslanoside is usually 0.8 to 1.6 mg intravenously, followed by 0.4 mg every 2 to 4 hours as needed.

Ouabain (G-Strophanthin): The usual initial dose of ouabain is 0.25 to 0.5 mg intravenously, followed by 0.1 mg every 30 minutes as needed.

Rapid Oral Digitalization (within 24 Hours). This method may be used when patients are suffering from acute congestive heart failure or supraventricular tachyarrhythmias, and when the clinical situation is not urgent enough to require very rapid parenteral digitalization. In these situations, therapeutic effect is reached within 24 to 48 hours:

Digoxin (Lanoxin): For this purpose, the preparation of choice is digoxin. The initial dose of digoxin is usually 1 to 1.5 mg by mouth followed by 0.5 mg every 6 hours until the patient is digitalized.

TABLE 7-2   *Methods of Digitalization[a]*

	Very Rapid Digitalization (within 12 Hours)	Rapid Digitalization (within 24 Hours)	Moderately Rapid Digitalization (within 2–3 Days)	Slow Digitalization (within 5–8 Days)
Digoxin	0.5–1 mg IV injection initially, then 0.25–0.5 mg q̄ 2–4 hr as needed	1–1.5 mg by mouth initially, then 0.5 mg q̄ 6 hr until digitalized	0.5 mg t.i.d. by mouth for 2–3 days until digitalized	0.25 mg t.i.d. by mouth for 5–8 days until digitalized
Deslanoside	0.8–1.6 mg IV injection initially, then 0.4 mg q̄ 2–4 hr as needed	—	—	—
Ouabain	0.25–0.5 mg IV injection initially, then 0.1 mg q̄ ½ hr as needed	—	—	—
Digitoxin	—	0.8 mg by mouth initially, then 0.2 mg q̄ 6 hr until digitalized	0.2 mg t.i.d. by mouth for 2–3 days until digitalized	0.1 mg t.i.d. by mouth for 5–8 days until digitalized
Digitalis leaf	—	0.8 g by mouth initially, then 0.2 g q̄ 6 hr until digitalized	0.2 g t.i.d. by mouth for 2–3 days until digitalized	0.1 g t.i.d. by mouth for 5–8 days until digitalized

[a] Reprinted with permission from Chung.[2]

Digitoxin: If the physician has chosen digitoxin, the initial dose is 0.8 mg by mouth, followed by 0.2 mg every 6 hours until the patient is digitalized.

Digitalis leaf: Digitalis leaf is now seldom used for this purpose.

Moderately Rapid Oral Digitalization (*within 2–3 Days*). This method is preferred when the patient shows well-developed but not acute signs of congestive heart failure. It is not usually recommended when congestive heart failure is associated with, or due to, supraventricular tachyarrhythmias. This method can be used either in the hospital or in the outpatient clinic.

Digoxin (Lanoxin): When digoxin is chosen, full digitalization can be accomplished with a dosage schedule of 0.5 mg three times daily for 2 to 3 days until digitalization is completed. If digoxin is given to an ambulant patient either at a clinic or in a private office, I prefer to see the patient after he has received a total of 3 mg in 48 hours rather than to prescribe routinely. This decision is made in order to prevent digitalis toxicity. After a careful evaluation of the patient, including interpretation of electrocardiograms, additional dosage will be prescribed.

Digitoxin: When digitoxin is chosen, 0.2 mg may be given in the same manner as digoxin.

Digitalis leaf: Digitalis leaf is now seldom used.

Slow Oral Digitalization (*within 5–8 Days*). This method is very useful for patients with mild congestive heart failure without any acute symptoms or supraventricular tachyarrhythmias. This method is frequently used for ambulant patients at clinics or in private offices. It can, of course, be used in the hospital as well.

Digoxin (Lanoxin): I often use digoxin in the dosage of 0.25 mg 3 times a day for 5 to 8 days. I prefer to see these patients after 5 days of digitalization. At that point, the amount of additional digoxin will be ordered as required after full evaluation of clinical and electrocardiographic findings. This method is quite safe for the treatment of uncomplicated mild congestive heart failure.

Digitoxin: If digitoxin is chosen, 0.1 mg may be given in the manner described for digoxin.

Digitalis leaf: Digitalis leaf is now seldom used for this purpose.

Full Digitalization and Maintenance Doses (Table 7-3). Although dosage varies markedly in different individuals and even in the same

Table 7-3   Full Digitalization and Maintenance Doses[a]

| | Digitalizing Doses within 24–48 hr | | | | Maintenance Doses | |
| | IV or IM Administration | | Oral Administration | | | |
	Average	Usual Range	Average	Usual Range	Average	Usual Range
Digoxin	1.5 mg	1–2.5 mg	2.5 mg	1.5–4 mg	0.25 mg	0.125–0.75 mg
Deslanoside	1.6 mg	1.2–2 mg	—	—	—	—
Ouabain	1 mg	0.5–1.2 mg				
Digitoxin	1.2 mg	1–2 mg	1.5 mg	1.2–2 mg	0.1 mg	0.05–0.2 mg
Digitalis leaf	—	—	1.5 g	1.2–2 g	0.1 g	0.05–0.2 g

[a] Reprinted with permission from Chung.[2]

individual at different times, extensive clinical experience enables us to set guidelines for average doses and usual ranges of dosage for full digitalization and maintenance use.

Digoxoin (Lanoxin): The average full digitalizing dose of digoxin by parenteral route is 1.5 mg with a usual range of from 1 to 2.5 mg. The average full digitalizing dose of digoxin by oral administration is approximately 2.5 mg, with a usual range of between 1.5 and 4 mg. The usual maintenance dose of digoxin is 0.25 mg, but some patients may require as little as 0.125 mg or as much as 0.75 mg daily as a maintenance dose.

Deslanoside (Cedilanid-D): The average full digitalizing dose of deslanoside is 1.6 mg, with a usual range of between 1.2 and 2 mg.

Ouabain (G-Strophanthin): The average full digitalizing dose of ouabain is 1 mg, with a usual range of between 0.5 and 1.2 mg.

Digitoxin: The average full digitalizing dose of digitoxin by parenteral route is 1.2 mg, with a usual range of 1–2 mg. The average oral digitalizing dose of digitoxin is 1.5 mg, with a usual range of 1.2–2 mg. The average maintenance dose of digitoxin is 0.1 mg, with a usual range of 0.05–0.2 mg.

Digitalis leaf: Digitalis leaf is little used because of the superiority of many other digitalis preparations.

Digitalization in Children. With a few exceptions, the fundamental principles, indications, and contraindications of digitalization in children are essentially the same as in adults.[20-22] The initial dosage of the cardiac glycosides varies markedly according to the patient's age. For example, patients below 2 years of age require significantly different amounts of digitalis than patients over the age of 2 years.[20-22] The manifestations of digitalis intoxication in children are somewhat different from those in the adult:[20-22] Ventricular premature contractions, the most common digitalis-induced arrhythmias in adults, are rather uncommon in children;[2,20-22] instead, AV block and SA block and marked sinus arrhythmia are commonly found. A detailed dosage schedule for parenteral and oral digitalization with digoxin (Lanoxin), the preparation most often used in children, is given below:

Parenteral Digitalization (Intravenous), Digoxin

1. *Initial dosage:* $\frac{1}{4}$–$\frac{1}{2}$ of estimated total digitalizing dose based upon:
    a.   0.02–0.03 mg/lb (under 2 years)
    b.   0.01–0.02 mg/lb (over 2 years)

2. *Full digitalization dosage:* Initial dosage is followed by ¼ of estimated total digitalizing dose every 8–12 hours until the child is digitalized.

Oral Digitalization, Digoxin

1. *Initial dosage:* ¼–½ of estimated total digitalizing dose based upon:
   a. 0.03–0.04 mg/lb (under 2 years)
   b. 0.02–0.03 mg/lb (over 2 years)
2. *Full digitalization dosage:* Initial dosage is followed by ¼ of estimated total digitalizing dose every 6–8 hours until the child is digitalized.
3. *Maintenance dosage:* ¼ of total digitalizing dosage.

Quinidine

For more than 50 years, quinidine has been the most valuable antitachyarrhythmic agent available. Quinidine has two major effects[1]: The direct effect of the drug is on the cell membrane, and the indirect effect is anticholinergic. The net clinical effect of the anticholinergic and direct actions is a marked prolongation of the refractory period in the atria and a lesser degree of prolongation in the ventricles. Quinidine also induces a shortening of the refractory period in the AV junction. The sinus rate tends to be slowed by the direct effect of quinidine, but the indirect (vagolytic) effect tends to counteract this effect. As a result, the sinus rate may not be altered significantly by quinidine, or it may even be accelerated.

Indications.   The primary use of quinidine has been to convert atrial fibrillation or flutter to sinus rhythm. Before DC cardioverters were available, large amounts of quinidine sulfate were necessary to restore sinus rhythm, but it is now used for this purpose only when a DC cardioverter is not available. At present, quinidine is largely used to prevent the recurrence of atrial fibrillation or flutter after restoration of sinus rhythm by either digitalization or DC shock.[1] It is also useful in the treatment of various acute supraventricular and ventricular tachyarrhythmias. In the treatment of atrial fibrillation or flutter with anomalous AV conduction in Wolff-Parkinson-White syndrome (Figure 7-10), a combination of digitalis and quinidine is often effective.[1] In the treatment of acute tachyarrhythmias, quinidine is found to be more effective in supraventricular tachyarrhythmias than in ventricular ones. Quinidine is also useful for the suppression of premature beats, especially those that are supraventricular in origin.

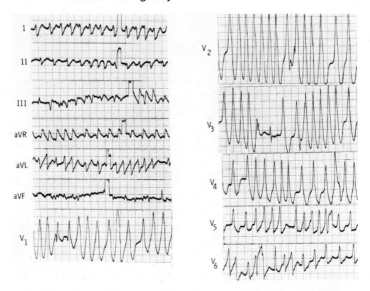

Figure 7-10. Atrial fibrillation with anomalous AV conduction and extremely rapid ventricular response (ventricular rate: 200–300 beats per minute) associated with Wolff-Parkinson-White syndrome, type A. The rhythm superficially resembles ventricular tachycardia. Note occasional normally conducted beats.

Full dosage.   For the treatment of acute tachyarrhythmias, quinidine gluconate 0.8 g diluted in 200 cc of 5% dextrose in water may be given intravenously at a rate of about 25 mg per minute, under continuous electrocardiographic monitoring. Intramuscular administration of quinidine gluconate may be carried out by giving 0.4 to 0.6 g initially, followed by 0.4 g every 2 to 4 hours as needed. Total dosage by intramuscular route should not exceed 2.4 g.

Maintenance dosage.   The usual maintenance dosage of quinidine sulfate for the prevention of recurrence of various arrhythmias is 0.3 to 0.4 g every 6 hours.

Side Effects and Toxicity.   Mild toxic manifestations include nausea, vomiting, diarrhea, tinnitus, slight impairment of hearing and vision, and slight widening of the QRS complex. When quinidine toxicity increases, tht above manifestations become more severe. Thus, the patient may develop blurring vision, disturbed color perception, photophobia, diplopia, abdominal pain, headache, confusion, and ventricular tachyarrhythmias. If the patient has an unusual sensitivity or idiosyncratic reaction to quinidine, respiratory depression, hypotension, convulsion, urticaria, macular or papular rashes, fever, thrombocytopenia, hemolytic anemia, and even sudden death may result.[1]

Lidocaine (Xylocaine)

The discovery of antiarrhythmic properties of lidocaine is probably the most important addition to the therapy of cardiac arrhythmias. The structure of lidocaine is similar to that of quinidine or procaine amide (see below), but its electrophysiologic properties are quite different.[14,15,17] Since it has little effect on the atria, lidocaine is of little use in the treatment of atrial tachyarrhythmias. Lidocaine depresses diastolic depolarization and automaticity in the ventricles. It is of interest that lidocaine, in standard doses, has no effect on conduction velocity and generally shortens both the action potential and the refractory period. Approximately 90% of an administered dose of the drug is metabolized in the liver, and the remaining 10% is excreted unchanged via the kidneys. The action of lidocaine is more transient than that of procaine amide, and it also penetrates the cardiac tissues more rapidly than does the latter drug.[14,15,17]

Indications.   Lidocaine is widely used, primarily for the treatment of ventricular tachyarrhythmias and ventricular premature contractions associated with acute myocardial infarction and cardiac surgery or cardiac catheterization (Figure 7-9).[14,15,17] In the past decade, lidocaine has gradually replaced procaine amide for parenteral use because of its greater effectiveness and the infrequency with which it produces hypotension when given properly. Lidocaine may also be indicated for the treatment of various supraventricular tachyarrhythmias if other arrhythmic agents are ineffective. However, the therapeutic effect of lidocaine in the treatment of supraventricular tachyarrhythmias is disappointing.

Administration.[14,15,17]   For the initiation of therapy, direct injection of 75 to 100 mg of lidocaine (1–1.5 mg/kg) is given slowly; the same dose may be repeated every 10 to 20 minutes until ventricular tachyarrhythmias are terminated. In general, the total dose should not exceed 750 mg, and it is advisable that no more than 300 mg be administered during an 1-hour period. When intravenous injection is not feasible, 200 to 250 mg of lidocaine may be given intramuscularly, and the same dose may be repeated once or twice every 10 to 20 minutes. It is recommended that lidocaine be administered under continuous electrocardiographic monitoring. Following the termination of ventricular tachyarrhythmia, continuous intravenous infusion at a rate of 1 to 5 mg/min is needed for 24 to 72 hours in most cases in order to prevent recurrence of the arrhythmia. If ventricular tachyarrhythmias do not recur, lidocaine may be replaced gradually with oral procaine amide. Oral use of lidocaine in clinical practice needs further investigation.

Side Effects and Toxicity. Toxicity of lidocaine is relatively uncommon but the drug may produce dizziness, drowsiness, confusion, muscle twitching, disorientation, euphoria, cardiac and respiratory depression, convulsion, and hypotension. Caution should be exercised in the repeated use of lidocaine in patients with severe liver or renal disease because accumulation may lead to toxicity.

Propranolol (Inderal)

Propranolol is a beta-adrenergic receptor blocking agent that has been widely used for the management of various tachyarrhythmias, including those induced by digitalis and those resistant to digitalis.[6,7] Antiarrhythmic actions of Inderal are produced in two ways: inhibition of adrenergic stimulation of the heart and direct action on the electrophysiologic properties of cardiac tissue. Thus, the overall effects of Inderal usually result in reduction of automaticity, including reduction of the sinus rate and prolongation of atrial and AV conduction time.[6,7]

Indications. Inderal is effective in terminating various tachyarrhythmias. The direct membrane actions of Inderal are primarily responsible for its effectiveness in the treatment of digitalis-induced tachyarrhythmias.[6,7] In addition, Inderal is very effective in the treatment of catecholamine-induced tachyarrhythmias, such as the arrhythmias precipated by exercise, emotional distress, or excessive sympathetic stimulation, and of supraventricular tachyarrhythmias related to Wolff-Parkinson-White syndrome.[6,7] In particular, Inderal is considered to be the drug of choice in the treatment of catecholamine-induced arrhythmias and supraventricular (usually atrial) tachycardia associated with Wolff-Parkinson-White syndrome in young individuals without demonstrable heart disease (Figure 7-4). In some cases of hyperthyroidism, tachyarrhythmias may be terminated by propranolol, but often large dosage is required.[6,7] Inderal is contraindicated in patients with bronchial asthma, allergic rhinitis, marked sinus bradycardia, second or third degree AV block, SA block, sinus arrest, cardiogenic shock, and congestive heart failure.

Full Dosage. Inderal should be administered slowly by intravenous injection, and the rate of administration should be 1 to 3 mg per minute under ECG monitoring. The second dose may be repeated after 2 minutes if needed. Additional medication should be withheld for at least 4 hours, and total dose should not exceed 10 mg.

Maintenance Dosage. In nonurgent situations, Inderal may be given orally in doses ranging between 10 and 30 mg 3 to 4 times daily before meals and at bedtime. The same dosage schedule is also recommended for long-term use or for prophylactic purposes.

Side Effects and Toxicity.   Side effects or toxic manifestations include nausea, vomiting, light-headedness, diarrhea, constipation, mental depression, asthma, hypotension, bradycardia, precipitation of congestive heart failure, and cardiogenic shock. In some patients, allergic manifestations such as erythematous rashes, paresthesias of the hands, and fever may be observed.

Procaine Amide (Pronestyl)

Procaine amide has been the traditional drug of choice in the treatment of ventricular tachycardia until the past decade, when lidocaine was proven to be a safer and more effective agent.[5,14,15] Large amounts of Pronestyl were often used in the treatment of ventricular tachycardia, especially before DC cardioverters became readily available.

The electrophysiologic effects of Pronestyl are very similar to those of quinidine. Pronestyl slows electrical conduction, increases the refractory period, and depresses diastolic depolarization and automaticity.[5,14,15] Pronestyl has an indirect vagolytic action, and AV conduction may be facilitated when low doses are used. However, the direct effect of Pronestyl produces depression of AV conduction with higher doses. The therapeutic levels are easily achieved by oral administration, since Pronestyl is almost completely absorbed from the gastrointestinal tract.[5,14,15] This drug should be administered with caution to patients with significant renal disease, because the drug is excreted primarily by the kidneys in unchanged form.

Indications.   Although the electrophysiologic actions of procaine amide are very similar to those of quinidine, the former drug has been used primarily in the treatment of ventricular tachyarrhythmias (Figure 7-11). At present, the primary indication for Pronestyl is to prevent the recurrence of ventricular tachyarrhythmias following their termination by DC shock or intravenous lidocaine.[14,15] Pronestyl is also effective for the treatment of supraventricular tachyarrhythmias, although it is not the drug of choice. Pronestyl has been used in place of quinidine when the patient is unable to tolerate the latter drug. At present, large dosage of parenteral Pronestyl is used only when a DC cardioverter is not available and lidocaine is found to be ineffective. Pronestyl is very effective in suppressing ventricular premature beats.

Full Dosage.   When intravenous Pronestyl has to be used, 1 to 2 g of the drug diluted in 200 cc of 5% dextrose in water is administered by continuous drip at a rate of 100 mg every 2–4 minutes under continuous ECG monitor. The total intravenous dose should not exceed 2 g. When the clinical situation is not urgent, Pronestyl may be given orally.

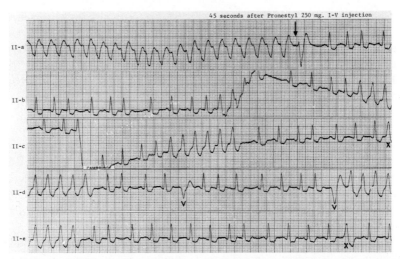

Figure 7-11. Leads II-*a,b,c,d*, and *e* are continuous. Bidirectional ventricular tachycardia is terminated by intravenous injection of Pronestyl, 250 mg. Note frequent ventricular premature contractions (marked *V* and *X*).

Initially, 1 g of Pronestyl may be given by mouth followed by 0.5 g every 2–3 hours as needed. The total oral dose should not exceed 3.5 g.

Maintenance Dose. Since the half-life of procaine amide is relatively short, the ideal maintenance oral dosage has been reported to be 250–500 mg every 3 hours.[5] However, simply because of the inconvenience such dosage would cause the patient, many physicians prescribe a maintenance dose of Pronestyl of 250–500 mg every 6 hours by mouth.

Side Effects and Toxicity. Toxic manifestations of Pronestyl include nausea, vomiting, fever, leukopenia, lymphadenopathy, lupus erythematosus-like syndrome, convulsion, AV and intraventricular block of varying degree, ventricular tachyarrrhythmias, and hypotension.[5,14,15] In some patients who are sensitive to Pronestyl, allergic manifestations such as eosinophilia, urticaria, and agranulocytosis may be observed.

Diphenylhydantoin (Dilantin)

The discovery of the antiarrhythmic properties of Dilantin provided another important tool for the management of various cardiac arrhythmias, particularly those induced by digitalis.[2,16] Dilantin has a structure similar to that of the barbituates, but the electrophysiologic properties are quite different from other antiarrhythmic agents. Atrial conduction velocity is accelerated by Dilantin as a result of a faster depolarization of the atria while the sinus rate is usually uninfluenced. While the AV conduction may not be influenced by Dilantin, it is often accelerated by the action of the drug. As a rule, intraventricular conduction is not altered significantly by Dilantin. One of the most important aspects of the use of Dilantin is that it counteracts the depressant effect on the AV conduction induced by digitalis or procaine amide. In addition, Dilantin depresses diastolic depolarization and automaticity and shortens the duration of the action potential and the effective refractory period.[2,16]

Indications. At present, Dilantin is considered to be the drug of choice in the treatment of various tachyarrhythmias induced by digitalis.[2,16] This is especially true in the management of digitalis-induced ventricular tachycardia (see Chapter 15). The drug is also a very useful substitute for Pronestyl or Xylocaine when these drugs are found to be ineffective.[1]

Full Dosage. The initial dose of Dilantin is between 125 and 250 mg intravenously for 1–3 minutes under ECG monitoring. Most patients respond within 3 seconds to 5 minutes. The same dose may be repeated every 10–20 minutes as needed, but a total dose should not exceed 750 mg per hour. Continuous intravenous drip is not practicable with Dilantin because the drug easily precipitates with various commonly used intravenous solutions. When the situation is not urgent, 200 mg of Dilantin may be given orally as an initial dose, followed by 100 mg every 4 to 6 hours as needed.[1]

Maintenance Dosage. After termination of the tachyarrhythmias, a maintenance dose of Dilantin, 100 mg 3 to 4 times daily, is often needed; the duration depends upon the clinical situation. Oral Dilantin is often useful in place of Pronestyl or quinidine for a long-term therapy.[1]

Side Effects and Toxicity. Toxic manifestations or side effects of Dilantin include respiratory and cardiac depression; skin reactions, such as urticaria and purpura; eosinophilia; drowsiness; ataxia; tremor; depression; nervousness; arthralgia; gingival hyperplasia; hypotension; and AV block of varying degree.[2,16] Fortunately, these manifestations are usually rare.

CAROTID SINUS STIMULATION

Carotid sinus stimulation is indicated for two major purposes—therapy and diagnosis.[9]

Therapy

Carotid sinus stimulation is extremely valuable in terminating paroxysmal atrial as well as AV nodal (junctional) tachycardia. In addition, regular and rapid (rate: 160–250 beats per minute) tachycardia is often terminated by carotid sinus stimulation even if the exact location of the ectopic focus is uncertain. Carotid sinus stimulation may be effective whether the QRS complex is normal or wide.

Diagnosis

It has been known for many years that carotid sinus stimulation is extremely useful in differentiating various tachyarrhythmias. This is particularly true for regular ectopic tachycardia and wide QRS complex. It should be emphasized that applying carotid sinus stimulation to patients with digitalis toxicity is dangerous and may induce ventricular fibrillation (see Chapter 15).

Various responses to carotid sinus stimulation may be observed, depending upon the type and nature of tachyarrhythmias.[4]

Sinus Tachycardia.   In general, it is not necessary to apply carotid sinus stimulation either diagnostically or therapeutically in cases of sinus tachycardia. However, the procedure is occasionally useful when the rate of sinus tachycardia is very rapid (around 150 to 160 beats per minute) and differentiation from atrial tachycardia is needed. Sinus tachycardia slows only transiently in response to carotid sinus stimulation.

Atrial Tachycardia.   Carotid sinus stimulation is extremely valuable in terminating paroxysmal atrial tachycardia (Figure 7-12). The patient with atrial tachycardia may respond to carotid sinus stimulation one of four ways: termination, no response, slowing of ventricular rate due to increased AV block, and increased atrial rate. When slowing of the ventricular rate occurs in atrial tachycardia because of increased AV block, the underlying cause is usually digitalis toxicity. (Figure 7-13).

Atrial Fibrillation or Flutter.   When carotid sinus pressure is applied

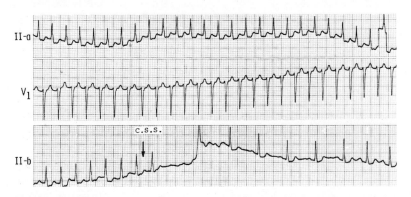

Figure 7-12. Leads II-*a* and *b* are not continuous. Supraventricular (probably atrial) tachycardia (rate: 187 beats per minute) is terminated by carotid sinus stimulation (indicated by arrow).

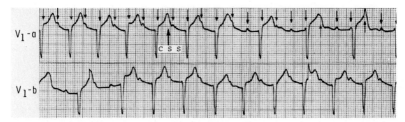

Figure 7-13. Leads V₁-a and b are continuous. Arrows indicate P waves. Note a transient slowing of the ventricular rate in atrial tachycardia by carotid sinus stimulation (indicated by CSS). Atrial tachycardia (atrial rate: 190 beats per minute) in this case is considered to be induced by digitalis.

to patients with atrial fibrillation or flutter, the ventricular rate invariably slows because of the increased atrioventricular block. Occasionally a long ventricular standstill may result when carotid sinus pressure is applied to an elderly patient with atrial fibrillation or flutter.

AV Nodal (Junctional) Tachycardia. It is often difficult, and at times impossible, to distinguish between paroxysmal atrial tachycardia and paroxysmal atrioventricular junctional tachycardia when only conventional electrocardiograms are available. The P wave may be superimposed on the S–T segment, T wave, or QRS complex or the preceding or succeeding beat. Therefore, the term "supraventricular tachycardia" is often used in this circumstance. It is believed that the response to carotid sinus stimulation is similar in paroxysmal atrioventricular junctional tachycardia and paroxysmal atrial tachycardia.

Paroxysmal atrioventricular junctional tachycardia may convert to sinus rhythm (Figure 7-14) or may not respond to the procedure. On the other hand, nonparoxysmal atrioventricular junctional tachycardia

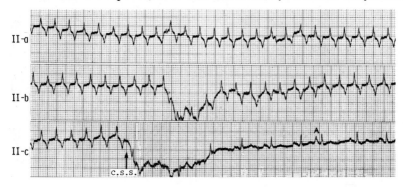

Figure 7-14. Leads II-a,b, and c are continuous. AV nodal (junctional) tachycardia is terminated by carotid sinus stimulation (indicated by arrow): Note one atrial premature beat (marked A) in lead II-c.

is usually unresponsive to carotid sinus stimulation, but ventricular fibrillation may ensue if the underlying cause is digitalis toxicity. Thus, carotid sinus stimulation is not recommended in the presence of nonparoxysmal atrioventricular junctional tachycardia, which is a common sign of digitalis toxicity (see Chapter 15).

Ventricular Tachyarrhythmias. Carotid sinus stimulation is often used to distinguish ventricular tachycardia from supraventricular tachycardia, especially when the QRS complex is wide and bizarre. In contrast to supraventricular tachyarrhythmias, ventricular tachycardia does not respond to carotid sinus stimulation. Therefore, any response to the procedure rules out ventricular tachycardia.

DIRECT CURRENT (DC) SHOCK

There are two major indications for DC cardioversion: treatment of acute tachyarrhythmias and elective cardioversion for chronic atrial fibrillation and flutter.

DC Cardioversion for Acute Tachyarrhythmias

In various supraventricular (atrial and AV junctional) and ventricular tachyarrhythmias with an acute onset, DC cardioversion is often a lifesaving measure. When the clinical situation is extremely urgent, as in the case of ventricular tachycardia or fibrillation (Figures 7-7 and 7-8), premedication for transient amnesia or anesthesia is not needed. Thus, 100–200 Wsec of DC shock can be applied directly. If the arrhythmia persists, DC shock of increased energy (200–400 Wsec) should be repeated immediately. On the other hand, if the clinical situation is not extremely urgent, small amounts of thiopental sodium or diazepam may be administered before the application of DC shock. Premedication may not be indicated when only a small energy discharge is required, particularly in the treatment of atrial flutter. Following termination of ventricular tachyarrhythmias, a continuous intravenous infusion of Xylocaine (less commonly procaine amide) is usually indicated and followed by oral maintenance therapy with procaine amide, diphenylhydantoin, or quinidine. When atrial flutter or fibrillation is terminated by DC shock (Figure 7-5), maintenance doses of oral quinidine after digitalization are needed in most instances. Direct current shock is often effective in terminating any tachyarrhythmia associated with Wolff-Parkinson-White syndrome (Figure 7-15).

Elective Cardioversion

Elective cardioversion is indicated for the treatment of chronic tachyarrhythmias, primarily atrial fibrillation or flutter, when restoration of sinus rhythm is considered to be beneficial. Less commonly, elective

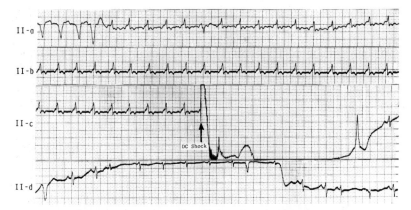

Figure 7-15. Leads II-a,b,c, and d are continuous. Atrial flutter with 2:1 AV response in Wolff-Parkinson-White syndrome is terminated by DC shock (indicated by arrow). Note two types of anomalous AV conduction during atrial flutter. There are occasional atrial as well as ventricular premature contractions.

cardioversion is applied to terminate other tachyarrhythmias such as atrial or AV nodal (junctional) tachycardia.

A detailed discussion of DC shock may be found in Chapter 9.

ARTIFICIAL PACEMAKERS

Although the primary use of the artificial pacemaker is in the treatment of slow rhythms, particularly complete AV block, artificial pacemakers may also be indicated for terminating and preventing drug-resistant refractory tachyarrhythmias.[11] In these circumstances, the

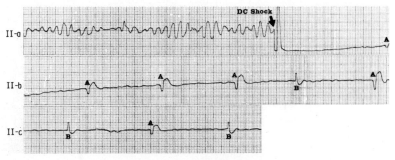

Figure 7-16. Figures 7-16 and 7-17 were obtained from the same patient on different occasions. In Figure 7-16, leads II-a,b and c are continuous. Ventricular fibrillation is terminated by DC shock (indicated by arrow). However, following DC shock, ventricular escape rhythms (idioventricular rhythms) originating from two foci (marked A and B) are observed in the presence of atrial fibrillation due to complete AV block. This ECG finding reflects a type of bradytachycardia syndrome.

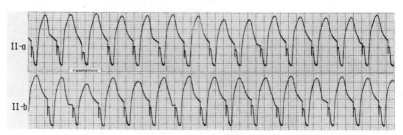

Figure 7-17. Leads II-a and b are continuous. These rhythm strips were obtained after insertion of a temporary artificial pacemaker with overdriving pacing (rate: 98 beats per minute).

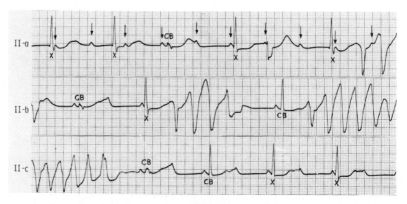

Figure 7-18. Figures 7-18 and 7-19 were obtained from the same patient on different occasions. In Figure 7-18, leads II-a,b, and c are continuous. The tracing shows sinus rhythm with intermittent ventricular escape rhythm (marked X) due to a high degree of AV block and frequent ventricular premature contractions with short runs of ventricular tachycardia. Note occasional ventricular captured beats (marked CB). This type of arrhythmia is called bradytachycardia syndrome.

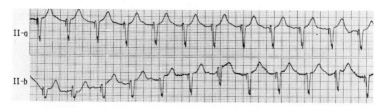

Figure 7-19. Leads II-a and b are continuous. These rhythm strips were obtained after insertion of a temporary artificial pacemaker with slight overdriving pacing (rate: 75 beats per minute).

overdriving pacing is necessary in order to suppress ectopic tachycardia. The primary indication for use of the overdriving pacemaker (rate: about 100–120 beats per minute) is in the management of refractory ventricular tachyarrhythmias[11] (Figures 7-16 and 7-17).

The overdriving pacing is also extremely useful in the treatment of bradytachyarrhythmia syndrome (Figures 7-18 and 7-19). In this case, only slight overdriving pacing (rate: about 80–100 beats per minute) may be sufficient. Occasionally, the overdriving pacemaker is indicated in the treatment of refractory supraventricular tachyarrhythmias (Figure 7-6).

A detailed discussion of artificial pacemakers is presented in Chapter 10.

SURGICAL APPROACHES

In the past several years, various surgical approaches to the management of drug-resistant refractory tachyarrhythmias have been developed.[23-28] Surgical management has been restricted primarily to the treatment of life-threatening ventricular tachyarrhythmias associated with coronary heart disease[23,24] and drug-resistant supraventricular tachyarrhythmias associated with Wolff-Parkinson-White syndrome.[25-28]

Recently, very favorable surgical results have been reported in eight patients with drug-resistant life-threatening ventricular tachyarrhythmias associated with documented coronary heart disease.[23] The surgical procedures in this study included a resection of the ventricular aneurysm or localized hypokinetic area in six patients and aortocoronary bypass grafting to at least one major coronary artery in all eight patients.

On the other hand, surgical management of drug-resistant supraventricular tachyarrhythmias associated with Wolff-Parkinson-White syndrome has not been always successful.[25-28] The surgical procedures include a ligation of the AV bundle and a surgical interruption of the anomalous pathway following an epicardial mapping study.[25-28] The surgical approaches to the WPW syndrome require further investigation.

Surgical approaches to the management of refractory tachyarrhythmias are discussed in detail in Chapter 17.

SUMMARY

The best therapeutic results can be obtained when a precise diagnosis of the tachyarrhythmia is made. In addition, underlying etiologic factors also significantly influence the therapeutic result. The first step in management is to eliminate the cause of the tachyarrhythmia if it is apparent.

Prevention of recurrence of tachyarrhythmias is another important aspect of management. Many patients require maintenance therapy with digitalis or other antiarrhythmic agents for long periods or even indefinitely. After the termination of the tachyarrhythmia by either carotid sinus stimulation or DC shock, one or more pharmacologic agents may be indicated in order to prevent recurrence of the arrthymia.

Digitalis is often the drug of choice in the treatment of supraventricular tachyarrhythmias, particularly atrial fibrillation or flutter with rapid ventricular response. Propranolol (Inderal) is considered to be the drug of choice in the treatment and prevention of catecholamine-induced tachyarrhythmias and supraventricular tachycardia associated with Wolff-Parkinson-White syndrome, especially in young individuals without demonstrable heart disease. Xylocaine (lidocaine) is the drug of choice in the treatment of ventricular tachyarrhythmias in almost all clinical situations, particularly in acute myocardial infarction. For digitalis-induced tachyarrhythmias, however, potassium or diphenylhydantoin (Dilantin) is the drug of choice. Dilantin is especially valuable in the treatment of digitalis-induced ventricular tachycardia.

At present, the primary indication for quinidine is the prevention of atrial fibrillation or flutter by oral administration following a restoration of sinus rhythm by digitalization or DC shock. Similarly, the main role of procaine amide (Pronestyl) is in the prevention of ventricular tachyarrhythmias by oral administration after termination of the arrhythmia by Xylocaine or DC shock.

In urgent situations, particularly in ventricular tachyarrhythmias, DC shock should be applied immediately. In refractory tachyarrhythmias, the artificial pacemaker with overdriving pacing rate is often lifesaving. The carotid sinus stimulation is the simplest and often the most effective way of terminating supraventricular tachycardia if it is applied properly. The procedure is also extremely valuable in the differential diagnosis of various tachyarrhythmias.

In refractory ventricular tachyarrhythmias, especially in the presence of coronary heart disease, surgical procedures should be seriously considered.

REFERENCES

1. Chung, E. K.: Cardiac Arrhythmias: Management. Baltimore, Williams & Wilkins Co., 1973.
2. Chung, E. K.: Digitalis Intoxication. Baltimore, Williams & Wilkins, 1969.
3. Chung, E. K.: Principles of Cardiac Arrhythmias. Baltimore, Williams & Wilkins Co., 1971.
4. Hurst, J. W., Paulk, E. A., Jr., Proctor, H. D., and Schlant, R. C.: Management of patients with atrial fibrillation. Am. J. Med. 37:728, 1964.
5. Koch-Weser, J., and Klein, S. W.: Procainamide dosage schedules, plasma concentrations, and clinical effects. JAMA 125:1454, 1971.

6. Gibson, D., and Sowton, E.: The use of beta-adrenergic receptor blocking drugs in dysrhythmias. Prog. Cardiovasc. Dis. 12:16, 1969.
7. Kosman, M. E.: Current status of propranolol hydrochloride (Inderal). JAMA 225:1380, 1973.
8. Day, H. W., and Bacaner, M.: Use of bretylium tosylate in the management of acute myocardial infarction. Am. J. Cardiol. 27:177, 1971.
9. Chung, E. K.: Use and abuse of carotid sinus stimulation. Postgrad. Med. 51:190, 1972.
10. Chung, E. K.: Use and abuse of direct current shock. Cardiology 55:310, 1970.
11. Furman, S., and Escher, D. J. W.: Principles and Techniques of Cardiac Pacing. Hagerstown, Md., Harper & Row, 1970.
12. Lister, J. W., Cohen, L. S., Bernstein, W. H., and Samet, P.: Treatment of supraventricular tachycardia by rapid atrial stimulation. Circulation 38:1044, 1968.
13. Chung, E. K.: Electrocardiography: Practical Applications with Vectorial Principles. Hagerstown, Md., Harper & Row, 1974.
14. Bigger, J. T., Jr., and Heissenbuttel, R. H.: The use of procaine amide and lidocaine in the treatment of cardiac arrhythmias. Prog. Cardiovasc. Dis. 11:515, 1969.
15. Harrison, D. C., Sprouse, J. H., and Morrow, A. G.: The antiarrhythmic properties of lidocaine and procaine amide. Circulation 28:486, 1963.
16. Damato, A. N.: Diphenylhydantoin: pharmacological and clinical use. Prog. Cardiovas. Dis. 12:1, 1969.
17. Wyman, M. G., and Hammersmith, L.: Comprehensive treatment plan for the prevention of primary ventricular fibrillation in acute myocardial infarction. Am. J. Cardiol. 33:661, 1974.
18. Beller, G. A., Smith, T. W., Abelman, W. H., et al.: Digitalis intoxication. A prospective study with serum level correlations. New Engl. J. Med. 284:989, 1971.
19. Doherty, J. E.: The clinical pharmacology of digitalis glycosides: a review. Am. J. Med. Sci. 255:382, 1968.
20. Hauck, A. J., Ongley, P. A., and Nadas, A. S.: The use of digoxin in infants and children. Am. Heart J. 56:443, 1958.
21. Levine, O. R., and Blumenthal, S.: Digoxin dosage in premature infants. Pediatrics. 29:18, 1962.
22. Neill, C. A.: The use of digitalis in infants and children. Prog. Cardiovas. Dis. 7:399, 1965.
23. Graham, A. F., Miller, D. C., Stinson, E. B., et al.: Surgical treatment of refractory life-threatening ventricular tachycardia. Am. J. Cardiol. 32:909, 1973.
24. Welch, T. G., Fontana, M. E. and Vasko, J. S.: Aneurysmectomy for recurrent ventricular tachyarrhythmias. Am. Heart J. 85:685, 1973.
25. Neutze, J. M., Kerr, A. R., and Whitlock, R. M. L.: Epicardial mapping in a variant of type A Wolff-Parkinson-White syndrome. Circulation. 48:662, 1973.
26. Dreifus, L. S., Nichols, H., Morse, D., Watanabe, Y., and Truex, R.: Control of recurrent tachycardia of Wolff-Parkinson-White syndrome by surgical ligation of the A-V bundle. Circulation. 38:1030, 1968.
27. Linsay, A. E., Nelson, R. M., Abildskov, J. A., and Wyatt, R.: Attempted surgical division of the preexcitation pathway in the Wolff-Parkinson-White syndrome. Am. J. Cardiol., 28:581, 1971. 1971.
28. Cole, D. D., Wills, R. E., Winterscheid, L. C., Reichenback, D. D., and Blackmon, J. R.: The Wolff-Parkinson-White syndrome. Problems in evaluation and surgical therapy. Circulation. 42:111, 1970.

Chapter 8
BRADYARRHYTHMIAS

EDWARD K. CHUNG

Bradyarrhythmia is defined as slow cardiac rhythm (usually slower than 60 beats per minute) that is due to various fundamental mechanisms.[1] Bradyarrhythmias may be divided into two major categories:

Disturbances of sinus impulse formation and conduction (sinus bradycardia, sinus arrest and sinoatrial block)
Atrioventricular (AV) block of various degrees

The therapeutic approaches will vary markedly, depending upon the fundamental mechanism responsible for the production of bradyarrhythmias, the ventricular rate, the underlying cause, and the symptoms, if present.[2]

DISTURBANCES OF SINUS IMPULSE FORMATION AND CONDUCTION

Mild sinus bradycardia (rate: 50–59 beats per minute) is not uncommon in healthy individuals, especially in young athletes and elderly persons. When the sinus rate is between 40 and 50 beats per minute, there may be some symptoms. Marked sinus bradycardia, with a rate below 40 beats per minute, often produces significant hemodynamic alterations, especially when it is associated with acute myocardial infarction.[2,3] Among the most common causes of sinus bradycardia are the therapeutic or toxic effects of various drugs, including digitalis, propranolol,

127

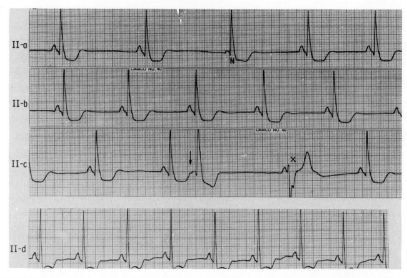

Figure 8-1. Leads II-*a*,*b*, and *c* are continuous. The first three rhythm strips show marked sinus bradycardia (rate 30–35 beats per minute), with AV nodal (junctional) and ventricular escape beats (marked *N* and *X*, respectively). Note a single atrial premature beat (indicated by arrow). The sinus rate has increased (rate: 56 beats per minute) immediately following intravenous injection of atropine, 0.4 mg (lead II-*d*).

reserpine, and guanethidine, and acute diaphragmatic myocardial infarction.[1-4] Drug-induced sinus bradycardia, sinus arrest, or SA block is best treated by discontinuing administration of that particular drug.[4]

Active treatment is indicated when marked sinus bradycardia persists and becomes symptomatic, and especially when it is associated with acute myocardial infarction (Fig. 8-1). The treatment of choice in this case is atropine, and the next commonly used agent is isoproterenol (Isuprel).[2,3] Essentially the same therapeutic approach may be used in the treatment of symptomatic sinus arrest and SA block.

In drug-resistant sinus bradycardia, sinus arrest, or SA block, a temporary or even a permanent artificial pacemaker is the treatment of choice (Figure 8-2). In most situations, only a temporary pacemaker is required.[5,6]

ATRIOVENTRICULAR (AV) BLOCK

It is important to remember that AV block *per se* does not require treatment. Whether the treatment of AV block is indicated depends primarily on the degree and the etiology of the AV block, the ventricular rate, and the presence or absence of symptoms.[2]

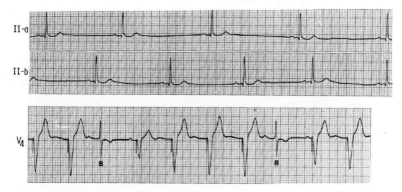

Figure 8-2. Leads II-*a* and *b* are continuous. The tracing shows sinus arrhythmia with marked sinus bradycardia (rate: 27–33 beats per minute). Because of symptomatic and drug-resistant sinus bradycardia, a permanent artificial (demand) pacemaker is implanted (lead V₄). In lead V₄, there are two sinus beats with long PR intervals (0.28 sec) in the presence of artificial pacemaker-induced ventricular rhythm (rate: 68 beats per minute). This patient has a definite evidence of "sick sinus syndrome," in which a markedly slow sinus mechanism fails to respond to any drug.

First-degree AV block usually requires no particular treatment, except that any apparent direct cause, such as digitalis intoxication, may be eliminated.[4] It has been reported that atropine is effective in abolishing digitalis-induced first- and second-degree AV block. Isoproterenol (Isuprel) may be effective in this situation, but the drug often produces untoward reactions such as increased ventricular irritability.

Wenckebach (Mobitz type I) AV block (Fig. 8-3) usually does not

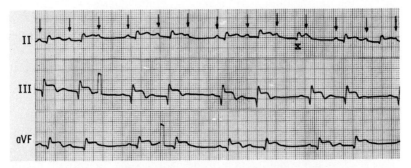

Figure 8-3. Arrows indicate sinus P waves. The tracing shows sinus rhythm (atrial rate: 98 beats per minute) with predominantly 3:2 Wenckebach AV block associated with acute diaphragmatic myocardial infarction. Unexpectedly conducted beat with long PR interval (marked *X*) is considered to represent a supernormal AV conduction.

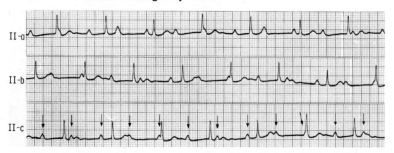

Figure 8-4. Leads II-*a,b,c,* and *d* are continuous. Arrows indicate P waves. The tracing reveals sinus rhythm (atrial rate: 87 beats per minute) with AV nodal (junctional) escape rhythm (ventricular rate: 55 beats per minute) due to complete AV block.

require active treatment unless significant symptoms are produced. On the other hand, Mobitz type II AV block often requires an artificial pacemaker, because it is considered to be a precursor of bilateral bundle branch block.[7]

In complete AV block, the therapeutic approach depends upon the ventricular rate and the magnitude of symptoms. Unless there are symptoms, active treatment is usually not indicated when the ventricular rate is relatively rapid (50–60 beats per minute) in AV nodal (junctional) escape rhythm due to complete AV block (Fig. 8-4), such as seen in acute diaphragmatic myocardial infarction. On the other hand, a temporary or often a permanent artificial pacemaker is indicated when the ventricular rate is slow (slower than 40 beats/min) in ventricular escape (idioventricular) rhythm due to complete AV block, as is seen in acute anterior myocardial infarction or in elderly individuals with degenerative changes in the conduction system[5,6,8] (Fig. 8-4). Bilateral bundle branch block of varying degrees often requires a permanent artificial pacemaker[7] (Fig. 8-5).

In urgent situations before the insertion of an artificial pacemaker, various agents such as isoproterenol (Isuprel) or epinephrine (Adrenalin) may be tried, particularly in ventricular standstill (Fig. 8-6). Extremely slow rhythm may be produced when an artificial pacemaker malfunctions, especially when the newer demand models are used.[5,6] The slow pacemaker rhythm is often associated with irregular pacing (Fig. 8-7). When a malfunction of the pacemaker is diagnosed, needless to say, a normally functioning pacemaker should be replaced immediately.[5,6]

A detailed description of artificial pacemakers may be found in Chapter 10.

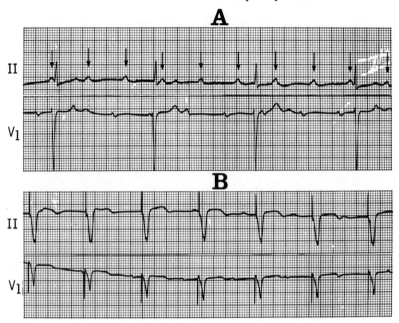

Figure 8-5. Tracings *A* and *B* were obtained from the same patient with Adams-Stokes syndrome. In tracing *A*, arrows indicate P waves. The tracing *A* shows sinus rhythm (atrial rate: 89 beats per minute) with ventricular escape (idioventricular) rhythm (rate: 35 beats per minute) due to complete AV block. Tracing *B*, taken after implantation of a permanent pacemaker, reveals artificial pacemaker-induced ventricular rhythm (ventricular rate: 63 beats per minute).

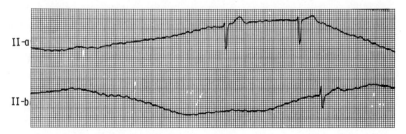

Figure 8-6. Leads II-*a* and *b* are *not* continuous. The rhythm is atrial fibrillation with areas of ventricular standstill.

ANTIBRADYARRHYTHMIC AGENTS (TABLE 8-1)

Because of ready availability of artificial pacemakers, the various antibradyarrhythmic agents have been much less commonly used in the past decade. Nevertheless, these agents are valuable for the management of milder forms of slow rhythms, such as marked sinus bradycardia and

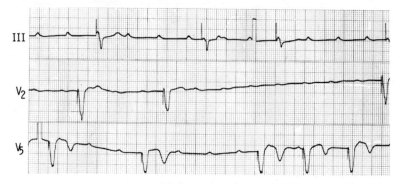

Figure 8-7. Sinus rhythm with markedly irregular and slow artificial pacemaker-induced ventricular rhythm due to malfunctioning unit.

sinoatrial block.[9-12] In addition, antibradyarrhythmic agents are extremely useful for urgent situations, such as in Adams-Stokes syndrome, when artificial pacemakers are not immediately available.[9-12] Of the antibradyarrhythmic agents, those most commonly used are probably atropine sulfate and isoproterenol.[2]

Atropine Sulfate[2,9-12]

Indications.   Atropine is used primarily to accelerate the sinus rate by vagal inhibition. Thus, this is the drug of choice for marked symptomatic sinus bradycardia (Fig. 8-1). Atropine is also effective in the treatment of sinus arrest or sinoatrial block. In first- or second-degree AV block (usually Wenckebach type), especially in acute diaphragmatic myocardial infarction or digitalis toxicity, atropine may also be used. It is usually not effective in the treatment of high-degree or complete AV block.

Administration.   Atropine is best administered intravenously in a dosage between 0.3 and 1 mg (up to 2.0 mg), and a similar dosage may be repeated every 10 to 15 minutes as needed. When the optimum dosage is determined, it may be repeated every 4–6 hours, but the total dosage of atropine should not exceed 4 mg. The effect of the drug is usually prompt. Atropine may be given subcutaneously if the intravenous route is not feasible. Atropine has been orally administered, but its effectiveness is less predictable.

Side Effects and Toxicity.   Serious toxic effects of atropine are uncommon, but ventricular premature contractions or ventricular tachyarrhythmias may be induced. Common side effects include a dry mouth, urinary retention, exacerbation of glaucoma, hallucinations, hyperpyrexia, and marked sinus tachycardia.

Isoproterenol (Isuprel)[2,9–12]

Before artificial pacemakers were available for clinical use, the treatment of choice for complete AV block was the administration of Isuprel. The drug is still very useful in the emergency treatment of Adams-Stokes syndrome or as a temporary measure until an artificial pacemaker can be implanted. Thus, Isuprel is still the drug of choice in the treatment of Adams-Stokes syndrome due to bradyarrhythmias, primarily complete AV block and ventricular standstill. Isuprel is capable of accelerating both the supraventricular and the ventricular pacemakers and of improving AV conduction. The drug possesses a potent inotropic action that increases the stroke volume, the amplitude of myocardial contraction, and the coronary blood flow.

Indications.   The primary indication for Isuprel is in the treatment of Adams-Stokes syndrome due to complete AV block or ventricular standstill (Fig. 8-6) until an artificial pacemaker is inserted. Isuprel may also be used, in place of atropine, in the treatment of symptomatic sinus bradycardia, sinus arrest, and SA block.

Administration.   Isuprel can be given by direct intracardiac, intravenous, intramuscular, or subcutaneous injection, or it may be given by intravenous infusion.

In emergency situations, such as in severe Adams-Stokes syndrome or ventricular standstill, Isuprel can be given by intracardiac or intravenous injection. The usual dosage is between 0.02 and 0.05 mg, but up to 0.1 mg may be administered. Otherwise, the drug can be given subcutaneously or intramuscularly in a dosage of 0.1 to 0.4 mg every 2–6 hours as needed. Continuous intravenous infusion of Isuprel is indicated in severe cases in order to maintain the ventricular rate around 50–60 beats per minute until an artificial pacemaker can be inserted. The usual method is to dilute 0.1 mg of Isuprel in 200 cc of 5% dextrose in water, and the initial infusion rate is 1 to 4 μg per minute. The infusion rate may be increased to 5 to 10 μg per minute, and up to 40 μg per minute may occasionally be required to maintain an ideal ventricular rate.

The most popular route for administration of this drug is sublingual, and the usual dosage is 10 to 30 mg every 1 to 6 hours. The drug can be given as often as every 30 minutes if needed.

Side Effects and Toxicity.   Side effects of Isuprel include tremor, nervousness, sweating, nausea, weakness, headache, dizziness, palpita-

Table 8-1   Antibradyarrhythmic Drugs

Drugs	Dosage	Onset of Action	Maximum Effect	Duration of Action	Indications	Side Effects and Toxicity
Atropine sulfate	0.3–2 mg q̄ 4–6 hr IV inj. as needed or the same dose may be given by SC inj. (total: 4 mg) or 0.4–0.8 mg q̄ 4–6 hr PO for mild form	1–5 min	Few minutes to 30 min	4–6 hr	Primary: Sinus bradycardia, sinus arrest, SA block Secondary: First-degree and occasionally second-degree AV block	Dry mouth, urinary retention, exacerbation of glaucoma, hallucinations, hyperpyrexia, postural hypotension, sinus tachycardia, VPC, ventricular tachycardia
Isoproterenol (Isuprel)	0.02–0.05 mg (up to 0.1 mg) IC or IV inj., or 0.1–0.4 mg SC or IM inj. q̄ 2–6 hr as needed or 1 mg/200 cc 5% D/W IV infusion, 1–4 μg/min initially and may increase to 5–10 μg/min as needed. 10–30 mg sublingually q̄ 1–6 hr (for mild cases)	At once / Irregular	At once / Irregular	Minutes / Irregular	Ventricular standstill, severe AS syndrome Primary: High-degree or complete AV block Secondary: Sinus bradycardia, sinus arrest, and SA block	Tremor, nausea, nervousness, sweating, weakness, dizziness, headache, palpitation, VPC, ventricular tachycardia and fibrillation, hypotension
Epinephrine hydrochloride (Adrenalin)	0.3–0.6 cc of 1:1000 solution IV, IM, SC, or IC inj., or 0.5–1 mg/250 cc 5% D/W IV infusion, 1–4 μg/min initially	At once	At once	Very short	High degree or complete AV block and ventricular standstill	Trembling, pallor, nervousness, hypertension, VPC, ventricular tachycardia and fibrillation

Drug	Dosage		Indications	Side effects/Toxicity
Ephedrine	and may increase to 4–8 µg/min as needed 30–60 mg PO q̄ 2–4 hr	—	High degree or complete AV block	Urinary retention, nervousness, vertigo, insomnia, hypertension, ventricular tachyarrhythmias
Corticosteroids	Hydrocortisone IV inj. 200–600 mg for 24 hr or Solu-Medrol 80 mg daily by IM inj. or Prednisone 40–60 mg daily PO	—	Primary: AV block with acute onset Secondary: Chronic AV block	Prolonged steroid therapy may induce sodium retention, Cushing's syndrome, dissemination of TB, aggravation of diabetes mellitus, glaucoma, and psychosis
Molar sodium lactate	5–7 cc/kg IV infusion over periods of hours. If urgent, 25–50 cc rapid IV drip initially	—	AV block in the presence of acidosis or hyperkalemia	Precipitation of CHF, alkalosis, hypokalemia, ventricular tachyarrhythmias
Chlorothiazide	0.5–2 g daily (PO) for 6–8 weeks	—	Sinus rhythm with intermittent AV block	Hypokalemia, precipitation of gout, predispose to digitalis toxicity

Key to the table: q̄: every; IV: intravenous; SC: subcutaneous; IC: intracardiac; IM: intramuscular; D/W: dextrose in water; PO: by mouth; AS syndrome: Adams-Stokes syndrome; VPC: ventricular premature contraction; TB: tuberculosis; CHF: congestive heart failure.

tion, and hypotension. A serious toxic effect is the production of ventricular tachyarrhythmias, a danger that is not dose-dependent.

Epinephrine Hydrochloride (Adrenalin)[2,9–12]

Adrenalin has been almost as popular as Isuprel in the treatment of Adams-Stokes syndrome. However, Adrenalin is considered to be definitely inferior to Isuprel because it produces significant hypertension and is likely to provoke ventricular irritability, particularly ventricular fibrillation.

Adrenalin is capable of accelerating the atrial rate as well as the ventricular rate. The degree of acceleration of the atrial rate has no relationship to the initial atrial rate, whereas the degree of acceleration of the idioventricular rate is closely related to the initial ventricular rate: The degree of acceleration of the idioventricular rate is greatest when the initial ventricular rate is very slow, and the enhancement of the ventricular rate is insignificant when the initial ventricular rate is relatively rapid.

Indications. The primary indication for Adrenalin is in the treatment of ventricular standstill, particularly associated with acute myocardial infarction. It is also indicated in the treatment of Adams-Stokes syndrome due to complete AV block until an artificial pacemaker is implanted.

Administration. In urgent situations, such as ventricular standstill, Adrenalin 0.3 to 0.6 cc of a 1:1000 solution may be given by intravenous, intramuscular, subcutaneous, or even intracardiac injection. Slow injection over a period of several minutes under ECG monitoring is recommended, and the rate of injection should be regulated according to the patient's response. For long-term therapy, 0.5 to 1 mg of a 1:1000 solution of Adrenalin diluted in 250 cc of 5% dextrose in water can be given by a continuous intravenous infusion. The initial rate of the intravenous drip is usually 1 to 4 μg per minute, and the rate may be increased to 4 to 8 μg per minute according to the patient's response.

Side Effects and Toxicity. Side effects of epinephrine include nervousness, trembling, pallor, and hypertension. A serious toxic effect is the production of ventricular tachycardia and fibrillation.

In general, the usefulness of epinephrine in the treatment of Adams-Stokes syndrome is limited by its serious toxic effects and its ineffectiveness in some cases.

Other Agents

The other agents listed in Table 8-1 (ephedrine, corticosteroids, molar sodium lactate, and chlorothiazide) are now little used in antibradyarrhythmic therapy.

ARTIFICIAL PACEMAKERS

Although a detailed description of artificial pacemakers is found in Chapter 10, the indications for short-term and long-term pacing will be briefly discussed here.

Indications for Short-Term Pacing

The precise criteria for use of a temporary or a permanent pacemaker vary slightly from institution to institution, but the following conditions are generally accepted for a short-term pacing[2,5,6,8,13]:

1. Symptomatic second-degree or third-degree AV block (Fig. 8-5), especially during acute myocardial infarction requires a temporary pacing. It should be noted that AV block *per se* does not require artificial pacing.
2. Symptomatic and drug-resistant sinus arrhythmias, including sinus bradycardia (Fig. 8-1), sinus arrest, and sinoatrial block.
3. Newly developed left or right bundle branch block and bilateral bundle branch block due to acute anterior myocardial infarction. Short-term pacing is usually required because these findings are often followed by a slow ventricular escape rhythm due to complete AV block.
4. Emergency treatment for Adams-Stokes syndrome and symptomatic bilateral bundle branch block.
5. Before or during implantation of a permanent pacemaker.
6. Therapeutic trial for intractable congestive heart failure, cardiogenic shock, or cerebral or renal insufficiency.
7. Prophylactic pacing during major surgery when Adams-Stokes syndrome is anticipated.
8. Drug-resistant tachyarrhythmias, which may be corrected by over-driving pacing rate.
9. Bradytachycardia syndrome.

Indications for Long-Term Pacing

The decision on long-term pacing should not be made lightly, because the patient must live with an artificial pacemaker all his life, taking the necessary precautions and caring for it daily. In addition, the battery should be changed every 18 to 24 months, (30–36 months in some newer models), depending upon the model. One of the most serious problems following permanent pacemaker implantation is malfunction of the unit; this may be fatal. At times, it is difficult to judge whether a permanent artificial pacemaker is required. In general, long-term pacing is considered to be indicated in the following situations[2,5,6,8,13]

1. Symptomatic, chronic second-degree (usually Mobitz type II or 2:1 AV block) or third-degree AV block.
2. Symptomatic, chronic, and drug-resistant sinus arrhythmias, including sinus bradycardia (Fig. 8–1), sinus arrest, and sinoatrial block.
3. Complete AV block in acute myocardial infarction (usually anterior wall involvement) lasting more than 2–3 weeks.
4. Symptomatic bilateral bundle branch block.
5. Recurrent Adams-Stokes syndrome due to various causes.
6. Intractable congestive heart failure or cerebral or renal insufficiency definitely benefited by temporary pacing.
7. Recurrent drug-resistant tachyarrhythmias benefited by temporary pacing.
8. Bradytachycardia syndrome benefited by temporary pacing.

SUMMARY

Bradyarrhythmias may be due to various fundamental mechanisms, and they may be found in many different clinical backgrounds. The therapeutic approaches vary markedly, depending upon the fundamental mechanism responsible for the production of bradyarrhythmia, the ventricular rate, the underlying cause, and the presence or absence of symptoms and their seriousness. It should be re-emphasized that electrocardiographic abnormality alone is not cause for treatment.

Because of the ready availability of artificial pacemakers, antibradyarrhythmic agents are much less used now than in the past. The most commonly used antibradyarrhythmic drug is atropine sulfate, particularly for treatment of a marked sinus bradycardia associated with acute myocardial infarction. Isuprel is the next most commonly used agent for treatment of bradyarrhythmias.

When complete AV block is due to a block below the bundle of His, a permanent artificial pacemaker is nearly always indicated. On the other hand, complete AV block associated with acute diaphragmatic (inferior) myocardial infarction usually does not require pacing because the ventricular rate is relatively fast (rate: 50–60 beats per minute) and the patient is often asymptomatic. Complete AV block associated with anterior myocardial infarction usually requires a permanent pacemaker, because the AV block is considered to be due to complete bilateral bundle branch block. Bradyarrhythmia induced by various drugs, particularly digitalis, is best treated by eliminating the direct causative agent. Antiarrhythmic agents are usually not effective in the treatment of bradytachycardia syndrome, and an artificial pacemaker with slightly overdriving pacing is considered to be the treatment of choice in this circumstance.

REFERENCES

1. Chung, E. K.: Electrocardiography: Practical Applications with Vectorial Principles. Hagerstown, Md., Harper & Row, 1974.
2. Chung, E. K.: Cardiac Arrhythmias: Management. Baltimore, Williams & Wilkins Co., 1973.
3. Rotman, M., Wagner, G. S., and Wallace, A. G.: Bradyarrhythmias in acute myocardial infarction. Circulation 45:703, 1972.
4. Chung, E. K.: Digitalis Intoxication. Baltimore, Williams & Wilkins, 1969.
5. Siddons, H., and Sowton, E.: Cardiac Pacemakers. Springfield, Ill., Charles C Thomas, 1967.
6. Furman, S., and Escher, D. J. W.: Principles and Techniques of Cardiac Pacing. Hagerstown, Md., Harper & Row, 1970.
7. Rosenbaum, M. B., Elizari, M. V., and Lazzari, J. O.: The Hemiblocks. Oldsmar, Fla., Tampa Tracings, 1970.
8. Cosby, R. S., and Bilitch, M.: Heart Block. New York, McGraw-Hill, 1972.
9. Gregory, J. J., and Grace, W. J.: The management of bradycardia, nodal rhythm and heart block for the prevention of cardiac arrest in acute myocardial infarction. Prog. Cardiovasc. Dis. 10:505, 1968.
10. Shillingford, J., and Thomas, M.: Treatment of bradycardia and hypotension syndrome with acute myocardial infarction. Am. Heart J. 75:843, 1968.
11. Adgey, A. A. J., Geddes, J. S., Mulholland, H. C., Keegan, D. A. J., and Pantridge, J. F.: Incidence, significance and management of early bradyarrhythmias complicating acute myocardial infarction. Lancet ii:1097, 1968.
12. Yu, P. N.: Prehospital care of acute myocardial infarction. Circulation 45:189, 1972.
13. Kaplan, B. M., Langendorf, R., Lev, M., and Pick, A.: Tachycardia-bradycardia syndrome (so-called "sick sinus syndrome"). Am. J. Cardiol. 31:497, 1973.

Chapter 9
DIRECT CURRENT SHOCK

LEON RESNEKOV

The management of cardiac dysrhythmias with drugs continues to have serious limitations in clinical practice. These may be summarized as follows:

1. An unstandardized dose, varying from patient to patient, has to be given.
2. The margin between what is therapeutic and what is toxic may be very small.
3. Current medical practice is to titrate dose against observed effect. This requires keeping the patient under close observation, often over several days.
4. Many antidysrhythmic drugs (see Chapter 7) are negatively inotropic. They may also be dromotropic.
5. Paradoxically, should toxic manifestations emerge following the use of a drug, these may be even more serious than the effects of the dysrhythmia being treated.
6. Drug overdosage may suppress the normal sinus mechanism, thereby actually inhibiting reversion to sinus rhythm.

An electric shock causes momentary depolarization of the majority of heart fibers, thereby terminating an ectopic tachycardia and allowing the sinus node to be re-established as the pacemaker of the heart. There is now abundant evidence that such therapy is both successful and safe, provided certain procedures are rigorously adhered to.

HISTORY

It was in 1850 that Hoffa and Ludwig described the rhythm disturbance we now call ventricular fibrillation. Shortly thereafter, the first fatal electrical accident was reported in the medical literature, but many years passed before the realization that fatal electrocution frequently resulted from ventricular fibrillation gained general acceptance. In 1900 Prevost and Battelli[1] observed that a direct current shock across the heart would terminate ventricular fibrillation in dogs. This important report, written as a postscript to an article on another subject, was generally unrecognized until the topic of electrical defibrillation was restudied by Kouwenhoven and his associates[2] in a series of experiments over many years and by Ferris and co-workers.[3] This latter group described a series of experiments undertaken between 1927 and 1935 on the effects of electricity on the heart, from which they reached the following important conclusions:

1. Current, rather than voltage, is the proper criterion for shock intensity.
2. The passage of an electrical current across the heart may precipitate ventricular fibrillation even in the absence of any recognizable myocardial damage.
3. Unless ventricular fibrillation is successfully treated by another shock within a few minutes, the animal will die.

Equally significant was the demonstration by King[4] that electrical shocks delivered in relation to the apex of the T wave of the electrocardiogram are more likely to cause ventricular fibrillation.

At about this time, workers in Europe, particularly in the Soviet Union, had been undertaking pioneer work in the applications of capacitor discharge (direct current) to clinical use. The studies of Gurvich and Yunyev[5] can be regarded as an important inspiration to later investigators, including Peleşka,[6] Tsukerman,[7] and Lown and co-workers.[8]

ELECTRICAL DEFIBRILLATION

Whether direct or alternating current is used, electrical defibrillation requires the passage of a high-energy impulse of short duration between two concave paddles closely applied to the heart (internal defibrillation) or between two flat paddles applied to the chest wall (external defibrillation). The total energy needed depends not only on the electrical current used but also on the resistance of the heart, the bony cage, and the skin. Hooker and associates[9] reported that a minimal current of 1 ampère is needed to bring all heart fibers instantaneously to the same refractory point. Delivery of this current requires about 100 volts and a power of 100 watts (voltage × current). Since the usual duration of an *alternating current* defibrillatory shock is ⅕ second, the energy used for internal defibrillation is about 20 joules. For external defibrillation, however, the change in resistance may require a sixfold increase in current rating: 1800 watts of electrical power are usually used for ⅕ second, i.e., 360 joules of electrical energy. The waveform for alternating current defibrillation is, of course, standard and is produced at the electrical power station as a sinusoidal impulse at a frequency of 60 Hz.

In contrast, *direct current* defibrillators discharge a single capacitor or a bank of capacitors that have been previously charged over a short period (2–10 seconds) from line current and a step-up transformer. The duration of the impulse is in the range of 1.5–4.0 msec. An unmodified capacitor discharge has a very characteristic waveform (Fig. 9-1), with an abrupt rise in voltage and current to a sharp peak, followed by an exponential decay to the baseline. This waveform may be shaped by adding varying amounts of inductance to the circuit, and an infinite variety of waveforms may thus be obtained. There is some experimental evidence to suggest that defibrillation is not only more successful but safer when inductance is introduced into the circuit.[10] Using a capacitor

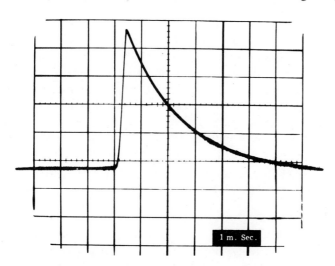

Figure 9-1. Spike capacitor discharge. No additional inductance in circuit. Note rapid rise time, sharp peak and exponential decay.

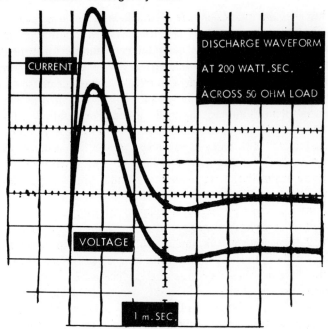

Figure 9-2. Monophasic slightly underdamped current and voltage waveform. Capacitor 16 μf, inductance 100 mh, 5 kV (Lown circuit). (Reprinted with permission from Resnekov and McDonald.[23])

of 16 microfarads charged to 7000 volts, stored energy for a 3.5 msec DC defibrillating waveform is equal to 392 joules, but it must be stressed that the setting on the moving coil meter of the apparatus reflects only the energy delivered to the skin. The true energy delivered to the heart muscle is influenced by the resistance of the skin and deeper tissues. Most commercially available DC apparatus use capacitors in the range of 10–20 microfarads, and the inductance of the circuit is about 100 millihenrys. Assuming a discharge of 400 joules energy lasting for 3 msec, the current delivered would be 19 ampères and the power, 133,000 watts. Its waveform is shown in Figure 9-2.

AC OR DC

Direct current develops many times the power of alternating current but requires less energy, since the shock lasts only 3–4 msec. Several investigators have reported that AC shocks are more harmful and produce greater deterioration of ventricular function than does direct current.[11,12]

The first successful human defibrillation was performed by Beck and co-workers in 1947,[13] using an alternating current discharge. For many years thereafter the convenience of AC defibrillation made it the standard method. (It must be appreciated, however, that since the waveform and duration of the current are so different in the two methods, any true comparison is extremely difficult.) Two important clinical observations stimulated further investigation of the use of direct current:

Alternating current was frequently unsuccessful when ventricular fibrillation was due to myocardial infarction.

There was a definite clinical need for the electrical conversion of rhythm disturbances other than ventricular fibrillation.

In regard to the latter observation, Lown and his colleagues[14] had reported terminating an organized dysrhythmia with alternating current, but the experience of others had already given clear warning of the risk of precipitating ventricular fibrillation and even death when alternating current was used in this way.[15] Although there are relatively few well-controlled defibrillation studies in which AC and DC have been compared, Nachlas and his colleagues[16] were able to show that direct current was unmistakably superior in terminating ventricular fibrillation.

From all this evidence, then, the following conclusions can be drawn: Alternating current is feasible for clinical treatment of ventricular fibrillation, but direct current is more effective. Alternating current cannot be recommended for elective treatment of atrial rhythm disturbances or ventricular tachycardia.

DC and Synchronized Shocks

Despite the fact that its waveforms are less likely to cause myocardial damage, DC shock is known to precipitate ventricular fibrillation on occasion. For many years, a vulnerable phase of ventricular excitability had been postulated,[17] and Wiggers and Wegria[18] were able to show that such a phase occurs 27 msec before the end of ventricular systole in dogs. It is due to nonuniform recovery from the refractory state, allowing re-entry of the depolarization wave and favoring self-sustained activity. That a similar phenomenon also occurs in the human heart has been shown by Castellanos and others.[19]

These animal and human investigations, therefore, indicate that in the treatment of rhythm disturbances other than ventricular fibrillation, the DC shock should be timed to avoid the apex of the T wave. It is almost impossible to avoid this vulnerable period when the longer-duration AC shocks are used (Fig. 9-3), but most DC defibrillators incorporate a synchronizer to allow triggering of the shock by the R or S wave of the electrocardiogram. When ventricular fibrillation is being treated, the synchronizer has to be switched out of the circuit.

The chance of occurrence of ventricular fibrillation following randomized unsynchronized shock is 2%.[20] Some workers, therefore, choose not to use a synchronizer in clinical practice, and they report no dire consequences.[21] It is most important when no synchronizer is used to ensure that sufficient energy is delivered, so that a current of at least 1.5–2 ampères passes across the heart; lower energy may well be danger-

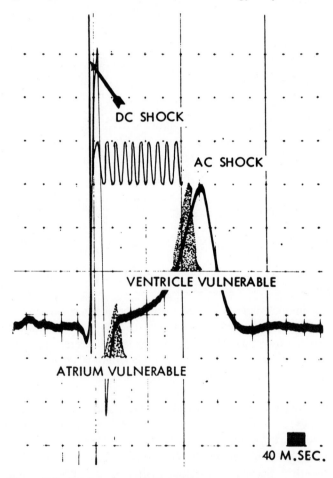

Figure 9-3. Atrial and ventricular phases of vulnerability. Note that an AC shock of $\frac{1}{5}$ second may end at the T wave even if synchronized with the R wave of the ECG.

ous. When no synchronizer is used, therefore, increased energy level settings are needed.

CLINICAL USE OF SYNCHRONIZED DIRECT CURRENT SHOCK

Lown and co-workers[8] were the first to use capacitor discharges with inductance in series for the treatment of ventricular tachycardia. Many thousands of patients have now been successfully treated by this method, and the total experience has completely justified initial confidence in the technique. The overall success rate for the termination of atrial and ventricular rhythm disturbances approaches 90%.[22,23] In addition, it has been shown that success rate of 86% occurs even after determined efforts at drug conversion have failed.[24] The correct choice of patients, meticulous attention to detail, including correction of electrolyte imbalance if present, postponement of treatment when overdigitalization occurs, proper synchronization, and the correct choice of antidysrhythmic agents (see Chapter 7) immediately before and after treatment[25] ensure both immediate success and a low incidence of complications.

Important aspects of the technique are summarized in the following sections.

Apparatus

The electrical integrity of the apparatus should be checked at least once a month, including an inspection of the waveform when the paddles are discharged across a 50-ohm load in the laboratory. At the same time, the actual delivered energy should be measured and compared with the setting of the apparatus.

The use of paddles of adequate size is mandatory, since during ventricular fibrillation the heart is subdivided into a large number of fibrillating segments. To succeed, the electrical current must stimulate the majority of myocardial fibers simultaneously. Equally important, small paddles will permit a very high current density in a localized pathway across the heart and may thus cause myocardial damage.

When external DC shock is used, two anterior paddles or, alternatively, an anterior and a posterior paddle may be employed. The latter method is more convenient since the patient lies on the flat posterior paddle, and it is only the anterior one that needs to be held by the operator—an important safety measure, particularly with apparatus in which one paddle is grounded. Although it has been reported that the anteroposterior paddle position significantly lowers energy needed for electroversion,[26] others could not confirm this finding.[23] Indeed, experimental work[16] has shown that anterior positioning of the electrodes as originally suggested by Kouwenhoven and co-workers[27] results in the delivery of approximately 2.5 times more current to the heart. The failure to note more striking clinical differences with variation in electrode placement is undoubtedly due to the excessive amounts of electrical energy that are consistently used in achieving electroversion. Thus, the anteroposterior position is recommended because of the added safety offered by a flat posterior paddle held in place only by the weight of the patient.

Drugs

Digoxin or any other digitalis preparation should be withheld for 24–48 hours before electroversion. If treatment cannot be postponed and has to be undertaken despite the presence of heavy digitalization, the initial energy setting should be reduced to 5–10 joules, and an intravenous injection of 50 mg lidocaine, 50–100 mg diphenylhydantoin, or 50–100 mg procaine amide should precede the shock (see below). There is little evidence that quinidine or other antidysrhythmic drugs (see Chapter 7) given orally, intramuscularly, or intravenously as a routine before direct current shock reduces the energy needed or helps to maintain long-term sinus rhythm afterward.[23] These drugs may help, however, in preventing premature beats following the shock that could precipitate a return to the dysrhythmia immediately after successful conversion (see below).

Anesthesia

Food should be withheld for some hours before treatment, lest vomiting occur. Premedication is not needed. Although general anesthesia is not mandatory,[28,29] amnesia produced by the use of 5–10 mg of diazepam intravenously is useful and can be recommended as the method of choice,[30] since it significantly reduces the complication rate.[31] Muscle relaxants, particularly halothane, which is known to predispose to rhythm disturbances, especially in the presence of CO_2 retention, and sympathomimetic drugs are specifically not recommended for electroversion.[32] The duration of action of diazepam is only 3–4 minutes, making it an ideal and safe drug for use in these circumstances, and additional doses may be given within a few minutes of the initial injection, should the first dose fail to induce drowsiness. It should be remembered, however, that patients with congestive heart failure should be given diazepam cautiously, and it is very unusual for more than 20 mg to be needed in any patient.[33] An added point in favor of diazepam is that its safety and speed of action mean that the skilled help of an anesthesiologist is not mandatory, nor is elaborate anesthetic equipment needed.

The Treatment Room

Treatment should be undertaken in an area fully equipped for cardiac monitoring and for resuscitation if needed, including emergency pacemaking. The heart rate should be displayed on a tachometer if one is available, and the electrocardiogram should be clearly visible on an oscilloscope throughout the procedure and should be recorded as needed.

Routine Preparation

A short strip of lead V_1 should always be recorded before the shock for comparison later, since P waves can be difficult to detect in the standard limb leads immediately after the shock. The skin of the chest should be prepared by the liberal application of electrocardiogram paste rubbed in well to reduce electrical resistance and prevent painful electrical burns. It is most important that this or any other substance used not be allowed to run between the two paddles. Current takes the path of least resistance, and most of the electrical energy may thereby be diverted away from the heart muscle, resulting in failure of the attempt at electroversion. Great care must also be taken to ensure that no part of the patient's skin is in direct contact with the metal of the trolley or the bed on which he is lying, nor must the patient, his bed, or any apparatus to which he is attached be touched by the operator, his assistant, or any bystander at the moment of the shock.

Levels of Electrical Energy

The shock may be administered across two anterior paddles or using an anterior–posterior position. Low energies should be used first. If these are unsuccessful, the shock may be repeated at an increased energy level setting. For an adult, an initial setting of 25–50 joules is satisfactory, increasing in 25–50-joule steps. In the presence of heavy digitalization, an initial setting of 5–10 joules is appropriate. Should extrasystoles follow the first shock and as a routine before treating a patient known to be heavily digitalized, 50 mg of lidocaine should be given intravenously before continuing to a high energy setting, as already described. The initial setting for a child is 5–10 joules delivered across appropriately sized pediatric paddles and then increased by 5–10-joule steps. There should be great reluctance to exceed an energy setting of 300 joules in an adult being treated for chronic rhythm disturbance, but where an acute dysrhythmia produces serious hemodynamic effects, maximum energy (400 joules) can be used. The initial setting for ventricular fibrillation (no synchronizer in circuit) is 200 joules, increasing by 100-joule steps to a maximum of 400. Appropriate settings for internal defibrillation (special spoon-shaped paddles) are 20–100 joules in 20-joule increments.

Following the Shock

With the reinstitution of sinus rhythm or if sinus rhythm should fail to occur after delivery of optimal energies, the amnesic drug is discontinued and a 12-lead electrocardiogram recorded. The ECG should be monitored for the next 24 hours, or longer if need be. Records of the blood pressure should be taken every half hour until the control value recorded before the shock, is regained.

TREATMENT OF RHYTHM DISTURBANCES

Atrial Fibrillation

This is the most common rhythm disturbance to be treated. Lone or idiopathic atrial fibrillation deserves special mention, since the success rate of electroversion is low, the incidence of complications high, and the length of time during which sinus rhythm persists disappointingly short.[34] For atrial fibrillation due to rheumatic heart disease, initial success is 87–90%,[23] but for idiopathic atrial fibrillation, it is less than 75%.[34] Initial success is not related to the age or sex of the patient, the type of heart disease (lone atrial fibrillation excepted), nor even to overall body size. An important factor on which success does depend is the duration of the rhythm disturbance (Fig. 9-4). When atrial fibrillation has been present for 5 years or longer, the rate of success is only 50%. In addition, overall increase in size of the heart and selective enlargement of the left atrium both lessen the chances of success.[23] It is clear, therefore, that every patient with chronic atrial fibrillation requires individual assessment to determine whether treatment is worthwhile; nevertheless, there is no doubt that hemodynamic benefit may be achieved by conversion to sinus rhythm,[35] particularly during exercise. Certain groups of patients can be kept free of cardiac failure only by repeated electrical termination of atrial fibrillation.

Although open chest electroversion is easy to achieve at the time of surgery, reversion to atrial fibrillation in the postoperative phase is almost universal. Atrial fibrillation with a ventricular rate controlled by digoxin is preferred to rapidly changing cardiac rhythms postoperatively, and it is recommended, therefore, that the electroversion of these patients be postponed until they are convalescent following open or closed valvular surgery.[25,36]

In addition, electroversion of atrial fibrillation should be attempted

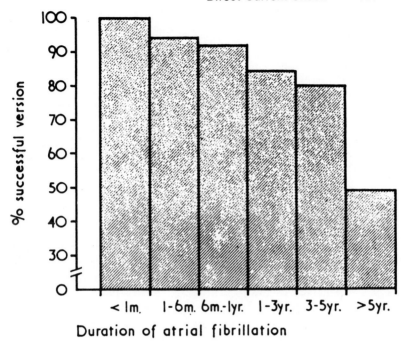

Figure 9-4. Percentage of successful electroversion and duration of atrial fibrillation before treatment (idiopathic atrial fibrillation excluded). (Reprinted with permission from Resnekov and McDonald.[23])

only under exceptional circumstances in the following groups of patients:

- Patients with idiopathic or lone atrial fibrillation.
- Patients with coronary heart disease and atrial fibrillation with a slow ventricular response in the absence of digoxin.
- Patients unable to maintain sinus rhythm for more than a very brief period of time, even when maintained on quinidine or other anti-dysrhythmic drug (see Chapter 7) in adequate doses.
- Patients who display varying atrial rhythm disturbances in rapid succession.
- Patients in the tachycardic phase of the tachycardia–bradycardia syndrome, unless emergency pacemaking is at hand, since dangerous asystole may well follow a transmyocardial shock in this condition.
- Those with long-standing atrial fibrillation (more than 5 years) with considerable enlargement of the heart (cardiothoracic ratio of more than 50%), unless cardiac surgery is contemplated.

• Patients with atrial fibrillation in association with conduction disturbances.

Atrial Flutter

A 90–95% success rate for the electroversion of atrial flutter is commonly reported. The electrical energy setting needed is usually much lower than that for atrial fibrillation, averaging 50 joules. Unlike idiopathic atrial fibrillation, atrial flutter not associated with detectable heart disease may still be successfully reverted by direct current shock at relatively low energy settings, and sinus rhythm may be maintained for significantly long periods.[34]

Paroxysmal Atrial Tachycardia

The success rate varies from 75–80%, depending on the underlying cause. Even so, electroversion is to be preferred to drug therapy. It should not be used, however, for digitalis-induced tachydysrhythmias such as atrial tachycardia with AV block of varying degree and nonparoxysmal AV junctional tachycardia (see Chapter 15) except under the most unusual circumstances, for the risk of precipitating ventricular fibrillation is very high.[37]

Paroxysmal AV Nodal (Junctional) Tachycardia

The success rate in the treatment of paroxysmal AV junctional tachycardia is similar to that for paroxysmal atrial tachycardia.

Ventricular Tachycardia

The initial success rate of electroversion exceeds 97%. The energies needed are low. Once more, great caution must be exercised when ventricular tachycardia is digitalis-induced (see Chapter 15), and under these circumstances electroversion is contraindicated except in rare instances.

Ventricular Fibrillation

Controlled clinical trials of unsynchronized direct current versus alternating current shock are difficult to design, but experimental animal studies have shown the superiority of direct current.[16] In clinical practice, successful resuscitation, as judged by the patient leaving the hospital, can be achieved in more than 60% of cases with direct current shock and proper application of the principles of resuscitation.[38]

COMPLICATIONS

Initially, complications were thought to be rare following electroversion, but an incidence of 14.5% among 220 patients has been reported.[39] These do not include minor complications such as superficial burns due to poor preparation of the skin or transient rhythm disturbances immediately after the shock. The following, however, were included:

Raised levels of serum enzymes (10%): The origin of the enzyme is still debated. Many consider damage to skeletal muscle to be the cause.[40] Nevertheless, other signs of myocardial damage are frequently seen,[39] and definitive studies are still awaited.

Hypotension (3%): A fall in blood pressure not related to the form of anesthesia used is more common when higher electrical energies are used. This hypotension may persist for several hours, but it usually requires no particular intervention.

ECG evidence of myocardial damage: ECG changes are found in 3% of patients treated, even in the absence of outward symptoms. Patterns of myocardial infarction may persist for many months, and are most common following electroversion at high energy settings (Fig. 9-5).

Pulmonary and systemic emboli: Embolism follows electroversion in 1.4% of patients; this indicates the need for anticoagulant cover (see below).

Ventricular dysrhythmias. Serious ventricular rhythm disturbances are common even at lower energy settings when the patient is heavily digitalized and at higher settings whether or not digoxin has been given. Their emergence requires an intravenous antidysrhythmic drug (see Chapter 7) before the energy level setting is increased.

Increase in heart size and pulmonary edema: Within 1 to 3 hours of treatment an increase in heart size and pulmonary edema may occur in 3% of patients.[39] This complication is unlike any other in that it seems to occur only in patients actually brought into sinus rhythm.[41] While Lown[22] considered pulmonary emboli to be a cause, others believe that there is considerable depression in the mechanical function of the heart following electroversion.[42] Despite the fact that sinus rhythm is recorded on the electrocardiogram, mechanical atrial systole in the left atrium may be depressed or absent. Any additional obstruction to flow across the mitral valve or any left ventricular dysfunction will aggravate the situation and result in pulmonary edema. As with other complications, its incidence is greatest following higher energy settings.

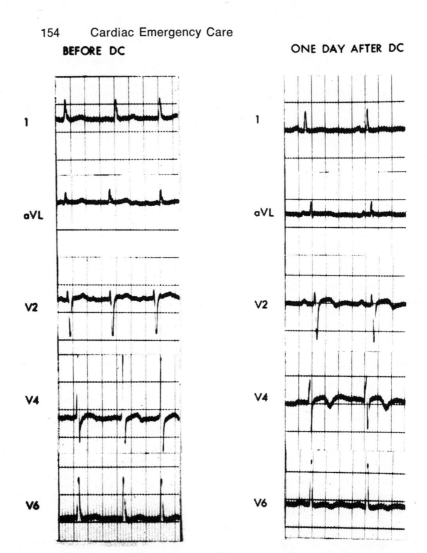

Figure 9-5. Idiopathic atrial fibrillation. ECG one day before and after electroversion. Note the deep T-wave inversion following the DC shock. This was associated with elevation of serum enzymes. (Reprinted with permission from Resnekov and McDonald.[39])

In the series already mentioned,[39] the incidence of complications was 6% when an electrical energy setting of up to 150 joules was used, but it increased to more than 30% at 400 joules (Fig. 9-6). It is usually patients being treated for atrial fibrillation who require high energy level settings, particularly those in whom atrial fibrillation has persisted for more than 3 years, those in whom the sinus rhythm disturbance is associ-

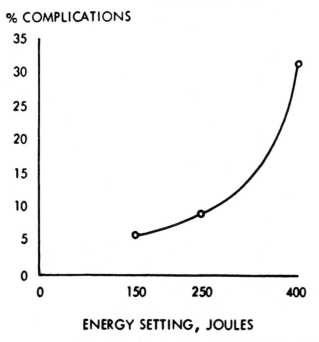

% COMPLICATIONS

ENERGY SETTING, JOULES

Figure 9-6. Percentage of complications in 220 patients treated by electroversion related to the maximal energy setting used. (108 patients were treated at an energy setting of <150 joules; 55 at <250 joules; and 37 at <400 joules.) (Reprinted with permission from Resnekov and McDonald.[39])

ated with cardiomyopathy or coronary heart disease, and those in whom idiopathic atrial fibrillation occurs.

From all this evidence, one may conclude that there rarely is an indication for exceeding an energy level setting of 300 joules in patients who present with long-standing atrial fibrillation. In addition, particular caution must be exercised in those who are heavily digitalized, in those whose dysrhythmia is due to cardiomyopathy or coronary heart disease, and in those with lone atrial fibrillation.

FOLLOW-UP STUDIES

While electroversion is highly successful, the number of patients who remain in sinus rhythm is disappointingly small, particularly when atrial fibrillation is treated.[25] A 36-month follow-up involving 183 patients successfully converted to sinus rhythm showed that less than 30% remained in sinus rhythm.[23] The majority who revert do so by the end of the first month of treatment (Fig. 9-7), but the highest incidence of reversion is actually within the first day (Fig. 9-8). Patients with

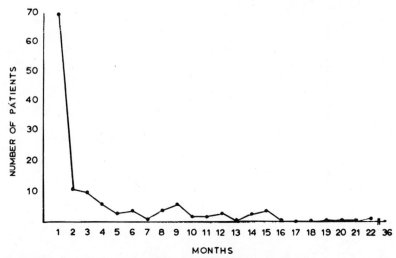

Figure 9-7. Thirty-six-month follow-up of 183 patients in whom electroversion succeeded: 131 (72%) reverted to their original dysrhythmia, 70 (53%) within the first month (see also Figure 9-8). (Reprinted with permission from Resnekov and McDonald.[23])

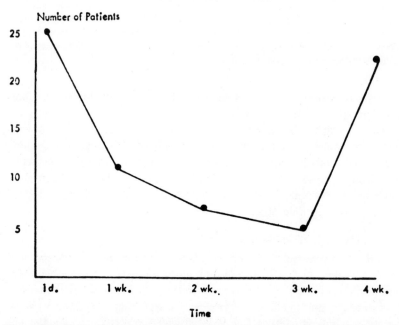

Figure 9-8. Of the 70 patients who reverted to their dysrhythmia within the first 4 weeks, 25 (35%) did so within the first day of electroversion (also see Figure 9-7). (Reprinted with permission from Resnekov and McDonald.[23])

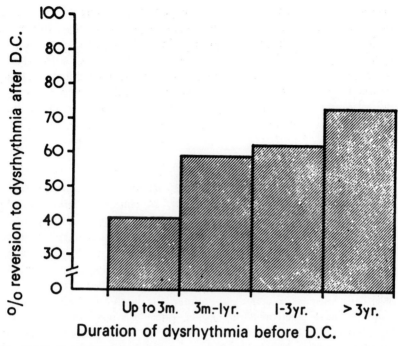

Figure 9-9. Percentage of patients who reverted to atrial fibrillation related to the duration of the dysrhythmia before electroversion. (Reprinted with permission from Resnekov and McDonald.[23])

significant underlying heart disease and radiographic evidence of cardiac enlargement are particularly prone to revert to their original rhythm disturbance, and in any patient in whom atrial fibrillation is of long duration (more than 3 years) a 70% chance of reverting back to that rhythm is to be expected (Fig. 9-9).

DRUGS AND DC SHOCK

Anticoagulants

The incidence of embolism following electroversion varies from 1.4% to 2.4%,[39,43] a figure similar to the reported incidence of emboli following quinidine conversion.[44] The need for anticoagulant protection has been the subject of much debate in the absence of any well-controlled study, but such a study has now been reported,[45] and the results indicate a statistical benefit in the group of patients who had electroversion under anticoagulant control. Where there is clear risk of embolism or thrombosis—as in patients with recent cardiac infarction, chronic coronary heart disease, mitral valvar disease, cardiomyopathy, prosthetic heart valves, or a previous history of embolism—anticoagulant therapy with a coumarin derivative should be given before electroversion, or heparin should be used when the need for DC shock is urgent. As the risk of reverting back to the dysrhythmia is highest within the first month of treatment (Fig. 9-8), it is wise to maintain anticoagulant therapy for at least 4 weeks, even after successful DC shock; it may be discontinued after 4 weeks unless the underlying heart disease requires its continuance.

Digitalis

In heavily digitalized dogs, the DC threshold for ventricular tachycardia fell by some 2,000% to $\frac{1}{5}$ joule.[46] The clinical importance of this observation is that digitalis effects not clinically apparent may be unmasked by an electrical shock, and any associated intramyocardial cell potassium deficit may enhance this effect. Conversely, administering potassium to raise the serum potassium level sharply may reverse the undesirable effect. The higher the electrical energy used, the greater the risk of serious ventricular dysrhythmia, and death has been reported to result.[37] Thus, electroversion should rarely be used in the management of a rhythm disturbance known to be digitalis-induced (see Chapter 15), for despite the occasional report of success,[47] fatal ventricular fibrillation may follow even when the shock is properly synchronized.

If electroversion is needed when the patient is known to be heavily digitalized, an intravenous injection of an antidysrhythmic drug, particularly diphenylhydantoin, should always precede the shock, and the initial energy setting should be 5–10 joules, with increments of 5–10 joules if further shocks are needed. Propranolol may also be helpful in reducing the dangerous myocardial sensitivity to high-energy electrical currents, but if used, it should be combined with intravenous atropine[48] to protect the patient against cardiac arrest, which may follow DC shock in patients primed with propranolol.[49] It is essential that a normal serum potassium level be achieved before electroversion, particularly in patients taking digoxin and using diuretic therapy, since hypokalemia may well precipitate serious ventricular rhythm disturbances even when only small amounts of digoxin are being used[50] (see Chapter 15).

Antidysrhythmic Agents

For electroversion to succeed, an energy level setting sufficient to depolarize the majority of the heart fibers instantaneously is needed. For sinus rhythm to follow, the sinus node must function adequately and must not be diseased or fibrosed. In addition, ectopic beats should be kept to a minimum immediately after the shock.[51] Excess electrical energy, as already indicated, may be harmful, and any interruption of the rhythm disturbance by the DC shock is good evidence that depolarization of the heart did occur, and that the level of electrical energy used was adequate. Should sinus rhythm fail to emerge or if it is short-lived despite adequate electrical energy, it is likely that either the sinus node is incapable of functioning as the pacemaker or that ectopic rhythms were precipitated by sudden catecholamine release following the electrical discharge.

To improve pacemaker function following DC shock, atropine 1–2 mg intravenously should be used routinely in patients in whom atrial fibrillation has been present for 5 years or longer, although it should be appreciated that the chance of these patients converting easily or maintaining sinus rhythm for an important length of time after conversion is small.[23] Similarly, any bradycardia after DC shock will enhance the likelihood of atrial or ventricular premature beats.[22] It must be remembered that although they are successful in suppressing ectopic beats, antidysrhythmic drugs, such as quinidine, procaine amide, lidocaine, and propranolol, all depress pacemaker function. Furthermore, since there is already a likelihood of intense parasympathetic stimulation immediately after DC shock,[52] their *routine* use is not advised, for they may well precipitate dangerous asystole.

Isolated ventricular premature beats or ventricular tachycardia immediately after DC shock frequently results from a combination of over-digitalization (see Chapter 15), the effect on the heart of the shock itself and a lowered myocardial potassium content. Such patients should be protected as previously indicated by postponing treatment if at all possible, ensuring an adequate serum potassium level and intramyocardial cellular potassium content, and administering antidysrhythmic drugs immediately before the shock.

Although there is good evidence in the literature that no antidysrhythmic agent now available, alone or in combination, can maintain sinus rhythm when sinoatrial function is faulty, when serious underlying myocardial or valvular heart disease is present, or when atrial fibrillation has existed for 5 years or longer, particularly when the heart is considerably enlarged, sinus rhythm may be hemodynamically important and can keep such patients free of cardiac failure. Under these circumstances, quinidine or procaine amide may be used in an attempt to maintain sinus rhythm over the long term.

If cardiac failure is not too severe, it may be possible to prolong sinus rhythm by combining quinidine and propranolol[53]; this combination will allow reduction of the dose of quinidine, thus lessening the incidence of its toxicity.

SUMMARY

Clinical electroversion with synchronized DC shock should be undertaken only by a medical team that understands the apparatus, the indications for the technique, and the potential risks, and only in a treatment area fully equipped for cardiac resuscitation, including emergency pacemaking. Except when ventricular fibrillation is being treated, a shock synchronized with the R or S wave to avoid the vulnerable phase of the ventricles should be used. Electrical energy should be kept to the minimum required to instantaneously depolarize the majority of the myocardial fibers, and the skin under the paddles should be carefully prepared to reduce its electrical resistance.

Anticoagulant therapy should precede the shock in most instances and should be maintained for at least 1 month in those treated successfully, for if reversion to the original rhythm disturbance is to occur, it is likeliest within the first month of treatment. Digitalis preparation should be stopped for 24–48 hours before treatment, and the procedure should be postponed in any patient with evidence of digitalis overdosage. If this is not possible, treatment should be modified to protect the patient against the very real risk of serious ventricular disturbances, including fibrillation. Any electrolyte imbalance should be corrected, with particular attention paid to potassium. Diazepam intravenously 5–10 mg is recommended instead of anesthesia. Lidocaine 50–100 mg, diphenylhydantoin 50–100 mg, or procaine amide 50–100 mg should be given intravenously as a routine before treating any patient known to be heavily digitalized and also if the first shock is followed by extrasystoles before continuing to a higher energy level setting. Any patient being given propranolol before the shock, any patient in whom atrial fibrillation has been present for 3 years or more, and any patient in whom atrial fibrillation with a ventricular rate of 70/min or less is being treated should have 1–2 mg atropine given intravenously to protect against serious bradycardia or asystole immediately after the shock.

The initial energy setting for adults not heavily digitalized should be 25–50-joules, increasing in 25–50-joule increments, if necessary, to 300 joules. There should be considerable reluctance to administer shocks at higher settings to patients with chronic rhythm disturbances, since complication rates are proportional to the energy used; however, when an acute rhythm disturbance producing severe cardiac dysfunction is being treated, maximal energies should be used if needed. In heavily digitalized patients the initial energy setting should be reduced to 5–10 joules and increments given in 5–10-joule steps. At the end of treatment, the rhythm should be confirmed by recording lead V_1 of the electrocardiogram. Ideally, all patients should be observed for any complications and the ECG monitored for 24 hours following treatment.

Complications are frequently multiple, including raised levels of serum enzymes, hypotension, ECG changes suggestive of myocardial infarction, pulmonary edema and increase in size of the heart in sinus rhythm, and pulmonary or systemic emboli. Other less serious complications are transient rhythm disturbances and superficial skin burns.

Electroversion succeeds in some 90% of patients, even when antidysrhythmic drugs have failed. It is the treatment of choice for all patients in whom an acute rhythm disturbance, supraventricular or ventricular, is causing circulatory depression; digitalis-induced rhythm disturbances, however, should not be treated by this means, unless all other forms of therapy have failed (see Chapter 15). Those with chronic dysrhythmias, particularly atrial fibrillation, require careful assessment before treatment is decided upon. Patients most likely to benefit are those in atrial fibrillation for 3 years or less in whom only mild overall enlargement of the heart and left atrium is present and in whom there is no hemodynamically important valvular heart disease. These patients are likely to remain in sinus rhythm for a significant period, whereas those who convert only on high energies are likely to revert within 1 month of treatment.

Synchronized DC shock should preferably not be undertaken at the time of cardiac surgery, but should be postponed until the patient is convalescent. No attempt should be made to convert patients with idiopathic atrial fibrillation, except under unusual circumstances, and the following groups are also generally unsuitable: those with slow ventricular rate, even in the absence of digitalis; those who do not maintain sinus rhythm despite antidysrhythmic drugs or who have varying atrial rhythm disturbances in rapid succession; those with atrial fibrillation of more than 5 years' duration, particularly if associated with considerable enlargement of the heart; and those with the bradytachycardia syndrome. Similarly, patients who have atrial fibrillation in association with conduction disturbances are, in general, unsuitable for electroversion.

At the time that synchronized DC shock is decided upon, a careful assessment of the drug regimen immediately before, during, and after the treatment is needed, and every effort should be made to reduce the emergence of premature beats, either atrial or ventricular, by using appropriate antidysrhythmic drugs and by ensuring an adequate heart rate by the judicious use of atropine.

Electrical defibrillation is an exciting advance, but greater effort is needed to uncover the basic mechanism of rhythm disturbances, thus encouraging the development of more physiologic approaches to their treatment and especially to the maintenance of sinus rhythm after treatment.

REFERENCES

1. Prevost, J. L., and Battelli, F.: Quelques effets des décharges electriques sur le coeur des mammifères. J. Physiol. Path. Gen. 2:40, 1900.
2. Kouwenhoven, W. B., Hooker, D. R., and Langworthy, O. R.: The current flowing through the heart under conditions of electric shock. Am. J. Physiol. 100:344, 1932.
3. Ferris, L. P., King, B. G., Spence, P. W., and Williams, H. B.: Effects of electrical shock on the heart. Elec. Eng. 55:498, 1936.
4. King, B. G.: The Effect of Electric Shock on Heart Action with Special Reference to Varying Susceptibility in Different Parts of the Cardiac Cycle. Aberdeen, Scotland, The Aberdeen University Press, 1934.
5. Gurvich, N. L., and Yunyev, G. S.: O vosstanovlenii normalnoi deyatel'nosti gibrilliroyuschego sevdtsa teplokrovaikh possedstrom kondensatornogo vazvyada. Byul. Eksp. Biol. Med. 8:55, 1939.
6. Peleşka, B.: Transthorákalni přimá defibrilace. Rozhl. Chir. 36:731, 1957.
7. Tsukerman, B. M.: Opit electricheskoi defibrillyatsii predserdii u 20 bol'nikh s mitralmini porokami sevdsta. Vestn. Akad. Med. Nauk SSSR 8:32, 1961.
8. Lown, B., Amarasingham, R., and Neuman, J.: New method for terminating cardiac arrhythmias. Use of synchronized capacitor discharge. JAMA 182:548, 1962.
9. Hooker, D. R., Kouwenhoven, W. B., and Langworthy, O. R.: The effect of alternating electrical currents on the heart. Am. J. Physiol. 103:444, 1933.
10. Kouwenhoven, W. B., and Milnor, W. R.: Treatment of ventricular fibrillation using a capacitor discharge. J. Appl. Physiol. 7:253, 1954.
11. Main, F. B., Aberdeen, E., and Gerbode, F. L. A.: Comparison of ventricular function subsequent to multiple defibrillations using the alternating current and the direct current defibrillators. Surg. Forum 14:258, 1963.
12. Yarbrough, R., Ussrey, G., and Whitley, J.: A comparison of the effects of AC and DC countershock on ventricular function in thoracotomized dogs. Am. J. Cardiol. 14:504, 1964.
13. Beck, E. S., Pritchard, W. H., and Feil, H. S.: Ventricular fibrillation of long duration abolished by electric shock. JAMA 135:985, 1947.
14. Alexander, S., Kleiger, R., and Lown, B.: Use of external electric countershock in the treatment of ventricular tachycardia. JAMA 177:916, 1961.
15. Zoll, P. M., and Linenthal, A. J.: Termination of refractory tachycardia by external countershock. Circulation 25:596, 1962.
16. Nachlas, M. M., Bix, H. H., Mower, M. M., and Siebano, M. P.: Observations on defibrillation and synchronized countershock. Prog. Cardiovasc. Dis. 9:64, 1966.
17. DeBoer, S.: On the fibrillation of the heart. J. Physiol. 54:400, 1921.
18. Wiggers, C. J., and Wegria, R.: Ventricular fibrillation due to single, localized induction and condensed shocks applied during vulnerable phase of ventricular systole. Am. J. Physiol. 128:500, 1940.
19. Castellanos, A., Jr., Lemberg, L., and Berkovits, B. V.: Repetitive firing during synchronized ventricular stimulation. Am. J. Cardiol. 17:119, 1966 (Abst.).
20. Peleşka, B.: Cardiac arrhythmias following condensed discharges and their dependence upon strength of current and phase of the cardiac cycle. Circ. Res. 13:21, 1963.
21. Kreus, K. E., Salokannel, S. J., and Waris, E. K.: Non-synchronized and

synchronized direct-current countershock in cardiac arrhythmias. Lancet ii:405, 1966.
22. Lown, B.: Electrical reversion of cardiac arrhythmias. Br. Heart J. 29:469, 1967.
23. Resnekov, L., and McDonald, L.: Appraisal of electroversion in treatment of cardiac dysrhythmias. Br. Heart J. 30:786, 1968.
24. McDonald, L., Resnekov, L., and O'Brien, K.: Direct current shock in treatment of drug resistant arrhythmias. Br. Med. J. i:1468, 1964.
25. Resnekov, L.: Synchronized capacitor discharge in the management of cardiac arrhythmias with particular reference to the haemodynamic significance of atrial systole. M.D. Thesis, University of Cape Town, 1965.
26. Lown, B., Kleiger, R., and Wolff, G.: The technique of cardioversion. Am. Heart J., 67:282, 1964.
27. Kouwenhoven, W. B., Jude, J. R., Knickerbocker, G. G., and Chestnut, W. R.: Closed chest defibrillation of the heart. Surgery 42:550, 1957.
28. Stock, R. J.: Cardioversion without anesthesia. N. Engl. J. Med. 269:534, 1963.
29. Lown, B.: Cardioversion without anesthesia. N. Engl. J. Med. 269:535, 1963.
30. Kahler, R. I., Burrow, G. N., and Felig, P.: Diazepam induced amnesia for cardioversion. JAMA 200:997, 1967.
31. Shephard, D. A. E., and Vandam, L. D.: Anesthesia for cardioversion. Am. J. Cardiol. 15:55, 1965.
32. Johnstone, M., and Nisbet, H. I. A.: Ventricular arrhythmia during halothane anaesthesia. Br. J. Anaesth. 33:9, 1961.
33. Nutter, D. O., and Massumi, R. A.: Diazepam in cardioversion. N. Engl. J. Med. 273:650, 1965.
34. Resnekov, L., and McDonald, L.: Electroversion of lone atrial fibrillation and flutter, including haemodynamic studies at rest and on exercise. Br. Heart J. 33:339, 1971.
35. Resnekov, L.: Haemodynamic studies before and after electrical conversion of atrial flutter and fibrillation to sinus rhythm. Br. Heart J. 29:100, 1967.
36. Yang, S. S., Maranhao, V., Monheit, R., Ablaza, S. G. G., and Goldberg, H.: Cardioversion following open-chest valvular surgery. Br. Heart J. 28:309, 1966.
37. Rabbino, M. D., Likoff, W., and Dreifus, L.: Complications and limitations of direct-current countershock. JAMA 190:417, 1964.
38. Gilston, A.: Clinical and biochemical aspects of cardiac resuscitation. Lancet ii:1039, 1965.
39. Resnekov, L., and McDonald, L.: Complications in 220 patients with cardiac dysrhythmias treated by phased direct-current shock and indications for electroversion. Br. Heart J. 29:926, 1967.
40. Mandecki, T., Biec, L., and Kargul, W.: Serum enzyme activities after cardioversion. Br. Heart J. 32:600, 1970.
41. Resnekov, L., and McDonald, L.: Pulmonary oedema following treatment of arrhythmias by direct current shock. Lancet i:506, 1965.
42. Logan, W. F. W. E., Rowlands, D. J., Howitt, G., and Holmes, A. M.: Left atrial activity following cardioversion. Lancet ii:471, 1965.
43. Sjorstein, D.: DC Cardioversion Session 18, p. 418. In E. Sandøe, E. Flensten-Jensen, and K. H. Olesen. (ed.), Symposium on Cardiac Arrhythmias. Sodertalje, Sweden, A. B. Astra, 1970.
44. Goldman, J.: The management of chronic atrial fibrillation: indications for and method of conversion to sinus rhythm. Progr. Cardiovasc. Dis. 2:465, 1959–1960.
45. Bjerkelund, C. J., and Orning, O. M.: The efficacy of anticoagulant therapy in preventing embolism following DC electrical conversion of atrial fibrillation. Am. J. Cardiol. 23:208, 1969.

46. Lown, B., Kleiger, R., and Williams, J.: Cardioversion and digitalis drugs: Changed threshold to electric shock in digitalized animals. Circ. Res. 17:519, 1965.
47. Corwin, N. D., Klein, M. J., and Friedberg, C. K.: Countershock conversion of digitalis associated paroxysmal tachycardia with block. Am. Heart J. 66:804, 1963.
48. Sloman, G., Robinson, J. S., and McClean, K.: Propranolol in persistent ventricular fibrillation. Br. Med. J. i:895, 1965.
49. Lown, B.: Discussion, p. 127. *In* D. G. Julian and M. F. Oliver (ed.), Acute Myocardial Infarction: Proceedings of a Symposium. Edinburgh, Livingstone, 1968.
50. Lown, B., and Wittenberg, S.: Cardioversion and digitalis. III. Effect of change in potassium concentration. Am. J. Cardiol. 21:513, 1968.
51. Resnekov, L.: Drug therapy before and after the electroversion of cardiac dysrhythmias. Prog. Cardiovasc. Dis. 16:531, 1974.
52. Childers, R. W., Rothbaum, D., and Arnsdorf, M.: The effects of DC shock on the electrical properties of the heart. Circulation 36:II-85, 1967 (Abstr.).
53. Byrne-Quinn, E., and Wing, A. J.: Maintenance of sinus rhythm after DC reversion of atrial fibrillation. Br. Heart J. 32:370, 1970.

Chapter 10

ARTIFICIAL PACING

LOUIS LEMBERG
AGUSTIN CASTELLANOS

The fundamental principles for the utilization of an artificial pacemaker were established as early as 1932 by Hyman[1] and later promulgated by Callaghan and Bigelow in 1951.[2] External cardiac pacing was introduced into clinical medicine in 1952 by Zoll.[3] In 1957, Weirich and associates introduced temporary direct myocardial stimulation in the treatment of complete AV block,[4] and a transistorized, self-contained implantable pacemaker for long-term correction of complete AV block was introduced in 1960 by Chardack and associates.[5] Since then, artificial pacemakers have become indispensable and are the most reliable method for treating Adams-Stokes syndrome.

At first, fixed-rate pacemakers were used, but they have been gradually replaced by demand pacemakers, which offer several advantages over the earlier type.

Artificial pacemakers are used primarily for the treatment of various bradyarrhythmias, particularly complete AV block. However, they also often provide a life-saving measure in the treatment of drug-resistant and refractory tachyarrhythmias, especially those of ventricular origin.

INDICATIONS FOR PACING

Artificial pacing is performed primarily for symptomatic arrhythmias.[6] Asymptomatic patients may be candidates for pacing when there are specific electrocardiographic alterations that are considered to be harbin-

165

gers of symptomatic arrhythmias. The indications for pacing are discussed here from the clinical viewpoint because it is symptoms and the clinical setting that determine the need for cardiac pacing.

Pacing in Symptomatic Patients

Adams-Stokes Syndrome. This is an attack of syncope, with or without a convulsive seizure, resulting from a sudden marked bradycardia, ventricular standstill, or transient ventricular repetitive beats associated with complete atrioventricular (AV) block. Brief episodes of faintness, dizziness, or weakness are variants of this syndrome.

Complete AV block in this clinical setting occurs in the elderly patient. There are no known predisposing diseases; however, the pathologic entities are known as Lev's disease and Lenegre's disease.[7] Lev described fibrosis or calcification of the connective tissue skeleton of the heart that envelops the conduction pathways, and Lenegre reported sclerodegenerative changes in the conduction pathways.

The first appearance of Adams-Stokes syndrome, corroborated by the presence of AV block, is an indication for immediate permanent pacemaker implantation.

Heart Failure. When congestive heart failure associated with a bradyarrhythmia is unresponsive to medical management, permanent cardiac pacing is indicated. Pacing at physiologic rates usually results in diuresis and compensation.

Altered Mentation. Altered mentation due to reduced cerebral blood flow may result from bradyarrhythmias. Pacing at physiologic rates augments the minute volume and cardiac output and thus improves cerebral perfusion.

Sick Sinus Syndrome. This is a syndrome of arrhythmias consisting of symptomatic bradycardia, alternating at times with symptomatic tachycardia. Recently, this syndrome was classified by DeSanctis[8] into three types:

1. Sinus bradycardia usually unresponsive to atropine sulfate or exercise
2. Sinoatrial block or arrest with long pauses
3. Alternating bradycardia and tachycardia

The bradycardia is due to (1) or (2) above, and it is followed by paroxysmal supraventricular tachycardia, which may be atrial fibrillation, atrial flutter, atrial tachycardia, junctional tachycardia, or any combination of these.[8] The pathology is idiopathic fibrosis or atherosclerotic coronary artery disease involving the SA node as well as the AV node.

However, AV conduction measured by the surface electrocardiogram is usually normal. His bundle electrograms may show alteration in either nodal conduction or His-Purkinje conduction.[9] Demand or standby pacing is indicated and can be accomplished by pacing the ventricle or the atrium, provided AV transmission is intact. Pacemaking insures against the development of bradycardia but has little effect in preventing the attacks of supraventricular tachycardia. However, suppressive doses of antiarrhythmic drugs can be used safely and effectively after pacemaker implantation in patients with supraventricular tachycardia. Both atrial and ventricular sequential pacing can also be employed by using a bifocal sequential demand pacemaker. This recently developed demand pacemaker can pace the atrium only or the atrium and ventricles in sequence or can remain dormant when normal sinus rhythm prevails.[10]

Bradycardia.   Patients with bradycardia-induced ventricular ectopic beats or ventricular tachycardia can benefit from overdrive suppression of the ventricular arrhythmias. The successful use of permanently implanted pacemakers for the control of recurrent ventricular tachycardia or ventricular fibrillation refractory to drug therapy has been reported extensively.[11] Demand or standby pacing has been effective in these cases. Pacemakers have also been employed in patients with atrial fibrillation or atrial flutter and slow ventricular response accompanied by congestive heart failure that was otherwise difficult to manage. Bradycardia resulting from hypersensitive carotid sinus reflex has at times required pacing.

After pacemaker implantation for symptomatic bradycardia, cardioactive drugs can be employed in therapeutic ranges without danger of added suppression of SA nodal discharge or AV nodal conduction.

Pacing in Asymptomatic Patients

The indications for electrical stimulation in the absence of any symptoms are less clear than when symptoms are present. The presence of Mobitz type II AV block is a definite indication for pacing. Correct electrocardiographic identification of this conduction disturbance is imperative. A diagnosis of Mobitz type II AV block is made when a nonconducted sinus P wave suddenly occurs and is preceded by conducted beats that have constant P–R intervals. Some patients may be symptomatic when the number of successively blocked P waves is significant. However, if the block is temporarily stabilized as a 2:1 or 3:1 AV block, symptoms may be absent or mild.

There are several processes that can simulate 2:1 AV block in the presence of fairly regular P–R intervals. Foremost amongst these are the recording of the end of a long run of Mobitz type I (Wenckebach)

AV blocks in which the increase in P–R interval is very slight before the blocked P wave. If Mobitz type II AV block emerges after a normal P–R interval, this possibility is less likely.

Concealed His bundle or fascicular extrasystoles can produce a similar phenomenon.[12,13] Mobitz type II AV block should be diagnosed with caution in patients having manifest AV junctional (His bundle) and fascicular beats.

The asymptomatic patient with right bundle branch block (RBBB) and left anterior hemiblock (LAH) or left posterior hemiblock (LPH) poses difficult problems of prophylactic therapy. According to Rosenbaum,[14] prophylactic pacemaker implantation is indicated whenever RBBB coexists with an abnormal right axis deviation due to LPH (other causes of right axis deviation have to be excluded).

Pacemaker therapy in patients who have RBBB and LAH due to chronic conducting system disease has also been a subject of debate and speculation.[9] Since the time of onset of symptomatic complete AV block in these patients is unpredictable, definite guidelines for prophylactic pacing have not been established.

Recent His bundle studies suggest that a prolonged H–V interval does not adversely affect the short-term prognosis in patients with RBBB and LAH. The implications are that His bundle electrograms may not be indicated for the evaluation of these patients. However, longer follow-up periods are required to prove this assumption. Some of these patients are prone to develop tachycardia-dependent or bradycardia-dependent AV block. Bradycardia-dependent AV block is precipitated by sinus slowing, which delays the subsequent P wave long enough that it falls during "phase 4" depolarization.[15] In other cases, the AV block is triggered by a premature beat when the postextrasystolic P-wave falls sufficiently late.[15] Continuous 12-hour electrocardiographic monitoring in patients with chronic RBBB and LAH can be used to reveal bradycardia-dependent AV block.

Atrioventricular Block in Acute Myocardial Infarction

There are special features and special therapeutic problems associated with atrioventricular block complicating acute myocardial infarction. Although AV block is an infrequent complication (7 to 10%), it has generated more controversy than any of the other arrhythmias occurring in the coronary care unit. The differences of opinion relate to the indications for the use of pacemakers and to the judgment of their beneficial effects.[16]

Knowledge of the site of the infarction is a critical factor in determining the prognosis as well as the management of AV block complicating acute myocardial infarction.[16] In Table 10-1 it is apparent that although AV block complicates diaphragmatic (inferior) infarctions more than twice as often as it does anterior wall infarctions, the mortality rate of AV block is three times greater in the latter than in the former.

The pathogenesis of acute AV conduction disturbances helps to explain these differences. Atrioventricular block in acute infarction of the inferior wall is located high in the AV node (above the bundle of His) and consists pathologically of edema or inflammation due to transient injury of the node or infarction of contiguous myocardium rather than involvement of the conduction tissue proper. The block is usually transient, and seldom is there a residual conduction defect. In anterior wall infarctions, AV block is secondary to destruction and necrosis of the bundle branches and distal parts of the conducting tissues, so that permanent damage results, with residual block of one or both bundles. Analysis of His bundle electrograms of patients with AV block following acute myocardial infarction have localized the conduction disturbance to an area above the bundle of His in inferior wall infarction and below the bundle of His in anterior wall infarction. Table 10-2 shows the other differences that characterize these two forms of AV block.

In general, first-degree AV block alone, regardless of the site of infarction, requires no treatment. In the presence of higher degrees of block complicating inferior wall infarctions, initial drug therapy is indicated if the existing ventricular rate is inadequate and symptoms of bradyarrhythmia develop. In this clinical setting, therefore, the critical factor is the heart rate and not the degree of block.[16,17]

In inferior wall infarctions, early acute AV block of any degree may result from excessive vagal discharge, and in these situations, sinus bradycardia is also present. Atropine sulfate improves AV conduction in more than half of these patients (Fig. 10-1). Intravenous infusion of isoproterenol may improve AV conduction when atropine is ineffective. Excessive sinus rates and ventricular rates should be avoided when using isoproterenol.

The clinical course and prognosis of AV block in inferior wall infarc-

Table 10-1   *Incidence and Mortality of Complete Atrioventricular Block Complicating Acute Myocardial Infarction*

Site of Infarction	Incidence of AV Block (%)	Mortality (%)
Inferior wall	7	30
Anterior wall	3	80

Table 10-2   *Atrioventricular Block Complicating Acute Myocardial Infarction*

	AV Block Complicating Inferior Wall Infarction	AV Block Complicating Anterior Wall Infarction
Pathogenesis	Edema or inflammation due to transient ischemia of AV node and contiguous myocardium	Destruction due to infarction of the bundle branches
Location of block	Above the bundle of His.	Below the bundle of His
Premonitory signs	Sinus bradycardia often. 1° AV block or 2° block. Wenckebach type often precedes complete AV block	RBBB plus LAH—often. RBBB plus LPH—infrequent. Alternating BBB or sudden asystole.
Adams-Stokes attacks	Rare (7% to 10%)	Almost always present
QRS complexes	Usually narrow, maintaining a supraventricular pattern	Usually wide (idioventricular)
Subsidiary pacemaker	Probably junctional	Ventricular
Mobitz II	Rare	Usual
Residual block	Very rare	BBB and/or fascicular block
Treatment	Drugs usually effective	Pacemaker
Prognosis	Good	Poor

tion are not significantly altered by endocardial pacing. Pacing in AV block due to acute inferior wall infarction is indicated in the following situations:

When the ventricular rate cannot be effectively maintained at optimal levels by drug therapy

In Mobitz type II AV block

In symptomatic complete AV block (usually ventricular rate slower than 50 beats per minute)

Early experiences in coronary care units showed that most patients who develop acute AV block following anterior wall infarctions have a poor prognosis even with artificial pacing. This was attributed to the extensive myocardial damage, frequently complicated by cardiogenic shock, heart failure, or myocardial rupture.

With recent advances in electrophysiology and after retrospective reviews of particular clinical situations, it has been noted that AV block with anterior wall infarctions is frequently ushered in by the appearance of block in any of the bundle branches. Specific ECG patterns are produced by interruption of the right bundle or the two fascicles (antero-

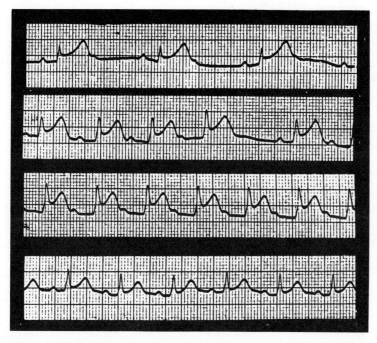

Figure 10-1. Regression of third-degree AV block to sinus rhythm with normal PR interval following intravenous administration of 0.6 mg of atropine sulfate in a patient with an acute inferior wall myocardial infarction. Wenckebach periods followed by first-degree AV block precede the return to normal sinus rhythm.

superior and posteroinferior) of the left bundle, or of any combination of these elements. With this knowledge, prophylactic insertion of a pacing catheter may improve prognosis when any two of these branches are blocked.

The approach to therapy for AV block complicating anterior myocardial infarction is quite different. Atropine is ineffective, but isoproterenol may be transiently helpful if advanced AV block or asystole occurs before a pacing catheter can be introduced. Therefore, in the following situations, a pacemaker catheter should be inserted prophylactically for demand or standby pacing:

Complete RBBB and LAH
Complete RBBB and LPH
Complete RBBB and first-degree AV block
Complete LBBB and first-degree AV block
Complete LBBB alternating with complete RBBB

Atrioventricular conduction disturbances that follow inferior myocardial infarctions are transient and seldom require permanent pacing. Because regular sinus rhythm may return at any time during the course of an acute myocardial infarction, the pacemaker of choice is the ventricular-inhibited, or demand pacemaker. This mode of pacing reduces the risk of repetitive ventricular beats or ventricular fibrillation. Figure 10-2 shows an episode of repetitive ventricular beating initiated by a stimulus from a continuous asynchronous pacemaker in a patient with an acute myocardial infarction.

Permanent demand pacemaker implantation is indicated in the few patients who survive transient AV block due to acute anterior myocardial infarction. Atkins et al.[18] reported that of 13 patients with RBBB and LAH who had transient AV block during the acute phase of myocardial infarction and survived, 11 died within 6 months after discharge. The posthospital mortality in this group is much higher than that of patients with otherwise uncomplicated myocardial infarction. The report continues with 8 similar patients in whom pacemakers were implanted prior to discharge. There were no deaths in this latter group during an 8- to 18-month follow-up.

Reciprocating Tachycardia

An increasing number of patients with reciprocating tachycardia are being treated by artificial pacing. Pacemaker therapy for reciprocating tachycardias is determined by the mechanism of the tachycardia. Knowledge of these mechanisms permits optimal therapy and avoids conceptual errors that may threaten the life of a patient. Modern use of pacemakers dictates the need for a discussion of these arrhythmias.

A classification of reciprocating tachycardia is presented in Tables 10-3 and 10-4. It is important to stress that the newer methods of intracardiac recording and stimulation have shown that multiple circuits can be involved in the origin and perpetuation of these arrhythmias.[19] The

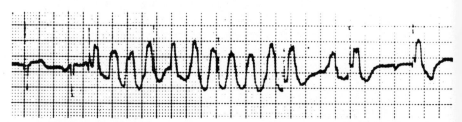

Figure 10-2. Continuous asynchronous (fixed rate) pacemaker stimulus artifact falling in the vulnerable period of a natural beat initiates repetitive ventricular beats.

Table 10-3   *Types of Reciprocating Atrial and Ventricular Tachycardias*

Sinus node–atrial reciprocation

Intra-atrial or interatrial reciprocation
  Reciprocating atrial flutter
  Rare cases of reciprocating atrial tachycardia

Intraventricular or interventricular reciprocation
  Reciprocation around the stimulating electrodes, as in classical "vulnerability"
  Reciprocation involving the bundle branches
  Reciprocation involving an area of acute myocardial infarction
  Reciprocation involving a scarred area
  Combinations of the above

---

mechanisms of reciprocating tachycardias in patients with pre-excitation Wolff-Parkinson-White (WPW) syndrome will be discussed first.

Pre-excitation is said to be present when a sinus (or atrial) impulse is conducted through pathways other than the normal AV route and activates a portion or all of the ventricle earlier than the impulse that is conducted through the normal AV pathways at the usual speed. From the clinical standpoint, any patient with recurrent, repetitive, supraventricular tachyarrhythmias can be considered to have a form (or variant) of the pre-excitation syndrome.[19] The resting electrocardiogram obtained during sinus rhythm may be deceiving because of the coexistence of congenital, atherosclerotic, or primary conduction system disease.

The short P–R interval with the wide QRS complex in Wolff-Parkinson-White syndrome is presumably due to a Kent bundle, but AV conduction time may be normal in the presence of atrial enlargement or intra-atrial conduction defects. A short P–R, narrow QRS complexes, and repetitive tachyarrhythmias suggest a Lown-Ganong-Levine (LGL) syndrome, perhaps due to total bypass of the area where the major AV nodal delay occurs. The P–R interval can be normal in the presence of atrial or bundle branch disease, but the ventricular complexes are wide and the A–H interval is short.

Table 10-4   *Types of Reciprocating AV Tachycardias*

Functional longitudinal dissociation of the AV node
Reciprocation involving AV node and Kent bundle
Reciprocation involving AV node and James bundle
Combinations of the above
When ventricular stimulation is performed at short coupling intervals, any of the
  reciprocating intraventricular or interventricular tachycardias described in
  Table 10-3 can be associated with any of the above reciprocating tachycardias

---

Some patients with recurrent tachyarrhythmias and normal P–R and A–H intervals but a narrow QRS complex may have a partial AV nodal bypass. These cases, as well as those with the LGL syndrome, are characterized by a dynamic response to atrial pacing at increasing rates and not by the measurement of conduction intervals at natural rates.[19] The A–H interval does not show the increase that is normally seen. At times, 1:1 AV conduction occurs at rates as high as 240/min. Adults with atrial flutter and 1:1 AV conduction are likely to have an AV nodal bypass.

A premature atrial beat with prolonged AV conduction time usually triggers the reciprocating tachycardia. However, the initiating event need not be an atrial extrasystole in the true sense, since retrograde atrial activation of ventricular extrasystoles or marked sinus arrhythmia may produce the same effect.

In WPW syndrome, the reciprocating arrhythmias appear when the premature atrial impulse is conducted to the ventricles through the AV node while being blocked at the Kent bundle. It can, nevertheless, return to the atria through the accessory pathway. Yet there is no reason a reciprocating tachycardia involving a single functionally dissociated anatomical pathway (AV node) cannot occur in these patients. Similar considerations apply to patients with LGL syndrome and its variants.

Various types of pacemakers have been implanted for the treatment of symptomatic patients with drug-resistant recurrent supraventricular tachycardias. There is no single mode of pacing that is appropriate for all forms of reciprocating tachycardias. Electrophysiologic evaluation is essential before selection of the optimal modality of stimulation.[19]

Specialized studies should be undertaken to distinguish among the types of reciprocating mechanisms that can be present (Table 10-3). These procedures can establish the presence or absence of pre-excitation and can evaluate the type of pre-excitation, as well as the functional properties of the normal and accessory pathways. Finally, these studies help in achieving understanding of the effects of electrical stimuli and the response to intravenously administered drugs.

Rapid Atrial Stimulation. This form of stimulation can transform an AV reciprocating tachycardia into atrial fibrillation or flutter, which, in the absence of atrial disease, is self-limited. Since the arrhythmia subsides promptly, sinus rhythm is generally re-established. However, in some patients with pre-excitation (usually those with WPW syndrome and rarely those with LGL syndrome or its variants) the effective refractory period of the accessory pathway is very short. In these patients (especially if they have organic disease), atrial fibrillation may be persistent and associated with clinically significant rapid ventricular rates. Cardioversion may be required in order to terminate the arrhythmia.

Stimulation of the Atria at Varying Coupling Intervals. Properly timed single or double atrial stimuli can break a reciprocating circuit, thus stopping the tachycardia. This type of pacing may at times induce vulnerability-related atrial fibrillation with the same potential hazards mentioned above. Such atrial fibrillation is generally triggered by stimuli delivered at short coupling intervals, immediately after the end of the atrial effective refractory period.

Ventricular Pacing. Stimulation of the ventricles can abolish a reciprocating tachycardia if the impulses are conducted retrograde to the atria, provided that the P wave falls in the moment of the cycle where it can break the tachycardia. At times, concealed retrograde conduction into the AV tissues collides with the oncoming supraventricular impulse, thus stopping the tachycardia.

However, premature ventricular stimuli delivered at short coupling intervals can produce additional reciprocating circuits (Table 10-4). The latter can be short-lived or persistent, at times interrupting (permanently or transiently) the original AV tachycardia.

As mentioned previously, several types of permanent pacemakers have been used in the treatment of reciprocating AV tachycardias.[19] Undesirable sinus bradycardia is prevented by QRS-inhibited ventricular demand pacemakers in patients receiving high doses of beta-blocking agents. Sequential AV bifocal units can abolish certain reciprocating circuits. Several authors have reported the use of an implanted pacemaker that can be activated externally by magnets or radiofrequency signals during bouts of tachycardia; conventional QRS-inhibited ventricular demand units, rapid atrial stimulators, and atrial- or ventricular-triggered pacemakers with preselected (fixed or varying) coupling (or triggering) intervals have also been employed in the treatment of reciprocating tachycardia.[19]

MODALITIES OF PACING

Since the advent of electronic cardiac pacemakers, a variety of pacing modalities have been developed. The physician who employs pacemakers in the care of the cardiac patient must understand the various types of pacing currently available in order to intelligently select the type best suited to the patient's needs.

A basic classification of the modalities of pacing is as follows[20]:

Stimulation of the ventricles only:
    Continuous asynchronous ventricular
    QRS-inhibited ventricular (demand)
    QRS-triggered ventricular (standby)
    P-wave-triggered ventricular

Stimulation of the atria only:
    Continuous asynchronous atrial
    P-wave-inhibited atrial
    P-wave-triggered atrial
    QRS-inhibited atrial
Stimulation of both atria and ventricles:
    Continuous sequential atrial and ventricular
    QRS-inhibited sequential atrial and ventricular (bifocal demand)

Stimulation of the Ventricles Only

Continuous Asynchronous Pacemaker. This pacemaker delivers stimuli to the ventricles continuously at rates that range between 60 and 80/min. The rate can be altered manually in some units, and since the output of the pacemaker is neither inhibited nor synchronized the term continuous asynchronous (Fig. 10-3) is more suitable than "fixed rate." During normal function, the interval between pacemaker stimuli does not change, even in the presence of natural beats (either sinus or ectopic). All stimulus artifacts except those appearing during the absolute refractory period of the ventricles result in propagated responses.

Transient appearance of natural beats occurs commonly in patients with pacemakers. Potential hazards due to competition are created as a result of the coaction of natural·and artificial pacemaker rhythm (Fig. 10-4). Summated heart rates are seen, and repetitive ventricular beats may occur when pacemaker stimuli fall during the vulnerable period of the cardiac cycle (Fig. 10-2). These problems led to the development and widespread use of noncompetitive (QRS-inhibited, QRS-triggered, and P-wave-triggered) pacemakers.[21] Because of the risks of competition, the continuous asynchronous pacemaker is not widely used today. The characteristics of this type of pacemaker are summarized in Table 10-5.

QRS-Inhibited Pacemakers. The QRS-inhibited pacemaker is the most widely used pacemaker. It has both a stimulating and sensing mechanism. When natural ventricular activity is sensed, the output of

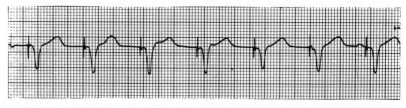

Figure 10-3. Continuous asynchronous (fixed rate) pacemaker functioning normally.

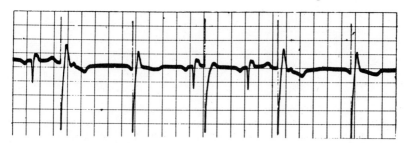

Figure 10-4. Summated heartbeats due to coaction of natural beats and pacemaker beats (continuous asynchronous pacemaker).

the pacemaker is suppressed. A stimulus is emitted only after a preset interval following a natural ventricular beat has been exceeded. Pacing automatically ceases when the natural rate exceeds that of the pacemaker (Fig. 10-5). In Table 10-5, the significant characteristics of this safe and useful pacemaker are outlined.[39]

Because of the difficulties of evaluating the stimulating properties of this pacemaker during periods of pacemaker inhibition, a magnetic reed switch was added to the pulse generator. Application of a magnet to the skin overlying the pulse generator activates the switch and causes a change to a continuous mode of operation at a fixed rate, which is not necessarily the same as its automatic rate. However, this additional feature introduced new problems. For instance, improper application

Table 10-5   *Pacemaker Characteristics*

Pacemaker	Type	Mode of Action	Stimulates	Senses	General Indications
Continuous asynchronous ventricular	Ventricular	Continuous asynchronous	Ventricles	—	SA arrest; AV block
QRS-Inhibited ventricular	Ventricular	QRS-inhibited (demand)	Ventricles	QRS	SA arrest; AV block electrical over-drive
QRS-triggered ventricular	Ventricular	QRS-triggered (standby)	Ventricles	QRS	SA arrest; AV block
P-wave-triggered ventricular	Ventricular	P-wave-triggered	Ventricles	P-waves	AV block in children
Continuous sequential atrial and ventricular	Atrial and ventricular	Continuous sequential	Atria and ventricles	—	AV block; Sinus bradycardia; AV synchrony when needed to enhance cardiac output
QRS-inhibited sequential atrial and ventricular	Atrial and ventricular	QRS-inhibited sequential (bifocal demand)	Atria and ventricles	QRS	Sick sinus syndrome; AV block over-drive; reciprocating tachycardia; AV synchrony when needed to enhance cardiac output

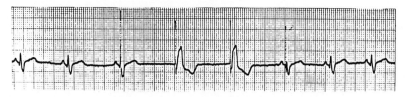

Figure 10-5. QRS-inhibited (demand) pacemaker pacing when the natural rate is below that of the pacemaker. With an increase in the natural rate shown at the right end of the trace, pacing stimulus artifacts are no longer seen.

of the magnet over the neck of pulse generators can lead to erratic firing in some normally functioning units (Fig. 10-6). In other units with component failure manifested by significant rate variations, the magnet can produce complete pacemaker inhibition.

Ventricular fusion beats result if portions of the ventricles are activated by the natural impulse and other portions by the pacemaker.[21] A true fusion beat appears when the pacemaker escape interval ends after the onset of ventricular depolarization but before the moment (within the QRS complex) at which inhibition would have occurred. This occurs if the perielectrode tissues have not been rendered absolutely refractory by the activation front propagating from the area first depolarized by the natural impulse.

Pseudofusion beats are due to electrocardiographic superimposition of an ineffective stimulus artifact upon a natural ventricular complex.[22] Pseudofusion beats appear when the pacemaker escape interval ends after the beginning of ventricular depolarization but before the moment (within the QRS complex) at which inhibition would have occurred.[20] However, the perielectrode tissues have been rendered absolutely refrac-

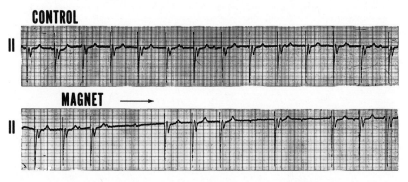

Figure 10-6. Erratic firing of a normally functioning QRS-inhibited ventricular pacemaker due to improper application of a magnet over the neck of the pulse generator. (Reprinted by permission of the American Heart Association.[20])

tory by the impulse propagating from the area first activated by the natural impulse. (Figure 10-7 is a diagrammatic representation of the mechanisms of true fusion beats and pseudofusion beats.)

The escape interval following a sensed ventricular beat is shorter or longer than, but rarely equal to, the interval between two consecutive stimulus artifacts (automatic interval). This occurs because the moment within the QRS complex at which inhibition starts cannot be determined from the surface electrocardiogram.[21,22] Moreover, the escape interval also changes with the morphology and origin of the ventricular beats.[23] Some manufacturers have preset the duration of the escape intervals

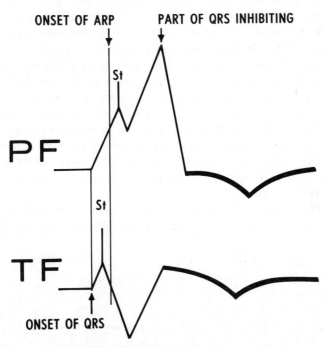

Figure 10-7. Diagrammatic representation of the mechanisms of true fusion beats (TF) and pseudofusion beats (PF). See text for explanation. *Onset of QRS* = the beginning of ventricular depolarization (in an area distant from the electrodes). *Onset of ARP* = the moment at which the muscle surrounding the electrodes is rendered refractory by the impulse propagating from its site of origin. *Part of QRS inhibiting* = the moment within the ventricular complex at which pacemaker inhibition would occur. *St* = pacemaker spike. For these events to occur, a built-in lag between *Onset of ARP* and *Part of QRS inhibiting* must be present. (Reprinted by permission of the American Heart Association.[20])

in demand pacemakers, thus adding the function of rate hysteresis. In rate hysteresis,[24] the escape intervals are intentionally longer than the automatic interval (Fig. 10-8). The clinical significance of rate hysteresis is that it can lead to an otherwise paradoxical situation in which a slower natural rhythm inhibits a faster artificial pacemaker. This phenomenon reflects a malfunction when it occurs in the units that do not have rate hysteresis.

The QRS complexes appearing after the end of the pacemaker refractory period may be sensed by normally functioning QRS-inhibited pacemakers. Since intracavity ventricular electrograms of 1 mV or less have been observed in the presence of myocardial infarction, non-sensing might occur in the absence of pacing system failure if the catheter electrodes are improperly positioned.[20] At times, unipolarization of a bipolar system is required. It should be emphasized that a good threshold for stimulation does not necessarily imply that sensing will be adequate. If voltages greater than 2.5 mV are not found, transvenous QRS-inhibited pacing should not be attempted. Contrary to commonly held assumptions, sensing is not an "all or none" phenomenon. It has been shown that borderline intracavity signals can produce an incomplete recycling of the sensing mechanism. This is characterized by escape intervals of longer duration than if the beat had not been detected at all. However, the escape interval is significantly shorter than that seen when normal sensing occurs.[25-28]

Partial sensing (Fig. 10-9) may occur in patients with normally functioning pacing systems if the intracardiac signals range between 1.5 and

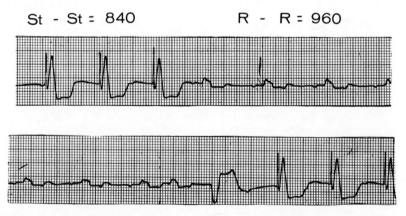

St - St = 840   R - R = 960

Figure 10-8. QRS-inhibited ventricular pacemaker with rate hysteresis. A slower natural rhythm (R–R cycle length of 960 msec) inhibits a faster automatic rate (St–St interval of 840 msec). St = stimulus artifact. (Reprinted by permission of the American Heart Association.[20])

S

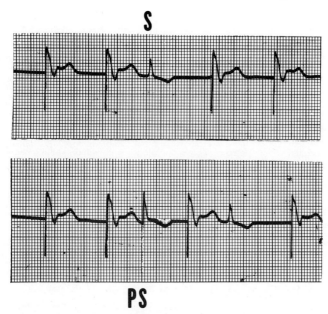

PS

Figure 10-9. Differences between "normal" and "partial" sensing. The escape intervals of "normally" sensed (*S*) beats are slightly longer (880 msec) and those of "partially" sensed (*PS*) QRS complexes are significantly shorter (610 msec) than the automatic intervals (840 msec). (Reprinted by permission of the American Heart Association.[20])

5 mV. The most frequent cause of partial sensing, however, is improper electrode placement. Thus, repositioning of the electrodes or unipolarization of the pacing system (and not pulse generator replacement) prevents partial sensing. This diagnosis (as with any problem involving sensing) can be confirmed by magnet conversion to continuous asynchronous pacing, which will differentiate between the stimulating and sensing functions of the pacing system.

QRS-Triggered Ventricular. The QRS-triggered ventricular pacemaker is similar to the QRS-inhibited type and has both stimulating and sensing mechanisms (Table 10-5). Unlike the ventricular-inhibited type, this pacemaker delivers an electrical stimulus during the formation of the patient's QRS complex when the natural rate exceeds that of the pacemaker (Figure 10-10). In addition, the pacemaker fires automatically after a preset escape interval, the duration of which is determined by the rate of the pacemaker. Triggered pacemaker stimuli falling within the QRS complexes are generally considered to be safe and ineffective.

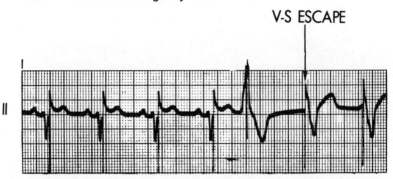

Figure 10-10. Pacemaker stimulus artifacts appear during the formation of the QRS as seen with the sinus conducted beats as well as with the ventricular premature beat. When a natural beat fails to appear, the pacemaker takes over ventricular-stimulus (V-S) escape and paces the ventricles.

A stimulus artifact seen in the middle of the QRS complex indicates that the sensing mechanism is functioning normally. However, it distorts the QRS morphology and in this way interferes with the evaluation of the ventricular complex. This introduces problems in the interpretation of certain acute conditions. At rates greater than 100/min firing will occur only after the second or third ventricular complexes. During atrial fibrillation, a chaotic arrhythmia results from the interplay of normal or aberrantly conducted supraventricular beats, pure pacemaker beats, and fusion and pseudofusion beats. In the presence of sinus rhythm, the function of capture can be tested by conversion to a continuous asynchronous mode of operation by the use of an external magnet. Improper application of the magnet over the neck of the pulse generator produces intermittent activation of the magnetic switch that is perceived by the corresponding circuit as an ectopic beat; as a result, a pacemaker stimulus is delivered. This causes irregular pacemaker firing not due to malfunction. The fact that this pacemaker makes electrocardiographic interpretation more difficult has resulted in a general decline in its use.

P-Wave-Triggered Ventricular. This pacemaker also has both stimulating and sensing mechanisms. The P-wave-triggered ventricular pacemaker functions as an artificial AV node. A sensing electrode in the atrium detects the P waves, and after a delay corresponding to the normal P–R interval, the ventricle is stimulated by a ventricular electrode (Fig. 10-11). If a P wave does not appear, the pacemaker will stimulate after a preset escape interval and maintain the ventricular output at a preset rate. It has been found useful in the management of chronic AV block in children. (The features of this pacemaker are summarized in Table 10-5.)

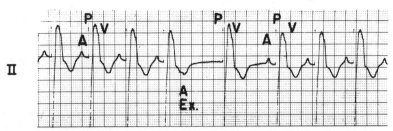

II

Figure 10-11. Wave-triggered ventricular pacemaker. An atrial extrasystole occurs during the refractory period of the pacemaker. In the absence of a P-wave, the pacemaker captures the ventricular after a present interval. A = P waves; P = pacemaker artifact; V = QRS; AEx = atrial extrasystole.

Stimulation of the Atria Only

The various modalities of atrial pacing are presented diagrammatically in Figure 10-12.[20,29-36]

Stimulation of Both Atria and Ventricles

Continuous Sequential Atrial and Ventricular.   Diagrams illustrating the electrocardiographic features of continuous sequential atrial and ventricular pacing and of QRS-inhibited sequential atrial and ventricular pacing (bifocal demand stimulation) are presented in Figure 10-13.[20]

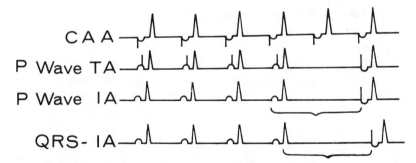

CAA

P Wave TA

P Wave IA

QRS- IA

Figure 10-12. Diagrammatic illustration of the modalities of pacing used for atrial stimulation. During continuous asynchronous atrial pacing (*CAA*) the stimulus artifacts precede and capture the atria; AV transmission is intact. With P-wave-triggered atrial pacing (*P Wave TA*) the stimulus artifacts appear during the formation of the sinus P-wave. When sinoatrial block occurs, the stimulus artifact appears at the end of the escape interval and precedes the P-wave. In P-wave-inhibited atrial pacemakers (*P Wave IA*) the faster atrial rates supress or inhibit the output of the atrial pacemaker. Pacemaker atrial escapes occur when a P-wave fails to appear before a preset interval. With QRS-inhibited atrial pacemakers (*QRS-IA*), faster ventricular rates supress the output of the pacemaker. A pacemaker atrial escape occurs when a QRS complex fails to appear before a preset interval. (Reprinted by permission of the American Heart Association.[20])

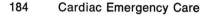

CS A-V

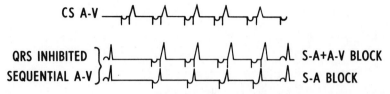

QRS INHIBITED ⎤   S-A+A-V BLOCK
SEQUENTIAL A-V ⎦   S-A BLOCK

Figure 10-13. Electrocardiographic features of implantable transvenous pacemakers that have been used for both atrial and ventricular stimulation. Continuous sequential atrioventricular pacemakers (CS AV) stimulate the atria and, after a preset delay, the ventricles. They are neither inhibited nor triggered by P waves or ventricular complexes. On the other hand, QRS-inhibited sequential AV (bifocal demand) pacemakers are inhibited by faster natural rates. Only the atria will be paced if intermittent pure sinoatrial (SA) block occurs. However, both atria and ventricles will be stimulated when intermittently coexisting SA and AV blocks appear. (Reprinted by permission of the American Heart Association.[20])

In the continuous sequential atrial and ventricular mode of pacing, electrodes in the atrium and in the ventricle stimulate at a continuous rate but with a sequential delay between the stimuli equal to that of the normally functioning AV node (Fig. 10-14). The competitive rhythms that often occur with continuous asynchronous pacemakers are potential problems in this mode of pacing. (See Table 10-5 for a summary of the characteristics of this pacemaker.)

QRS-Inhibited Sequential Atrial and Ventricular (Bifocal Demand). This pacemaker, like the ventricular demand pacemaker, monitors ventricular electrical activity but programs both atrial and ventricular stimulation (see Table 10-5). It consists of two demand units, a conventional QRS-inhibited demand pacemaker and a QRS-inhibited atrial demand pacemaker.[10,37] The escape interval of the atrial pacemaker is shorter than the escape interval of the ventricular pacemaker. The difference between the two escape intervals defines the AV sequential interval, i.e., the P–R interval. Both pacemakers acting in synchrony provide QRS-inhibited AV sequential stimulation (Fig. 10-15).

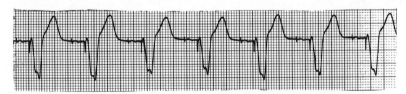

Figure 10-14. Continuous sequential atrial and ventricular pacing. Stimulus artifacts capture the atria and the ventricles with a delay equal to the normal P–R interval.

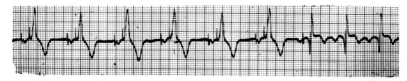

Figure 10-15. QRS-inhibited AV sequential pacing (bifocal demand). At the right end of the trace, when normal sinus rhythm returns, the ventricular pacemaker stimulus artifact is inhibited first, and then both atrial and ventricular pacemaker stimuli are inhibited.

The ventricular electrodes have a dual function. They sense the ventricular signal and also stimulate the ventricles when required. The atrial electrode stimulates the atrium but does not have a sensing function. Therefore, the signal detected by the ventricular electrode is responsible for both atrial and ventricular pacing.

COMPLICATIONS OF PACEMAKERS

Pacemaker Arrhythmias

Pacemaker arrhythmias were discussed in the preceding section, since different modes of pacing have their characteristic rhythm problems.

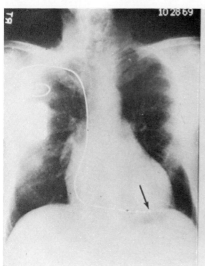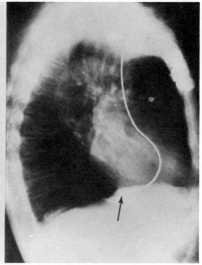

Figure 10-16. Posteroanterior view on the left shows the catheter tip position to be in the area of the right ventricular apex. However, the lateral view on the right indicates the true position of the catheter tip, in the inferior and posterior region of the cardiac shadow—probably in the middle cardiac vein.

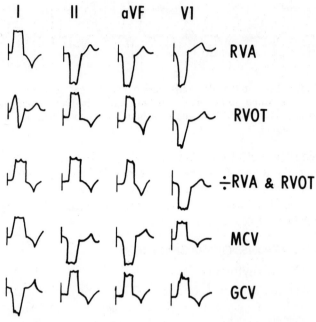

Figure 10-17. QRS patterns produced by pacing from different ventricular sites. RVA, right ventricular apex; RVOT, right ventricular outflow tract; ÷, between; GCV, great cardiac vein; MCV, middle cardiac vein. Right chest lead V1 is the best single lead to determine whether the catheter electrodes induce beats arising in the right ventricular cavity (top three rows) or at the epicardial left posterior wall (bottom two rows) stimulated through the corresponding veins (GCV and MCV) entering the coronary sinus. On the other hand, the direction of the electrical axis as determined from leads I, II and aVF is a function of the caudal (first and fourth rows), cephalic (second and fifth rows) or intermediate (third row) location of the catheters.

Only those arrhythmias related to the most commonly used pacemakers have been presented.

Malposition of Transvenous Pacemaker Catheters

Proper positioning of the electrode catheter in the apex of the right ventricle is not always achieved. Misplacement of the catheter tip can be avoided by (1) radiographic localization using both posteroanterior (PA) and lateral views and (2) recording at least two electrocardiographic leads. Exclusive reliance on the posteroanterior view is to be discouraged, since the catheter tip may appear to be located in the right ventricular apex on the PA film when it actually lies in the middle cardiac vein, as can be seen in a lateral view (Fig. 10-16). To arrive at this location, the electrode catheter must have been passed through the coronary sinus.

The position of the pacing catheter can be determined by the QRS pattern produced by the stimulus artifacts (Fig. 10-17). Right chest lead V_1 is the best single lead to determine whether the impulse is produced by an electrode located within the right ventricular cavity or in the coronary sinus or great and middle cardiac vein.[37] The superior or inferior location of the stimulating electrode is determined by the inferior or superior orientation of the frontal plane electrical axis of QRS as determined from leads I, II, and aVF.[38]

Displacement of Electrode Tip and Perforation of Electrode Catheter Tip into the Pericardial Space

These complications of permanent transvenous pacing are infrequent. Loss of pacemaker capture, either intermittent or permanent, during normal pacemaker battery life should alert the physician to these possible complications. Pericardial irritation or diaphragmatic stimulation may occur because of perforation of the catheter tip into the pericardial space.

SUMMARY

Pacemaker implantation was initially employed for the treatment of AV block resulting from chronic conduction system disease. With experience gained in coronary care units, basic principles have been established that serve as guidelines for therapy of AV block following acute myocardial infarction. Since very few patients develop chronic AV block as a result of acute myocardial infarction, the need for permanent pacing in this setting is rare.

The indications for pacing have been extended to include arrhythmias other than AV block. Artificial pacing has been established as a useful therapeutic measure in the management of reciprocating tachycardias, which may be initiated and perpetuated by a variety of mechanisms. Effective pacemaker therapy demands understanding of the electrophysiologic aspects of reciprocating tachycardias. These aspects have been discussed in detail.

The sophisticated use of pacemakers requires knowledge of the various types of pacing modes currently available. This permits intelligent selection of the mode of pacing best suited to each patient. Various types of artificial pacemakers have been described in detail.

Familiarity with complications of pacemakers is vital for those who treat patients with artificial pacemakers. Electrocardiographic criteria have been established that allow precise location of the tip of the pacemaker electrode catheter, since malposition of transvenous pacemaker catheters can be responsible for pacemaker failures. Radiographic localization requires two views, the posteroanterior and the lateral. Reliance on the posteroanterior view alone is unacceptable.

REFERENCES

1. Hyman, A. S.: Resuscitation of the stopped heart by intracardiac therapy: Further use of the artificial pacemaker. JAMA 99:1888, 1932.
2. Callaghan, J. C., and Bigelow, W. G.: An electrical artificial pacemaker for standstill of the heart. Ann. Surg. 134:8, 1951.
3. Zoll, P. M.: Resuscitation of the heart in ventricular standstill by external electric stimulation. N. Engl. J. Med. 247:768, 1952.
4. Weirich, W. L., Gott, V. L., and Lillehei, C. W.: Treatment of complete heart block by combined use of myocardial electrode and an artificial pacemaker. Surg. Forum 8:360, 1957.
5. Chardack, W. M., Gage, A. A., and Greatbatch, W.: A transistorized self-contained, implantable pacemaker for the long-term correction of complete heart block. Surgery 48:643, 1960.
6. Zoll, P. M.: Development of electrical control of cardiac rhythm. JAMA 266:881, 1973.
7. Rosenbaum, M. B., Elizari, M. V., and Lazzari, J. O.: The Hemiblocks. Oldsmar, Fla., Tampa Tracings, 1970, p. 107.
8. DeSanctis, R. W.: Sick sinus syndrome. ACCEL, Vol. 6, No. 1, 1974.
9. Narula, O. S.: Advances in clinical electrophysiology: Contribution of His bundle recordings. In P. Samet (ed.), Cardiac Pacing. New York, Grune & Stratton, 1973.
10. Castellanos, A., Jr., Berkovits, B. V., Castillo, C. A., and Befeler, B.: Sextapolar catheter electrode for temporary sequential atrioventricular pacing. Cardiovasc. Res. 8:712, 1974.
11. Haft, J. I., Treatment of arrhythmias by intracardiac electrical stimulation. Prog. Cardiovasc. Dis. 16:539, 1974.
12. Langendorf, R., and Mehlman, J. S.: Blocked (non-conducted) A-V nodal premature systoles imitating first and second degree A-V block. Am. Heart J. 34:500, 1947.
13. Castellanos, A., Befeler, B., and Myerburg, R. J.: Pseudo A-V block produced by concealed extrasystoles arising below the bifurcation of the His bundle. Br. Heart J. (in press).
14. Rosenbaum, M. B., Elizarin, M. V., and Lazzari, J. O.: Los Hemibloqueos. Buenos Aires, Paidos, 1968, p. 19.
15. Corrado, G., Levi, R. J., Nau, G. J., and Rosenbaum, M. B.: Paroxysmal atrioventricular block related to phase 4 bilateral bundle branch block. Am. J. Cardiol. 33:553, 1974.
16. Lemberg, L., Castellanos, A., Jr., and Arcebal, A. G.: The treatment of arrhythmias following acute myocardial infarction. Med. Clin. N. Am. 55:273, 1971.
17. Lemberg, L., Arcebal, A. G., Castellanos, A., Jr., and Claxton, B. W.: Cardiac Drugs in the Coronary Care Unit. Chest 59:289, 1971.
18. Atkins, J. M., Leshin, S. J., Blomquist, G., and Mullins, C. B.: Ventricular conduction blocks and sudden death in acute myocardial infarction. N. Engl. J. Med. 288:281, 1973.
19. Castellanos, A., Jr., and Myerburg, R. J.: Recurrent supraventricular arrhythmias in context. Am. Heart J. (in press).

20. Castellanos, A., Jr., and Lemberg, L.: Pacemaker arrhythmias and electrocardiographic recognition of pacemakers. Circulation 47:1382, 1973.
21. Castellanos, A., Jr., and Lemberg, L.: Electrophysiology of Pacing and Cardioversion. New York, Appleton-Century-Crofts, 1969.
22. Spitzer, R. C., Donoso, E., Gadboys, H. L., and Friedberg, C. K.: Arrhythmias induced by pacing on demand. Am. Heart J. 77:619, 1969.
23. Kastor, J. A., Berkovits, B. V., and DeSanctis, R.: Variations in discharge rate of demand pacemakers not due to malfunction. Am. J. Cardiol. 25:344, 1970.
24. Medtronic, Chardac: Model 5943 implantable unipolar demand pulse generator. Minneapolis, Medtronic Inc., 1971.
25. Barold, S. S., and Gaidula, J. J.: Evaluation of normal and abnormal sensing functions of demand pacemakers. Am. J. Cardiol. 28:201, 1971.
26. Barold, S. S., and Gaidula, J. J.: Failure of demand pacemaker from low voltage bipolar electrogram. JAMA 215:923, 1971.
27. Barold, S. S., Gaidula, J. J., Lyon, J. L., and Carbol, M.: Irregular recycling of demand pacemaker from borderline electrographic signals. Am. Heart J. 87:477, 1971.
28. Barold, S. S., Pupillo, G. A., Gaidula, J. J., and Linhart, J. W.: Chest wall stimulation in evaluation of patients with implantable ventricular-inhibited pacemakers. Br. Heart J., 32:783, 1970.
29. Silverman, L. F., Mankin, H. T., and McGoon, D. C.: Surgical treatment of an inadequate sinus mechanism by implantation of a right atrial pacemaker electrode. J. Thorac. Cardiovasc. Surg. 55:264, 1968.
30. Harris, P. D., Malm, J. R., Bowman, F. O., Hoffman, B. F., Kaiser, G. A., and Singer, D. A.: Epicardial pacing to control arrhythmias following cardiac surgery. Circulation 37(Suppl. II):II-178, 1968.
31. Kastor, J. A., DeSanctis, R. W., Leinbach, R. L., Harthorne, J. W., and Wolfson, I. N.: Long term pervenous atrial pacing. Circulation 40:535, 1969.
32. Lister, J. W., Cohen, L. S., Hildner, F. J., Bernstein, W. H., Linhart, J. W., and Samet, P.: Electrical stimulation of the atria in patients with an intact conduction system. Ann. N.Y. Acad. Sci. 167:785, 1969.
33. DeSanctis, R. W.: Diagnostic and therapeutic uses of atrial pacing. Circulation 43:748, 1971.
34. Kramer, D. H., and Moss, A. J.: Permanent pervenous atrial pacing from the coronary vein. Circulation 42:427, 1970.
35. Nathan, D. A., Lister, J. W., Castillo, R., Keller, W., and Gosselin, A.: Current status of atrial pacing. Ann. Cardiol. Angeiol. 20:451, 1971.
36. Siddons, H.: Long term sequential and atrial ventricular pacing. Ann. Cardiol. Angeiol. 40:431, 1971.
37. Castillo, C. A., Berkovits, B. V., Castellanos, A., Jr., Lemberg, L., Callard, G., and Jude, J. R.: Bifocal demand pacing. Chest 59:360, 1971.
38. Castellanos, A., Jr., and Lemberg, L.: A Programmed Introduction to the Electrical Axis and Action Potential. Oldsmar, Fla., Tampa Tracings, 1974.
39. Lemberg, L. and Castellanos, A., Jr., Berkovits, B. V.: Pacemaking on demand in A-V block. JAMA 191:12, 1965.

Chapter 11
CARDIOPULMONARY RESUSCITATION

PAUL WALINSKY
EDWARD K. CHUNG

Sudden and unexpected cessation of effective cardiopulmonary performance is a cardiac emergency requiring immediate recognition and rapid and effective institution of measures to maintain delivery of oxygen to vital tissues and to reverse the initiating pathophysiologic derangements. Although the techniques of sustaining critical tissues and returning cardiac performance to a level adequate to sustain life are now universally practiced, they have been generally accepted and practiced only within the past 15 years.[1] Before that time, cardiac resuscitation was performed, if at all, primarily by thoracotomy with open chest cardiac massage. The demonstration by Kouwenhoven and associates[2] in 1960 of the effectiveness of closed-chest cardiac massage freed cardiac resuscitation from the requirement of proximity to trained surgical hands and made it possible for all appropriately trained physicians and paramedical personnel to successfully perform cardiac resuscitation.[2] Even before the demonstration of the efficacy of closed-chest cardiac massage, the development of an external alternating current cardiac defibrillator capable of reverting ventricular fibrillation to a normal rhythm was reported by Zoll and associates.[3] Since then, the DC defibrillator has been demonstrated to be the preferred mode of cardiac defibrillation[4] (see Chapter 9).

Appropriate utilization of these techniques has saved countless lives.

Perhaps the most important factor, aside from considerations related to the underlying etiology, in determining the outcome of a sudden cardiac catastrophe is the presence of personnel skilled in cardiac resuscitative techniques. Every physician, regardless of subspecialty or interest, should make the acquisition and maintenance of these skills an essential part of his training. Were all medical and paramedical personnel so trained, even more people could be successfully resuscitated.

ETIOLOGY OF CESSATION OF CARDIAC PERFORMANCE

The sudden and unexpected cessation of effective cardiac performance and cessation of spontaneous respiratory activity has many potential etiologies, but the primary causes are neurologic, pulmonary, and cardiovascular disorders. In a review of 552 patients in whom cardiopulmonary resuscitation was attempted, Johnson and co-workers demonstrated the etiology of the cardiovascular collapse to be coronary artery disease in 239 patients, respiratory failure in 55 patients, pulmonary embolism in 18 patients, Adams-Stokes syndrome in 11 patients, cardiomyopathy in 7 patients, reaction to angiography in 6 patients, and uremia in 32 patients.[5] The remainder, 184 patients, had cardiopulmonary collapse of various etiologies. Similar distributions of etiology have been reported by others.

The likelihood of recovery is determined by the underlying primary pathophysiologic derangements, even when immediate and effective cardiopulmonary resuscitation (CPR) is instituted. Although cardiovascular stability may be attained following anatomic damage, the phenomena most likely to be reversible are those associated with abnormal cardiac electrical events. However, it is often unclear what the initiating cardiac rhythm was, for by the time electrocardiographic monitoring becomes available there may have been a significant change in cardiac rhythm. When it can be determined, the nature of the cardiac arrhythmias causing cardiopulmonary collapse is found to be either a tachyarrhythmia or a bradyarrhythmia, ventricular tachycardia or fibrillation being the most common tachyarrhythmia and ventricular standstill the most common bradyarrhythmia. It is possible, but less common, for a rapid supraventricular tachyarrhythmia to cause cardiovascular collapse; likewise, a severe degree of bradyarrhythmia of various potential mechanisms may result in cardiovascular collapse.

The inciting cardiac arrhythmia may have disparate etiologies. Recent experience with cardiac care units has demonstrated a high incidence of such arrhythmia related to acute myocardial infarction or ischemia. However, catastrophic arrhythmia may develop de novo or in the presence of chronic, but self-limited, arrhythmia. Thus, chronic ventricular ectopic beats may be observed before the development of ventricular tachycardia and may be related to myocardial fibrosis, cardiomyopathy, click prolapse syndrome, electrolyte disturbance, or drug toxicity, particularly digitalis intoxication (see Chapter 15).

INDICATIONS

The indication for institution of CPR is the sudden cessation of effective cardiopulmonary performance and may be recognized by a loss of carotid and femoral pulses, heart tones, respirations, and the development of unconsciousness. The rapidity of recognition of such status often depends on a patient's location. Thus, in a cardiac or intensive care unit, where continuous monitoring is available, the need for CPR should be immediately recognized. In a general hospital bed, the recognition of cardiovascular collapse depends on the presence of medical personnel, who may be alerted by hospital personnel or visitors. In this setting, the recognition of cardiovascular catastrophe may be delayed by lack of an observer.

Outside the hospital, even more critical delays are encountered. It is unusual, indeed, for adequately trained personnel to be available for the emergency that occurs on the street, in the office, or at home. It is important, therefore, that those individuals recognized to be at high risk of developing serious cardiac arrhythmias or cardiac catastrophe be hospitalized under appropriate monitoring systems. The recent experience with precoronary care has been an attempt to decrease the incidence of arrhythmic death in myocardial infarction by ensuring that patients are monitored and thus can be treated as soon as possible following symptoms suggestive of myocardial infarction[6] (see Chapter 4).

ORGANIZATION

Cardiopulmonary resuscitation can be performed by one person, but may also be performed by a team if necessary. In the hospital setting, where a team is likely to be present, there must be a plan so that the individuals needed for CPR can be immediately summoned to the scene. There must be an organized effort in which one individual, the most senior and experienced member of the team, directs the entire procedure. The other members of the team should be assigned specific duties with which they are well acquainted. With appropriate organization, the greatest efficiency may be attained in the resuscitative efforts.

CANDIDATES

In whom should CPR be performed? This can be a difficult question, not readily resolved by strict categorization, because different philosophical views will be involved. In patients with incurable or terminal disease, such as terminal cancer patients, and patients with severe neurologic disturbances, particularly those involving loss of higher cortical function, CPR would seem to be inappropriate. CPR should primarily be aimed at the patient in whom restoration of cardiopulmonary stability will result in a potential for continued life and not perpetuation of preterminal agony or a vegetative existence. In the hospital setting if there is sufficient reason not to resuscitate a patient, this should be clearly noted as part of the orders, in order to prevent possible medicolegal problems. However, if the medical status of a patient is not known before cardiopulmonary collapse, it is best to proceed without hesitation.

INITIAL MEASURES AND TECHNIQUES

The goal of initial emergency measures is to maintain ventilation of the lungs and to deliver adequate amounts of oxygenated blood to tissues. These initial measures have been described as the ABC of therapy[7]: (A) clearing the airway, (B) instituting breathing, and (C) restoring circulation.

Because it has been reported that a direct blow to the sternum can revert ventricular fibrillation and tachycardia and cardiac asystole to normal sinus rhythm, it is appropriate to attempt this maneuver first; this should take only 1–2 seconds.[8–10] A forceful blow should be delivered to the sternum with the heel of the hand. It may be repeated once or twice if there is no response. If this maneuver is not successful one should immediately proceed to other measures required to support life.

Clearing the Airway

The first step, of securing an airway, is performed by placing the patient in a supine position (Fig. 11-1). One hand is placed behind the neck, and the other is placed on the forehead. The head is tilted back; this maneuver lifts the tongue from the back of the throat and results in an intrinsically unobstructed airway. At the same time, any obvious foreign body or obstruction in the mouth or nasal passages should be removed. These maneuvers alone may sometimes lead to a restoration of breathing and to recovery.

Institution of Ventilation

Institution of ventilation may be performed by a variety of techniques, including mouth-to-mouth, mouth-to-nose, mouth-to-oral or nasal airway, and bag-and-mask. With the *mouth-to-mouth technique,* the resuscitator maintains the backward tilt of the head with one hand, and the

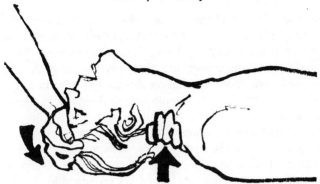

Figure 11-1. Head tilt method of opening airway. (Reprinted with permission from *Journal of the American Medical Association.*[1])

other hand pinches the nostrils closed. The mouth is placed over the patient's mouth with complete seal so that there is no leak of air. At end inspiration, the resuscitator exhales a larger than normal breath into the patient's mouth. If appropriately performed, one should note a rise in the patient's chest as intrathoracic volume is increased. There should be no loss of air through the nose or mouth as the lungs are being inflated. Following inflation of the lungs, the resuscitator should remove his mouth, allowing exhalation to occur. Following a successful inflation, one should hear air escaping.

The *mouth-to-nose technique* may also be used with the patient in the supine position and with backward head tilt maintained with one

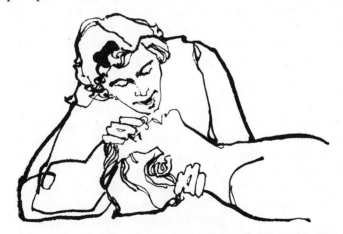

Figure 11-2. Mouth-to-mouth resuscitation. (Reprinted with permission from *Journal of the American Medical Association.*[1])

hand. With the other hand the jaw is closed and the mouth is sealed. The resuscitator places his mouth over the patient's nose and following a deep inhalation again exhales through the patient's nose. The indications of a successful maneuver are the same as those described for mouth-to-mouth technique. Ventilation should be performed at the rate of 12 per minute whether the mouth-to-mouth or the mouth-to-nose technique is used.

If there is resistance to inflation of the lungs when either of these techniques is used, a foreign body in the airway should be suspected. In this case, the patient should be rolled onto his side, and firm blows should be delivered over the spine between the shoulder blades in an attempt to dislodge the foreign body. The patient's mouth and oropharynx should then be explored for a foreign body. These maneuvers should be repeated if there is continued evidence of a foreign body.

Vomiting may have occurred at some time in the course of events. Therefore, it is imperative that adequately functioning suction equipment be readily available. Gastric distention is best managed by insertion of an indwelling nasogastric tube. If this equipment is not available, however, it may be corrected by pressure over the epigastrium. Recurrence of gastric distention may be prevented by intermittent epigastric pressure. Caution must be exercised with this maneuver since it may induce reflex of gastric contents.

The first two steps of CPR relate to the institution of ventilation. They may be performed in any setting, even by a single individual. In the hospital setting, where more help and more facilities may be available, there may be some modifications, but the basic approach is the same. In the hospital, a *bag-and-mask technique* may be utilized instead of either of the expired-air techniques. The prime advantages of this technique are that oxygen may be added to the intake and that it is aesthetically less distressing to some physicians.

Restoration of Circulation

The final step of the initial resuscitative measures is the institution of *cardiac massage*. Except when the patient is already in the operating room or where chest wounds may preclude it, there is virtually no situation where one would not perform closed-chest cardiac massage rather than open-chest massage.[7]

In order for *closed-chest cardiac massage* to be effective, the patient's back must be on a firm surface. If he is in bed, a hard board placed under the back will be sufficient. The resuscitator should be at the patient's side. The heel of one hand should be placed over the lower third of the sternum (but not on the xyphoid process). Except for the heel,

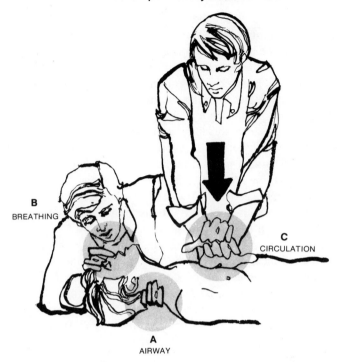

Figure 11-3. Two-rescuer cardiopulmonary resuscitation. (Reprinted with permission from *Journal of the American Medical Association.*[7])

that hand should not be in contact with the chest. The other hand may rest on the first hand. The sternum is then depressed $1\frac{1}{2}$–2 inches (approximately one fifth of the AP thickness). The heart, encased in the pericardiac sac, is compressed between the sternum and spine, and blood is ejected through the aorta. The pressure should be smooth and uninterrupted. Following compression, the sternum should be released and the hand readied for the next compression. The duration of chest compression should approximately equal the duration of relaxation. How effective is closed-chest cardiac massage? Although cardiac output has been demonstrated to be quite low during cardiac massage,[11] a significant improvement in EEG pattern has been documented.[12] Thus, the goal of maintaining the viability of vital tissue may be achieved with cardiac massage.

The rate of compression should be approximately 60 per minute. Although it is not an ideal measure of the efficiency of closed-chest cardiac massage, palpation of peripheral pulses following chest compression may provide a rough guide. If an indwelling arterial line is present, the contour of the pressure pulse obtained may be of value in assessing the efficiency of the chest compression.

Although cardiac massage is a safe procedure, one must not be overly vigorous in sternal compression, particularly in children. Reported complications, primarily caused by inappropriate application of cardiac massage techniques, include fractures of the ribs and sternum, hemothorax, hemopericardium, pneumothorax, bone marrow emboli, gastric rupture, lacerations of the spleen and liver, and rupture of the aorta.[13]

It is to be emphasized that both lung ventilation and cardiac compression must be performed in coordination. If either phase is lacking, resuscitative efforts will be doomed to failure. If only one resuscitator is present, it is recommended that fifteen chest compressions be performed, followed by two quick lung ventilations. If two or more resuscitators are present, every fifth chest compression should be followed by a lung inflation.

A number of mechanical devices, some manual and some automatic, are available for closed-chest cardiac massage. In the hands of trained individuals, they may make cardiac massage easier and facilitate resuscitative efforts. They should never be utilized by inexperienced personnel, whose misapplication of these devices may result only in ineffective resuscitation.

Evaluation of Success

During these emergency measures one must monitor several signs that may yield an indication of the success or failure of one's efforts. These parameters are essentially those which were the initial signs of cardiovascular collapse: the presence or absence of pulses in the femoral or carotid arteries, of heart tones, of spontaneous respiratory efforts, and any change in neurologic status. If there is evidence that resuscitative efforts have been successful, one may stop and observe for several seconds. If a reversal of cardiovascular collapse has been achieved, the patient should continue to be closely observed and the etiology of the episode be determined. If however, there is no change in status, then artificial ventilation and cardiac massage must be continued, while further, more sophisticated diagnostic and therapeutic approaches are sought. During this period cardiac massage and ventilation must be continuous and should not be halted for longer than 5 seconds.

SECONDARY MEASURES

If there is no response to the initial resuscitative measures, there are a number of secondary diagnostic and therapeutic measures that should be performed while artificial support is continued. If the patient is not known to the resuscitating team, the chart should be quickly reviewed to extract any relevant information. An electrocardiogram should be taken in order to assess the cardiac rhythm and to evaluate the possibility of any abnormality, such as myocardial infarction, pulmonary embolism, electrolyte imbalance, or digitalis intoxication. An arterial blood gas sample should be obtained to assess acid–base balance and the adequacy of ventilation. Venous or arterial blood should be drawn for the determination of serum electrolytes. An intravenous infusion site should be established. When these steps have been taken, further therapeutic intervention may be instituted.

Determination of cardiac rhythm is based on either a conventional electrocardiogram or an oscilloscopic monitored tracing. Various cardiac arrhythmias, with appropriate therapeutic intervention, are described below.[14]

Ventricular Fibrillation

Ventricular fibrillation and tachycardia have been reported to respond to a sharp precardial blow to the sternum.[8,9] However, this maneuver is usually unsuccessful. An immediate attempt at electrical cardioversion should be made with any standard DC defibrillator. Because of the urgency of the situation, the current delivered should be the maximum the defibrillator can deliver, usually 400 Wsec. The electrode paddles should be well coated with either saline or electrode gel and firm contact should be made between skin and paddles. The paddles may be applied to either anterior and posterior chest or diagonally across the anterior chest wall alone.

Following discharge of the defibrillator, an immediate assessment of cardiac rhythm is required. If ventricular fibrillation persists, a second DC shock may be applied. If a second DC shock is unsuccessful, the type of fibrillatory wave should be determined. If fine fibrillatory waves are present, they may be made coarser and of higher amplitude by administration of epinephrine (0.2–1.0 cc of a 1 to 1,000 dilution, i.e. 200–1,000 μg) either by intravenous or intracardiac injection. Calcium chloride (10 cc intravenous or intracardiac) may have a similar effect on the amplitude of the fibrillation waves. A word of caution must be heeded regarding intracardiac injections. It is important to demonstrate by aspirating blood into the syringe that the needle tip is in a cardiac chamber. Injection into the myocardium may precipitate intractable ventricular tachycardia or fibrillation. Following the development of higher-amplitude fibrillation waves, electrical cardioversion should be repeated.

Attempts at defibrillation should be repeated if initial attempts are unsuccessful. Correction of acidosis may enhance the possibility of cardioversion. Direct current shock is described in detail in Chapter 9.

Ventricular Tachycardia

Ventricular tachycardia may be the underlying cardiac rhythm or it may be noted before deterioration to ventricular fibrillation. Attempts should be made to electrically convert to a sinus rhythm as with ventricular fibrillation. Appropriate pharmacologic agents (see Chapter 7) should also be administered in the presence of ventricular tachycardia. The agent of choice is lidocaine (Xylocaine). It should be given as an initial bolus of 100 mg intravenously. At the same time, an intravenous infusion should be started at a rate of administration of 2–5 mg/min. If ventricular tachycardia persists or recurs, repeated boluses of 100 mg should be given, up to a total of 300–400 mg. If ventricular tachycardia is refractory to lidocaine, procaine amide (Pronestyl) may be administered in intravenous boluses of 100 mg administered slowly. A procaine amide drip of 2–4 mg/min may likewise be instituted if ventricular irritability persists. Other agents that may be effective for persistent ventricular tachycardia include quinidine, propranolol (Inderal) and bretylium tosylate. Diphenylhydantoin (Dilantin) is the drug of choice for digitalis-induced ventricular tachycardia (see Chapter 15). Overdrive pacing with a ventricular pacemaker may sometimes be effective in refractory ventricular tachycardia (see Chapter 10).

Supraventricular Tachyarrhythmias

In elderly patients with underlying impairment of cardiovascular performance, a rapid supraventricular tachycardia may be sufficient to cause profound hypotension and cardiovascular collapse. If a profound degree of cardiovascular decompensation is caused by this arrhythmia, DC cardioversion is appropriate. If, however, in the presence of such arrhythmia there is no evidence of lack of organ perfusion, no significant neurologic change, and an adequate blood pressure, one may use appropriate pharmacologic agents that may require a modest period of time to take effect. Such agents include digitalis, propranolol, and quinidine. It is of interest that, on a number of occasions, a rhythm that on rapid inspection during emergency circumstances has been interpreted as ventricular tachycardia and has been treated with lidocaine has, on closer analysis, been found to be a supraventricular tachycardia with aberrant ventricular conduction. It should be remembered that lidocaine has little or no effect on atrial tachyarrhythmias (see Chapter 7).

Bradyarrhythmias

Mild sinus bradycardia may respond to atropine 0.3 to 1.0 mg intravenously. The more profound sinus bradycardias associated with hypotension, second-degree or complete AV block with slow ventricular rate, and hypotension or complete cardiac asystole are more ominous rhythms and are initially approached in the same manner. The initial pharmacologic maneuver with these arrhythmias should be administration of a chronotropic agent, either epinephrine 100 μg or isoproterenol 100 μg intravenously. The choice of agent may depend on whether one would prefer the accompanying vasoconstricting effect of epinephrine or the vasodilating effect of isoproterenol. If 100 μg of epinephrine or isoproterenol is not successful in restoring cardiac rhythm, a drip of epinephrine or isoproterenol may be instituted. At the same time, repeated boluses of larger doses of isoproterenol or epinephrine (200–1,000 μg) may be administered intravenously. If these are not effective, 1 mg of epinephrine or isoproterenol may be given by intracardiac injection. The administration of calcium chloride by intravenous or intracardiac injection may have a synergistic chronotropic effect. During administration of these potent chronotropic agents, one must watch carefully for any signs of ventricular irritability. When ventricular irritability is observed, dosage of these agents should be reduced. If an inadequate ventricular response persists in spite of pharmacologic stimulation, one must consider the insertion of an artificial pacemaker electrode. This may be accomplished via cutdown on a medial vein in the antecubital fossa and blind advancement of a standard bipolar electrode catheter. This technique, however, has a significant incidence of failure if there is no fluoroscopic guidance. Alternatively, there are several commercially available pacing catheters that may be inserted directly into the heart by thoracic puncture. Once adequate electrode contact is made, pacing should be instituted (see Chapter 10).

If sinus rhythm is restored or is present initially, attention must be directed to ensuring adequate perfusion. Palpation of the carotid or femoral pulses may be utilized as a gross indication of cardiac mechanical activity. The level of cuff blood pressure or directly monitored intraarterial blood pressure is, of course, a more satisfactory measure of cardiac performance. If there is no mechanical activity associated with sinus rhythm or if hypotension is present, pharmacologic stimulation with an inotropic agent is required. Additionally, a vasoconstrictor is often required to obtain a high enough head of pressure to perfuse the brain and myocardium. Epinephrine, which has inotropic, chronotropic, and peripheral constrictive effects, is an ideal agent in this circumstance. It may be administered as a 500–1,000-μg intravenous bolus. An epinephrine drip of 2–8 μg min should also be started. Other inotropic agents that may be of value include isoproterenol, norepinephrine, dopamine, metaraminol, and calcium chloride. Isoproterenol may be given as a bolus of 100–300 μg and then administered as a drip of 1–4 μg/minute. Isoproterenol may be of value in situations where vasodilation is desirable. Norepinephrine is of value where profound vasoconstriction is desirable; it also has a moderate chronotropic effect. Dopamine produces inotropic stimulation while causing only a modest decrease in peripheral resistance, but its most significant attribute is its production of an increase in renal blood flow.[15] Metaraminol possesses modest chronotropic and inotropic effects as well as peripheral vasodilation. Calcium chloride may be administered as an intravenous bolus along with the above agents and may act synergistically following administration of the other sympathomimetic agents.

Other sympathomimetic agents that cause vasoconstriction alone are sometimes required. Phenylephrine, methoxamine, and mephentermine have little or no inotropic or chronotropic effect and may be of value in the presence of hypotension and vasodilation, particularly if there is associated ventricular irritability.

OTHER THERAPEUTIC MEASURES

Ventilation

If continued resuscitative efforts are required following the initial institution of artificial ventilation, consideration should be given to insertion of an endotracheal or nasotracheal tube. Such a tube permits more effective pulmonary expansion, administration of oxygen in high concentration, and removal of secretions or vomitus from the bronchi by suction. Although such an airway is desirable, it should be inserted only by someone who can do so quickly. It should not be inserted by a novice whose fumbling efforts may stop resuscitation for a prolonged period. Following insertion of a tracheal airway, the cuff should be inflated. This will prevent any further aspiration of vomitus. Ventilation should continue to be manual and co-ordinated with cardiac massage. Self-triggering ventilators should not be used unless they are fully co-ordinated with cardiac massage. The adequacy of ventilation should be determined by serial assessment of arterial blood gases.

Treatment of Acidosis

Metabolic acidosis occurs as a result of inadequate tissue perfusion and oxygenation. Respiratory acidosis occurs if there is significant underlying pulmonary disease, airway obstruction, or inadequate artificial ventilation. If resuscitative efforts can be initiated without any delay, there may be only minimal metabolic acidosis. The best way to assess the need for bicarbonate replacement is to sample arterial blood to determine pH, HCO_3^-, pCO_2, and pO_2. Acidosis and elevated pCO_2 and a normal or slightly decreased HCO_3^- indicate respiratory acidosis. In this case, bicarbonate replacement will not be of major value, and more effective ventilation is required.[16] If, however, acidosis is accompanied by a normal pCO_2 and a decrease in bicarbonate metabolic acidosis is present bicarbonate should be administered with serial determination of arterial blood gas to assess the efficacy of treatment and continuing needs. If arterial blood gas values cannot be determined, it is difficult to assess the need for bicarbonate. Several regimens are prescribed in the literature as guides to bicarbonate therapy.[17,18] Sodium bicarbonate should be given if arrest is longer than 1 minute. The initial amount will be 100 cc (89.2 mEq) $NaHCO_3$ followed by 50 cc every 10 minutes. It is important to correct acidosis because it decreases cardiac and peripheral responses to catecholamines, lowers the threshold of ventricular fibrillation, and may induce cardiac asystole.

Electrolytes

Significant derangements of serum electrolytes may lead to cardiac arrhythmias. Either hyperkalemia or hypokalemia may cause various cardiac arrhythmias, including ventricular irritability. In particular, hypokalemia frequently predisposes to digitalis-induced arrhythmias (see Chapter 15). Serum electrolytes should be determined, and appropriate replacement therapy is essential.

ABANDONMENT OF CARDIOPULMONARY RESUSCITATION

There are two reasons to terminate resuscitative efforts. The first is inability to restore appropriate cardiac rhythm and adequate pump performance. The second is evidence of severe and irreversible cerebral damage. Resuscitative efforts should be continued until all potential means of restoring cardiopulmonary stability have been attempted. If at that point the heart appears unable to maintain an adequate rhythm and mechanical performance, resuscitation should be terminated.

Determination of the severity of neurologic damage is often difficult and can be a medicolegal dilemma. However, severe neurologic damage is suggested by unconsciousness, lack of spontaneous movement, lack of spontaneous respiration, and pupillary dilatation without response to light and "boxcarring" of the retinal vessels. Although these are not absolute signs of permanent neurologic impairment, they are suggestive of severe, potentially irreversible damage and point toward discontinuation of CPR.

CARE AFTER CARDIOPULMONARY RESUSCITATION

Following successful cardiopulmonary resuscitation, assessment of the initial etiology and recognition of any persistent risk factors are essential. If any premonitory abnormalities of cardiac rhythm are present, they should be treated prophylactically. If there is evidence of myocardial infarction, assessment of hemodynamic status and cardiac rhythm should be continued in a cardiac care unit. If there is evidence of pulmonary insufficiency, careful attention should be directed to assuring adequacy of ventilation by monitoring blood gases. If pulmonary embolism is suspected, the patient must be anticoagulated with heparin (see Chapter 2).

A complete assessment of the degree of recovery should be part of post-CPR care. Particular attention should be directed to the patient's neurologic status. If cerebral edema is suspected, intravenous dexamethasone should be given, 10 mg initially and 4 mg every 12 hr for 3 to 6 days.

All patients who have survived CPR should be observed for several weeks to ensure their stability. During this time emergency resuscitative facilities must be immediately available should they be required.

RESULTS OF CARDIOPULMONARY RESUSCITATION

Many factors determine the success of CPR. The speed with which CPR is instituted and the underlying etiology causing cardiopulmonary collapse are of major importance in determining ultimate recovery. The best survival statistics seem to occur in coronary artery disease, cardiomyopathy, pulmonary embolism, and respiratory insufficiency.[5] Although one would expect the best results to be noted in an intensive or coronary care unit because of the constant attention given to the patients, this has actually not been noted.[19] Because only the sickest patients are in the intensive care unit, survival has been found to be as good, if not better, in a well-staffed medical ward, where patients are generally less acutely ill.

There is no universal agreement as to the rhythm disturbance that is most amenable to CPR. However, most reviews of CPR results indicate that ventricular fibrillation is more amenable than asystole to reversion. Age and sex have not been found to be major determinants of success in CPR.

Survival figures vary from series to series and are difficult to compare because of different criteria of inclusion and different criteria of success.[19-22] However, a majority of studies have demonstrated that 4–15%

of patients who undergo CPR are discharged from the hospital. However, there are few long-term studies of CPR survivors once they have left the hospital; also lacking is some assessment of the quality of the life that has been preserved.

SUMMARY

Unexpected cardiopulmonary collapse is a medical emergency requiring immediate institution of artificial measures to support life and to reverse the initiating pathophysiologic event. In order to approach this problem efficiently, one must have a predetermined plan that can be implemented on a moment's notice. The initial goals of CPR are to establish an open airway, to institute artificial breathing, and to restore circulation. If these measures do not result in immediate recovery, assessment of cardiac rhythm, cardiac pump performance, ventilatory adequacy, acid–base balance, and serum electrolytes is required. The primary therapeutic modalities are DC defibrillation, intervention to restore normal sinus rhythm and normal blood pressure, and restoration of normal oxygenation and acid–base balance. If CPR is successful, continued surveillance of the patient is required for complete assessment and for immediate intervention if cardiopulmonary collapse recurs. Successful resuscitation, as defined by hospital discharge, has been reported in various series to occur in 4–15% of all patients in whom CPR is initiated.

Detailed descriptions of antiarrhythmic therapy, direct current shock, and artificial pacemakers are found elsewhere in this book (see Chapters 7, 8, 9, and 10).

REFERENCES

1. Kouwenhoven, W. B.: The development of the defibrillator. Ann. Intern. Med. 71:449, 1969.
2. Kouwenhoven, W. B., Ing, Jude, J. R., and Knickerbocker, G. G.: Closed-chest cardiac massage. JAMA 173:94, 1960.
3. Zoll, P. M., Paul, M. H., Linenthal, A. J., Norman, L. R., and Gibson, W.: The effects of external electric currents on the heart. Circulation 14:745, 1956.
4. Lown, B., Neuman, J., Amarasingham, R., and Berkovits, B. V.: Comparison of alternating current with direct current electroshock across the closed chest. Am. J. Cardiol. 10:223, 1962.
5. Johnson, A. L., Tanser, P. H., Ulan, R. A., and Wood, T. E.: Results of cardiac resuscitation in 552 patients. Am. J. Cardiol. 20:831, 1967.
6. Pantridge, J. F., and Geddes, J. S.: A mobile intensive-care unit in the management of myocardial infarction. Lancet ii:271, 1967.
7. Standards for cardiopulmonary resuscitation (CPR) and emergency cardiac care (ECC). JAMA 227(Suppl.):833, 1974.
8. Harwood-Nash, D. C. F.: Thumping of the precordium in ventricular fibrillation. S. Afr. Med. J. 36:280, 1962.
9. Pennington, J. E., Taylor, J., and Lown, B.: Chest thump for reverting ventricular tachycardia. N. Engl. J. Med. 283:1192, 1970.

10. Scharf, D., and Bonnemann, C.: Thumping of the precordium in ventricular standstill. Am. J. Cardiol. 5:30, 1960.
11. Del Guercio, L. R. M., Coomaraswamy, R. P., and State, D.: Cardiac output and other hemodynamic variables during external cardiac massage in man. N. Engl. J. Med. 269:1399, 1963.
12. Pappelbaum, S., Lang, T., Bazika, V., Bernstein, H., Harrold, G., and Corday, E.: Comparative hemodynamics during open vs. closed cardiac resuscitation. JAMA 193:93, 1965.
13. Nelson, D., and Ashley, P. F.: Rupture of the aorta during closed-chest cardiac massage. JAMA 193:115, 1965.
14. Zoll, P. M.: Rational use of drugs for cardiac arrest and after cardiac resuscitation. Am. J. Cardiol. 27:645, 1971.
15. Goldberg, L. I.: Use of sympathomimetic amines in heart failure. Am. J. Cardiol. 22:177, 1968.
16. Chazan, J. A., Stenson, R., and Kurland, G. S.: The acidosis of cardiac arrest. N. Engl. J. Med. 278:360, 1968.
17. Gilston, A., and Leeds, M. B.: Clinical and biochemical aspects of cardiac resuscitation. Lancet ii:1039, 1965.
18. Goldberg, A. H.: Cardiopulmonary arrest. N. Engl. J. Med. 290:381, 1974.
19. Hollingsworth, J. H.: The results of cardiopulmonary resuscitation. A 3-year university hospital experience. Ann. Intern. Med., 71:459, 1969.
20. Saphir, R.: External cardiac massage. Prospective analysis of 123 cases and review of the literature. Medicine 47:73, 1968.
21. Linko, E., Koskinen, P. J., Siitonen, L., and Ruosteenoja, R.: Resuscitation in cardiac arrest. An analysis of 100 successful medical cases. Acta Med. Scand. 182:611, 1967.
22. Wildsmith, J. A. W., Dennyson, W. G., and Myers, K. W.: Results of resuscitation following cardiac arrest. Br. J. Anaesth. 44:716, 1972.

Chapter 12
INFECTIOUS HEART DISEASE

ALBERT S. KLAINER

Infectious diseases involving the three basic anatomic compartments of the heart—the pericardium, the myocardium, and the endocardium—uncommonly present as acute emergencies that necessitate the immediate institution of therapy without affording the physician time to obtain the information necessary for an adequate presumptive or definitive diagnosis. Some, such as *acute* bacterial endocarditis, require urgent attention in that they will need to be treated before culture results are available. In contrast, more slowly progressive infections, such as subacute bacterial endocarditis, allow the luxury of time to obtain specific bacteriologic information to aid the physician in making the correct diagnosis and choosing the proper therapy. Still others, such as viral infections, should not be treated because there are no effective drugs available. In other words, there is no parallel in infectious heart disease to the immediate urgency precipitated by such entities as the acute, potentially fatal arrhythmias, e.g. ventricular tachycardia or fibrillation. It is imperative, then, that any discussion of infectious heart disease be preceded by the admonition that the diagnostic and therapeutic approach to infections primarily or secondarily involving the heart be accomplished in an orderly, rational manner based upon clinical judgment and that therapy be instituted only when the available evidence suggests that a treatable disease is present.

Infectious diseases involve the heart in two basic ways: (1) the pericardium, myocardium, and endocardium, together or separately, may be the site of primary infection or of infection resulting from bacteremia or contiguous spread from surrounding structures; (2) the heart may be affected not by infection *per se* but by hemodynamic abnormalities resulting from extracardiac infection, especially septic shock.

In this chapter, an attempt will be made to provide the physician with a practical, orderly approach to the diagnosis and treatment of infection involving the heart as well as noncardiac infection that ultimately affects the heart via a variety of pathophysiologic events.

PERICARDITIS

Pericarditis is an inflammatory state involving the parietal and/or visceral pericardium, including the pericardial space. Diseases of the pericardium usually do not affect heart function unless tamponade or constrictive pericarditis develops to cause restriction of ventricular filling or unless cardiac arrhythmias occur. (See Chapter 13 for a complete discussion of pericardial tamponade.)

Almost any infectious agent may result in pericarditis (Table 12-1), but, since a myriad of noninfectious diseases also may affect the pericar-

Table 12-1   *Etiology of Pericarditis*

Infectious
Bacterial
Staphylococcus aureus
Diplococcus pneumoniae
Streptococcus pyogenes
Neisseria meningitidis, N. gonorrheae
Haemophilus influenzae
Salmonella
Coliforms
Mycobacterium tuberculosis
Viral
Coxsackie A,B
ECHO
Adenoviruses
Influenza
Infectious mononucleosis
Varicella
Mumps
Rubeola
Fungal
Histoplasma
Coccidioides
Blastomyces
Aspergilli
Rickettsial
Typhus
Q fever

Table 12-1   (Continued)

Other
   Actinomyces
   Nocardia
   Psittacosis–lymphogranuloma venereum group
   Echinococci
   Amoebae
   Toxoplasma
   Trypanosomes
Noninfectious
   Acute rheumatic fever
   Collagen disorders
      Systemic lupus erythematosus
      Rheumatoid arthritis
      Scleroderma
      Polyarteritis nodosa
   Hypersensitivity reactions
      Postbacterial infections
      Drugs (hydralazine, procainamide)
      Serum sickness
      Allergic vasculitis
   Neoplastic
      Primary
         Benign (Lipoma, Fibroma, Angioma)
         Malignant (Mesothelioma, Sarcoma)
      Metastatic
         Lymphoma, leukemia
         Carcinoma (breast, lung, pancreas, ovary, esophagus)
         Thymoma
         Undifferentiated carcinomas
   Other
      Uremia
      Myxedema
      Myocardial infarction (post-MI syndrome)
      Trauma
      Postcardiotomy syndrome
      Radiation
      Rupture of aortic aneurysm into pericardium
      Chylopericardium
  Acute idiopathic or nonspecific pericarditis

dium, a differential diagnosis is necessary if proper therapy is to be instituted. In infectious pericarditis, involvement of the heart may occur via the blood or by contiguous spread of infection of neighboring structures, such as pneumonia and mediastinitis.

Signs and Symptoms

The signs and symptoms of pericarditis (Table 12-2) can be arbitrarily divided into those due to inflammation, effusion, tamponade (if it occurs), and constriction. Pain is usually sudden in onset; although

Table 12-2   *Clinical Features of Acute Pericarditis*

Chest pain
  Precordial
  Increased by lying flat
  Decreased by sitting up and bending forward
  May be referred to neck, shoulders, upper arms
Pericardial friction rub
Ewart's sign if pericardial effusion is present
Low pulse pressure, paradoxical pulse if large effusion or tamponade present
Cardiac arrhythmias may be present (paroxysmal supraventricular tachycardia,
    premature contractions, atrial flutter or fibrillation, especially if myocarditis
    present)
Heart sounds distant or muffled if effusion present
Chest x-ray showing normal heart (enlarged if effusion present)
ECG
  Elevation of S–T segments
  T-wave inversion
  S–T segment vector points toward apex
  T vector tends to point upward and to the right shoulder
  S–T and T changes may change from day to day; S–T segment alterations usu-
    ally disappear with clinical improvement; T-wave inversions may persist.

---

it is the most common symptom, it may be absent. It is usually severe and may mimic myocardial infarction. It is precordial in nature; it is made worse by lying flat, relieved by sitting up and leaning forward, and may be referred to the neck, shoulders, and upper arms. If pleuropericarditis is present, the pain may be pleuritic in nature and aggravated by deep inspiration. If tamponade or constriction occurs, right upper quadrant, epigastric, and abdominal pain may result from congestion.

Signs and symptoms of congestive heart failure are usually absent unless tamponade or constriction is present. Ewart's sign is not diagnostic but is common in patients with large pericardial effusions; this sign consists of an area of dullness in the region of the inferior angle of the left scapula and is accompanied by bronchial breathing, whispered pectoriloquy, and egophony; these findings are due to compression of the lung and bronchi by the accumulating pericardial fluid, which forces the heart and great vessels backward.

Pulse pressure may be low in the presence of tamponade or constriction; a paradoxical pulse may be elicited. Cardiac arrhythmias, especially paroxysmal supraventricular tachycardia, premature contractions, atrial flutter, or fibrillation may occur, especially if myocarditis accompanies pericarditis. Jugular venous pressure is elevated when tamponade or constriction alters ventricular filling. Heart sounds are distant and muffled in the presence of a significant effusion. In constrictive pericarditis, a "pericardial knock," an early diastolic sound, may be heard. The pericardial friction rub is diagnostic of pericarditis. It may be diffuse or localized, persistent or transitory. It may persist or disappear with the development of a significant pericardial effusion. Classically, the rub consists of three components: (1) that caused by ventricular systole (this component may sound like a click and occurs in early, middle, or late systole or may occupy all of systole); (2) that coinciding with ventricular diastole occurring during early diasystole or mid-diastole; and (3) a presystolic component due to atrial contraction. Characteristically, all three components blend to cause the usual to-and-fro sound.

Diagnosis and Therapy

Clinical evaluation of the patient with pericarditis is outlined in Table 12-3. The basic responsibility of the physician is to decide, using all available data, whether an infectious etiology exists, and if so, whether it is treatable. Since viral pericarditis is most common, the large majority of patients with acute pericarditis need not be given specific therapy. On the other hand, every effort must be made to determine whether treatable infection exists, especially in acute bacterial pericarditis; if so, the appropriate antimicrobial agent should be administered. Therefore, any approach to the diagnosis of pericarditis must include a careful history and physical examination and those laboratory tests (Table 12-3) necessary to define the presence of pericarditis and the most probable

Table 12-3 *Clinical Evaluation of the Patient with Acute Pericarditis*

1. History and physical examination
2. ECG to document changes of acute pericarditis and examine for presence of (a) Q waves and reciprocal changes to suggest acute myocardial infarction and (b) AV block suggestive of acute rheumatic fever
3. Chest x-ray for heart size and silhouette and for presence of evidence for bacterial pneumonia, TB, fungus disease, neoplasm
4. Hb, Hct, WBC, differential to evaluate possibility of leukemia, lymphoma, or other blood dyscrasia
5. Urinalysis
6. LE preps, antinuclear antibody, rheumatoid factor, appropriate serologies available for the common infectious agents (acute and convalescent sera 2 to 4 weeks later should be obtained)
7. PPD, histoplasma skin tests
8. ASLO titer
9. Serum creatinine to exclude uremia
10. Thyroid function tests to exclude myxedema
11. Blood, throat, sputum, urine, stool cultures to evaluate for presence of possible etiologic infectious agents
12. Pericardiocentesis for cell count, differential, protein, sugar (to be compared to simultaneous blood sugar), gram stain, acid-fast stain, cultures (for aerobes, anaerobes, fungi, mycobacteria), viral studies, cytology
13. Consider open pericardial biopsy for culture and histology

Table 12-4   *Characteristics of Pericardial Fluids*

	Suppurative	Viral	Tuberculous	Rheumatic	Neoplastic
Cells	Many (polymorpho-nuclear leukocytes, RBC)	Moderate no. (lymphocytes, RBC)	Moderate no. (lymphocytes, RBC)	Moderate no. (polymorphonuclear leukocytes, RBC)	Moderate no. (mixed cells, RBC)
Specific gravity	>1.016	Usually <1.016	>1.016	>1.016	>1.016
Protein	>3.0 g	Usually <3.0 g	>3.0 g	Usually >3.0 g	Usually >3.0 g
Stains for micro-organisms	Etiologic agent may or may not be seen	Negative	Occasionally seen by acid-fast stain	Negative	Negative
Routine culture	May or may not be positive	Negative (virus isolation possible)	Cultures for mycobacteria may be positive	Negative	Negative
Cytology	Negative	Negative	Negative	Negative	Positive

cause for it. Specific diagnosis most commonly rests on diagnostic procedures not involving the pericardium. Appropriate cultures of the throat,
nasopharynx, sputum, and blood should be obtained in search of an
etiologic agent. If these tests are unrewarding and the illness is not self-
limited but progressive, pericardiocentesis and pericardial biopsy will
be necessary. If pericardial fluid is obtained (Table 12-4), gram-stain,
stain for acid-fast bacteria, and culture may provide sufficient evidence
for a presumptive and definitive diagnosis. A pericardial biopsy will be
of additional help for histologic examination as well as culture. Depending upon the most likely etiology, therapy may or may not need to be
instituted as outlined in Table 12-5.

Idiopathic benign pericarditis is a common but inexact term suggesting the lack of an absolute diagnosis. It should not be used synono-
mously with viral pericarditis, a term that should be used for cases of

Table 12-5   *Suggested Specific Antimicrobial Therapy for
Acute Pericarditis*[a]

Bacterial
   Staphylococcus aureus (penicillin-sensitive)
      1.   Aqueous penicillin G: 2.0×10^6 U IV q̄ 4 hr $\times$ 14–28 d.[b]
      2.   In the penicillin-allergic patient: Clindamycin 900 mg IV q̄ 8 hr $\times$ 14–28 d.
   Staphylococcus aureus (penicillin-resistant[c])
      1.   Semisynthetic penicillin (penicillinase-resistant), e.g. methicillin 2.0 g IV
          q̄ 4 hr $\times$ 14–28 d.
      2.   Cephalothin 2.0 g IV q̄ 4 hr $\times$ 14–28 d.
      3.   Clindamycin 900 mg IV q̄ 8 hr $\times$ 14–28 d.
   Diplococcus pneumoniae and *Streptococcus pyogenes*
      1.   Aqueous penicillin G: 2.0×10^6 U IV q̄ 4 hr $\times$ 14–28 d.
      2.   In the penicillin-allergic patient: Clindamycin 900 mg IV q̄ 8 hr $\times$ 14–28 d.
   Neisseria meningitidis, N. gonorrheae
      1.   Aqueous penicillin G: 2.0×10^6 U IV q̄ 4 hr $\times$ 14–28 d.
      2.   In the penicillin-allergic patient: Chloramphenicol 1.0 g IV q̄ 6 hr $\times$
          14–28 d.
   Salmonella: Chloramphenicol 1.0 g IV q̄ 6 hr $\times$ 14–28 d.
   Mycobacterium tuberculosis: Isoniazid, ethambutol, and streptomycin
Viral: None
Fungal: Amphotericin B
Rickettsial
      1.   Chloramphenicol 1.0 g IV q̄ 6 hr $\times$ 10–14 d. or
      2.   Tetracycline 500 mg q̄ 6 hr $\times$ 10–14 d.
Other types of infectious pericarditis should be treated with antimicrobial agents
   known to be effective by sensitivity testing.

---

   [a] There are a variety of therapeutic regimens that are acceptable; those noted
are the author's preferences
   [b] The duration of therapy is dictated by clinical response; the author feels that
a minimum of 2 weeks' therapy is necessary
   [c] Until sensitivities are available, all staphylococci should be considered to be
penicillin-resistant

proven viral etiology. Idiopathic pericarditis apparently is just a waste-basket term encompassing many types of pericarditis for which no etiology has been found. Many cases are probably due to undetected or undiagnosed viral infection; however, other causes may also produce this picture. Proper management necessitates a careful search for the etiologic agent, and this term should be used only when no agent can be found; pericardial biopsy is particularly necessary before the label of "idiopathic" should be applied. Although the course is usually benign, it may be complicated by pericardial effusion or constriction or relapsing subacute disease. Pericardiectomy can benefit the patient with tamponade, constriction, or prolonged smoldering or recurrent disease.

Cardiac tamponade, which is discussed in detail in Chapter 13, presents a more acute emergency because of its potential effect on cardiac function. It may be the presenting feature of pericardial disease caused by infection, tumor, trauma, or connective tissue disease. The diagnostic features of acute cardiac tamponade are listed in Table 12-6. The diagnostic and therapeutic approach is similar to that for pericarditis, but if cardiac function is impaired, a drainage procedure should be carried out during which pericardial fluid and biopsy should be obtained.

Constrictive pericarditis, usually a chronic disease, still warrants discussion because of its effect on cardiac function. Although often no obvi-

Table 12-6   *Diagnostic Features of Acute Cardiac Tamponade*

Signs and symptoms
   History of acute pericardial disease or chest or heart trauma or surgery
   Dyspnea
   Orthopnea
   Tachypnea
   Normal, distant, or absent heart sounds and precordial movements
   Expanding precordial flatness or dullness
   Ewart's sign
   Decreased systolic pressure with narrow pulse pressure
   Pulsus paradoxus
   Elevated venous pressure and hepatic engorgement
   Exaggerated venous pulsation
   Pericardial rub (may or may not be present)

X-ray and other diagnostic procedures
   Rapid enlargement of cardiopericardial silhouette (especially if lung fields are clear)
   Cardiac pulsations normal or diminished by fluoroscopy
   Positive angiocardiogram (gas or opaque)
   Positive radioisotope scan
   Positive echocardiogram
   ECG: low voltage (especially if decrease is recent), electrical alternans, S–T segment elevation or nonspecific T-wave changes; preceding electrocardiographic evolutionary change typical of pericarditis is helpful

---

ous cause is found, it may be the result of previous bacterial infection, tuberculosis, fungus disease (especially histoplasmosis), or viral infection, as well as connective tissue disease, neoplasm, trauma, or x-radiation. The signs and symptoms are insidious in onset and are usually those related to congestive heart failure. On exertion dyspnea is common, orthopnea and paroxysmal nocturnal dyspnea less so, but abdominal and peripheral swelling is usually prominent. Physical examination may reveal an elevated venous pressure, hepatomegaly and ascites, peripheral edema, paradoxical pulse, narrow pulse pressure, and pericardial knock. The electrocardiogram is usually characterized by low voltage with flat or inverted T waves; there is a high incidence of atrial fibrillation. On chest x-ray, the lungs are usually clear with a normal to slightly enlarged heart, but pericardial calcification may be seen in over half the patients. Cardiac catheterization may show no specific abnormalities, but diminished stroke volume, elevated right atrial mean pressure, and ventricular tracings with early diastolic dip and an elevated diastolic plateau are common. The treatment of constrictive pericarditis is surgical removal of the pericardium.

BACTERIAL ENDOCARDITIS

Endocarditis, infection of the endocardial surface of a valve, the ventricular wall, or septum is an infrequent, but important, disease entity whose recognition is of major importance because the proper diagnosis and treatment have greatly improved the morbidity and mortality characteristic of the preantibiotic era. In addition, if endocarditis is allowed to progress unabated, it may result in permanent cardiac damage that ultimately may cost the patient his life or necessitate cardiac surgery.

Although there is considerable overlap between acute and subacute bacterial endocarditis, the acute form does represent a potential cardiac emergency that necessitates rapid diagnosis and treatment to preserve cardiac integrity and to halt unremitting infections that may be fatal.

Acute Bacterial Endocarditis

Acute bacterial endocarditis results from bacteremia with organisms that have the capability to induce an acute, necrotizing, ulcerating lesion on the endocardial surface and, therefore, may rapidly destroy the infected structure. Infections caused by such invasive species as *Staphylococcus aureus, Diplococcus pneumoniae, Haemophilus influenzae,* group A beta-hemolytic streptococci, meningococci, or gonococci can result in the invasion of both normal and damaged endocardium. It should be emphasized that acute bacterial endocarditis occurs very often in persons with previously normal hearts. Because the bacteria involved are usually highly invasive, even small numbers can invade the endocardium and establ.sh infection.

The prototype and the most virulent form of acute endocarditis is that due to *Staphylococcus aureus*. The underlying event is staphylococcal bacteremia, most commonly originating from skin infection, although it can be precipitated by wounds or any other type of minor or major staphylococcal infection. Fever is by far the most common sign and is usually accompanied by myalgia, arthralgia, leukocytosis, and signs of metastatic infection. The changing cardiac murmur is typical of acute endocarditis, but a small number of patients may have no detectable murmur at the onset, the murmur first appearing during the course of the disease or even during or after therapy. Signs of metastatic infection usually, but not always, appear and are characterized by abnormalities in whatever organ system is involved by the bacteremia. The following sites of metastatic infection are common and their involvement is helpful in making the diagnosis: the meninges (staphylococcal meningitis); the lungs (staphylococcal pneumonia, usually bilateral); the joints (acute staphylococcal arthritis); the skin (petechiae, septic infarcts, subungual hemorrhages, and microabscesses); the eyes (subconjunctival and retinal hemorrhages); the kidneys, liver, and brain, where multiple microabscesses may coalesce to form a large nephric or perinephric, hepatic, or brain abscess, respectively; and bone, where osteomyelitis results, with more than one bone usually being involved.

The most vital anatomic area involved is the heart. The endocardium, myocardium, and/or pericardium may be involved, resulting in acute staphylococcal pericarditis, acute myocarditis or discrete myocardial abscesses, or acute endocarditis. The endocarditis is usually characterized by the rapidly changing murmur, which may progress to signs and symptoms of intractable congestive heart failure secondary to valve rupture or fenestration.

Diagnosis. Diagnosis on clinical grounds alone may be difficult. Patients usually appear acutely ill and may or may not present with the signs and symptoms of metastatic infection listed above. Fever is usually spiking in nature, but it may be minimal or absent, especially in the neonate, the elderly, or the patient with altered host defense mechanisms. The most important laboratory aid is the blood culture, from which information critical to an etiologic diagnosis is obtained. Meticulous care must be exercised in obtaining blood cultures because contaminat'on of the sample may result in considerable confusion and possibly inappropriate therapy; this is especially true in staphylococcal endocarditis since *S. aureus* is a normal inhabitant of many parts of the body. At least three, and preferably six, blood cultures should be drawn to avoid misinterpretation when only a single culture is positive; at least two, and preferably three, positive cultures are necessary to confirm the presence of bacteremia. If the patient has previously been treated with penicillin G, penicillinase should be added to the blood culture bottles, although several commercially available types of media contain penicillinase. Occasionally, blood cultures may be negative; among the factors that may be responsible for this are the use of antibiotics in etiologically undefined febrile illnesses; inappropriate culture techniques; the presence in the blood of factors that inhibit microbial growth; and right-sided endocarditis.

In addition to blood cultures, all sites of obvious metastatic infection, such as sputum, spinal fluid, joint fluid, material obtained from aspiration of skin lesions, and urine should be similarly cultured. Recovery of the same organism from several sites is extremely helpful in documenting the diagnosis.

Therapy.   The patient with acute endocarditis is acutely ill. Left untreated, the infection may do permanent damage to the endocardium in a very short time, so therapy should be instituted when the *clinical* diagnosis has been made and then substantiated with cultural data when it becomes available. This means that one chooses antibiotic therapy based upon immediately available information, bacteriologic statistics, and examination of body fluids with gram or other appropriate stains that frequently provide sufficient information to make a presumptive etiologic diagnosis. Examination of spinal fluid, joint fluid, urine, and even a buffy coat preparation of peripheral blood may demonstrate the organism and be of significant help in choosing therapy.

The specific choice of antibiotics for the management of endocarditis is often based upon personal experience. The only requirement, whatever the agent employed, is that the organism be highly sensitive to it. In general, bactericidal compounds appear to be more effective than bacteriostatic ones. There is insufficient data at present to indicate optimal doses, duration of therapy, or route of administration of any of the antibiotics used to treat endocarditis, but the author feels that all patients should be treated for a minimum of 4 weeks with parenteral antibiotics. The regimens listed in Table 12-7 have been found to be successful.

Subacute Bacterial Endocarditis

Subacute bacterial endocarditis is not a cardiac emergency because it is a slowly progressive disease, with the interval between the onset of symptoms and diagnosis frequently exceeding 3 months. Nevertheless, a discussion of subacute bacterial endocarditis is appropriate to contrast

Table 12-7   *Regimens for Treatment of Bacterial Endocarditis*

Organism	Sensitivity	Antibiotic	Dose per day	Duration (wk)
Streptococcus viridans	Penicillin G-sensitive (<0.2 μ/ml)	Penicillin G IM;	6–12 million units	4
	Penicillin G-sensitive (>0.2 μ/ml)	IV	12-20 million units	
Group A β-hemolytic streptococcus Pneumococci Gonococci Meningococci		Penicillin G IM; IV	12–20 million units	4
Staphylococcus aureus *S. epidermis*	Penicillin-G-sensitive	Penicillin G IM; IV	12–24 million units	6
	Penicillin-G-resistant	Oxacillin IV Keflin IV Clindamycin IV	1 g q̄ 4 hr 2 g q̄ 4 hr 900 mg q̄ 8 hr	
Streptococcus faecalis		Penicillin G or ampicillin IV and streptomycin IM Chloramphenicol Vancomycin	20–40 million units 12 g 1 g 6 g 3 g	6
Haemophilus influenzae		Ampicillin IV	8–12 grams	6

it to the acute form (Table 12-8); untreated, it too may result in permanent cardiac damage that will necessitate urgent intervention.

This discussion will specifically emphasize aspects other than the classical clinical picture to ensure that diagnosis and treatment of the disease as it is seen today will be approached in a rational manner. Diagnosis on clinical grounds is difficult: the possibilities may not be considered; the presenting manifestations include many syndromes other than the ones thought of as "typical" for endocarditis; and the presence of the infection may be indicated by none of the special features but rather by certain combinations of often minor ones.

Etiology. The valvular disease is a consequence of the bacteremia, and many of the subsequent signs and symptoms are a combination of those arising from the systemic infection and those related to the damage produced in the afflicted valve.

Subacute bacterial endocarditis is due to infection with less invasive bacteria, such as those occurring in the oral cavity, especially in gingival crevices or in apical abscesses; these are mainly streptococci, including many nontypable strains, *Streptococcus viridans*, and microaerophilic and anaerobic streptococci, but they may also be of other species, such as *Staphylococcus epidermidis* and diphtheroids. Subacute bacterial endocarditis can follow cardiac surgery, upper respiratory tract infection, and dental manipulation. Abdominal sepsis and genitourinary

Table 12-8   *A Comparison of Major Features of Acute (ABE)*
and Subacute (SBE) Bacterial Endocarditis

Feature	*ABE*	*SBE*
Etiologic agents	*Staphylococcus aureus* *Streptococcus pyogenes* *D. pneumoniae* *H. influenzae* *N. meningitidis* *N. gonorrheae*	*Streptococcus viridans* Enterococci Anaerobic streptococci *Staphylococcus epidermidis* Gram-negative bacilli
Valve most commonly involved	Aortic	Mitral
Previously damaged endocardium	Unnecessary	Necessary
Valve pathology	Ulcerative; necrotizing	Indolent
Constitutional reaction	Mild to severe	Mild
WBC	N or ↑	N or ↑
Change in murmur	Rapid	Not rapid
Valve rupture	Not uncommon	Uncommon
Duration of symptoms before diagnosis	1–2 weeks	≥3 months
Primary focus	None found; wounds; skin infection	None found; teeth; GU tract

infection can lead to heart valve infection with such organisms as *Escherichia coli, Proteus mirabilis,* Klebsiella, and Pseudomonas. Surgical procedures, urinary tract instrumentation, parturition, abortion, and trauma may also be associated with its inception. The disease produced is usually slow in evolution and is comprised of many different manifestations because it is a combination of both slowly progressive destruction and early healing in the same lesion, with the former process exceeding the latter.

Five factors are involved in the development of subacute bacterial endocarditis:

1. A previously damaged valve (not always manifested by a detectable murmur).

2. The specific hemodynamics that favor deposit of fibrin clots—high-velocity flow through a small conduit (as in the regurgitant flow through a mitral valve or a ventricular septal defect) into a low-pressure sink (as into the left atrium or right ventricle).

3. The development of a sterile platelet fibrin thrombus. Fibrin slowly but gradually deposits on the surface of the leaflet, forming a sterile platelet fibrin thrombus over a variable period of time.

4. The presence of antibody, which serves to agglutinate bacteria

. within fibrin clots without killing them. The fact that the organisms involved are usually indigenous and that bacteremia precedes endocardial localization assures antibody development.

5. Bacteremia that establishes infection of the endocardial surface. This is usually asymptomatic. Whether it follows a tooth extraction, for example, is deduced by the history of such manipulation in many with the infection, but it is of importance to recognize that, rather than a single episode of bacteremia, there may have been many.

Although rheumatic heart disease and congenital heart disease are still the most common underlying disorders on which subacute infective endocarditis is superimposed, their frequency has decreased, and arteriosclerotic heart disease has become a significant antecedent lesion predisposing to the development of bacterial endocarditis. The introduction of various types of surgery of the heart has added a group of iatrogenic lesions that may serve as foci for the development of both acute and subacute valvular infections. There also has been an increase of endocarditis in patients with acute myocardial infarction; the infection may be subacute or acute, depending on the nature of the organism involved, and may involve either the right or left side of the heart.

Signs and Symptoms

Fever is by far the most common sign in infective endocarditis. Under certain circumstances, the febrile response may be minimal or absent for variable periods. Fever may be absent in patients with endocarditis who also have severe heart failure, uremia, or a ruptured mycotic aneurysm or who have received antimicrobial therapy. The increasing incidence of endocarditis in older persons may account for the greater frequency with which fever is absent. Repeated short courses of antibiotic therapy in patients with undiagnosed endocarditis produces a characteristic clinical pattern of repetitive episodes of remission and relapse of fever; even small quantities of antibiotic may mask the fever as well as other manifestations of endocarditis.

A cardiac murmur was once the *sine qua non* for the diagnosis of infective endocarditis, and the change in its quality and intensity was common in the acute but not the subacute type of infection. However, it is now accepted that as many as 15% of patients may have no detectable murmurs when they present with endocarditis. Murmurs can first appear during therapy or some time after therapy has been completed, or they may fail to develop at any time.

Petechiae are the most common cutaneous manifestation of endocarditis. They are seen in 20–40% of patients; in the preantibiotic era, they were seen in 85%. Subungual hemorrhages are presently uncommon in patients with bacterial endocarditis. Osler's nodes are seen in only 10% of cases of subacute bacterial endocarditis and are rare in acute endocarditis. The incidence of splenomegaly has decreased and is now seen in 20–55% of patients. "Roth spots," located in the retina and having the appearance of cotton wool exudates or oval or boat-shaped hemorrhages with a central white area, are uncommon. Neuropsychiatric complications are common in bacterial endocarditis and, if sought, may be found in up to 50% of patients. Any acute neurologic syndrome or psychiatric illness arising in a patient with fever and a cardiac murmur in the absence of arrhythmia should suggest subacute bacterial endocarditis. Acute glomerulonephritis developing as a complication of endocarditis is a form of immune complex disease. Glomerulonephritis complicating endocarditis is partially reversible with effective antimicrobial therapy. Renal insufficiency secondary to endocarditis is seen in about 10% of cases. Hematuria is common, occurring in 25–90% of patients. Uremia can develop and is generally accompanied by absence of hypertension, little or no fever, and a high incidence of sterile blood cultures. Careful and frequent urinalysis early in the disease may show red cells, red cell casts, white cells, and albuminuria.

Elevation of the sedimentation rate is the most common abnormal laboratory finding in patients with bacterial endocarditis. Although the leukocyte count may be elevated and there may be a shift to the left, these findings are frequently absent. Abnormality of serum proteins, namely hyperglobulinemia, with inversion of the albumin/globulin ratio, is also common and is accompanied by an increase in numbers of plasma cells in the bone marrow. Anemia is common, occurring in 50–80% of cases. The degree of anemia is generally related to the duration of infection, although in more acute cases it may develop rapidly. It is usually normocytic and normochromic. The serum iron level and the total iron-binding capacity may be reduced. Rheumatoid factor is present in the serum of 50% of patients and decreases or entirely disappears after successful treatment. Recent studies of subacute bacterial endocarditis have indicated that most patients develop higher titers of agglutinating, complement-fixing, and opsonizing antibodies specific for the invading organisms.

Diagnosis: Classical signs and symptoms of fever, murmur, anemia, and petechiae with an illness of 6 weeks' to 3 months' duration are easily recognized, and allow a diagnosis. Clubbing, hematuria, and history of dental disease and/or manipulation are also helpful.

Nonspecific presenting features of this disease are listed in Table 12-9, and some of them are discussed below:

Table 12-9   *Nonspecific Presenting Clinical Features in Endocarditis*

Unexplained fever
Arrythmias and congestive heart failure
Pulmonary infarction
Mental confusion
Sterile meningitis
Unexplained uremia
Hemiplegia
Subarachnoid hemorrhage
Acute abdomen
Night sweats
Joint or back pain

Prolonged unexplained fever, especially accompanied by high sedimentation rate, anemia, hyperglobulinemia. Especially important is the response of "fever" to short-course antibiotic trials when treatment is chosen empirically.

Arrythmias and congestive heart failure. The incidence of atrial fibrillation or cardiac failure or both, previously rare in the early stage of subacute endocarditis, is now relatively common. This is probably related to the empiric administration of short courses of antimicrobial therapy without a diagnosis. Such ineffective treatment may go on for weeks or months and lead to progressive cardiac damage with the establishment of congestive heart failure and/or arrhythmias.

Pulmonary infarction as a direct result of bacterial endocarditis is limited almost entirely to cases involving the right side of the heart. In fact, the lung is the most common site for deposition of emboli in this form of bacterial endocarditis.

Mental confusion. Psychiatric changes range from minor aberrations in personality and behavior to major psychiatric breakdowns necessitating the patient's admission to a psychiatric ward. Psychiatric complications are more common in older patients; those presenting with mental aberrations have a poorer prognosis. In some cases, abnormalities in the cerebrospinal fluid may suggest an underlying cause, but many patients who present with psychiatric features have no localizing cerebral signs and no significant cerebrospinal fluid changes. The presence of fever and a cardiac murmur should be given respectful attention in such instances.

Sterile meningitis. An episode of sterile meningitis is not uncommon as the initial manifestation of subacute bacterial endocarditis. Because viral or partially treated bacterial infections of the meninges are more common causes of sterile meningitis, the association with endocarditis is often not considered.

Unexplained uremia. Renal failure may be a major factor in the failure to establish a diagnosis of endocarditis for several reasons: Blood cultures are often sterile, and the physician is so concerned with kidney dysfunction that he overlooks the cardiac disease.

Blood cultures are the most important laboratory aid in establishing an etiologic diagnosis of endocarditis. The author's experience, as well as that of others, has indicated that the best time to draw blood for culture is about 2 hours before the temperature begins to rise, but this is not always feasible. Monitoring the temperature at 30–45-minute intervals, beginning at the time an increase is expected, may be helpful. Frequently, the rise in temperature can be predicted on the basis of the previous 24 hours. Blood is cultured as soon as it is evident that fever is developing. Six separate cultures are obtained at 10–30-minute intervals. A single positive culture, however, must be interpreted with great caution because of the possibility of contamination. This is true even when the organisms are those usually not considered contaminants. Two positive blood cultures are necessary to confirm that the bacteremia is continuous rather than transient. One would not want to commit a patient to 4–6 weeks of hospitalization on the basis of one positive blood culture. For this reason, it is our policy to obtain at least two, and preferably three, positive blood cultures to establish the diagnosis of infective endocarditis.

All blood cultures should be incubated at 37°C; room temperature may be required for some yeasts and fungi. The cultures should be incubated for at least 2 to 3 weeks and as long as 4 weeks if Brucella is suspected.

Recent studies have shown that blood cultures are negative in about 20% of patients with subacute infective endocarditis. Among the factors that may be responsible for negative blood cultures are the use of antibiotics in etiologically undefined febrile illnesses, inappropriate culture techniques, the presence in the blood of factors that inhibit microbial growth, right-sided endocarditis, the presence of renal disease, and the prolonged duration of subacute bacterial endocarditis ("bacteria-free state").

Therapy. An acceptable outline for the treatment of subacute endocarditis is shown in Table 12-7, but the choice of antibiotics for therapy of endocarditis due to such unusual species as Mimeae, Escherichia, Enterobacter, Klebsiella, Alcaligenes, Pseudomonas, Hafnia, anaerobic diphtheroids, and *S. epidermidis* is based on the *in vitro* sensitivity of the organism recovered from the blood. The drug chosen should be bactericidal and should be given in maximal tolerated dose.

Amphotericin is presently the most effective drug for the management of endocarditis caused by fungi and yeast. Several dosage schedules have been used:

1.5 mg/kg every other day for the entire course of treatment.

0.25 mg/kg for the first day, 0.5 mg/kg the second, 0.75 mg/kg the third, and 1 mg/kg the fourth and subsequent days until therapy is completed.

The administration of quantities of the drug necessary to produce and maintain blood levels 2 to 4 times greater than *in vitro* inhibitory concentration. In general, a total of 2 g, or, preferably, 3 g, of amphotericin B is desirable, although larger doses may be necessary.

Surgery has been recently added to the therapy of infective endocarditis. This new dimension may be lifesaving in cases in which chemotherapy fails to produce total cure, or when potentially lethal complications develop in the area of the infected valves. The indications for surgery in endocarditis are as follows:

Infections that fail to respond after treatment with appropriate doses of the proper antimicrobial agent(s)

Recurrence of infection following two or more courses of therapy with an effective antibiotic

A single recurrence of fungal endocarditis

Development of aneurysms of the sinus of Valsalva or the atrioventricular junctional tissues

Intractable or rapidly progressive heart failure despite specific medical therapy

The presence of an infected prosthetic valve or patch (if initial treatment is followed by cure, removal of the prosthesis may not be necessary; if, however, relapse occurs after completing one course of therapy, replacement of the intracardiac foreign body is usually indicated)

Recurrent systemic or pulmonary emboli

When surgery is otherwise indicated, the presence of active infection is not a contraindication. It is probably a mistake to wait until the infectious process seems to be under control because, during the delay, tissue destruction may proceed so far that surgery becomes technically difficult or impossible. Antimicrobial therapy must be maintained before and after surgery.

Infection Following Cardiac Surgery

The advent of cardiac surgery or surgery on the great vessels has introduced a new class of acute life-threatening infections involving the heart. This is particularly true in cases where an artificial prosthesis has been inserted. Infection of an artificial valve, for example, may be a catastrophic event not only because of the infectious process *per se* but also because it is extremely difficult to treat the infection successfully without removing the infected foreign body. It is of paramount importance, therefore, that infection arising after cardiac surgery be diagnosed immediately and that appropriate treatment be instituted without delay to prevent infection on the prosthesis and to ensure that infection arising elsewhere is not misinterpreted as cardiac infection, giving rise to unnecessary further surgical procedures.

Infection occurring during cardiac surgery is more likely related to high-grade rather than low-grade contamination. Sources of a contamination include blood transfusion, the pump-oxygenator (uncommon with newer sterilizing techniques), devices used for pressure recordings, septic thrombophlebitis resulting from indwelling catheters, and minor or major breaks in aseptic surgical techniques. Staphylococci are the organisms most commonly involved; they may enter the operative field from the environment or from infected personnel or carriers, but usually the patient himself is the source. The prostheses themselves may be contaminated, as may the surgical suture materials, but newer equipment has reduced this risk. Systemic factors in the host such as altered defense mechanisms, shock, and corticosteroid therapy may also predispose to infection.

Post-cardiac-surgery infection generally occurs early (immediately or 1 to 4 weeks after surgery) or late (several months postoperatively; some of these late infections may be coincidental and unrelated to the surgical procedure).

Symptoms may be obvious or occult, with high fever and positive blood cultures being the most prominent features. Diagnosis may be difficult, however, when fever is low-grade, especially since the characteristic features of endocarditis may be lacking.

The microbiology of post-cardiac-surgery endocarditis is varied. The most common organisms involved are *Staphylococcus aureus* (coagulase-positive) and *S. epidermidis* (coagulase-negative); the latter infections are particularly difficult to treat. Though they are rare in other types of endocarditis, gram-negative organisms such as *E. coli,* Proteus species, Klebsiella, Enterobacter, and *Pseudomonas aeruginosa* are not uncommonly seen in post-cardiac-surgery endocarditis. Other uncommon bacteria are seen occasionally and therefore should not be automatically dismissed as contaminants; these include species of diphtheroids, chromobacteria, flavobacteria, and even the tubercle bacillus.

Fungal endocarditis is a particularly difficult post-cardiac-surgery problem, in which species of Candida and Aspergillus are most commonly implicated. Although the sources of contamination are similar to those involved in bacterial endocarditis, antibiotic and steroid therapy and debilitation appear to be particularly important predisposing factors. Because fungal endocarditis is usually characterized by larger vegetations than those due to bacteria, emboli to large arteries are seen with impressive frequency and are, in fact, a common presenting symptom. Thus, any post-cardiac-surgery patient who presents with an embolus to a major vessel should be suspect, and it is imperative that at the time of embolectomy gram stains and cultures be obtained to look for the offending organism. It is also of interest that fungal endocarditis generally occurs later after surgery than does bacterial endocarditis.

Because of the life-threatening nature of post-cardiac-surgery endocarditis, any such patient with unexplained fever, and with any of the peripheral manifestations of endocarditis described above, should be rapidly and vigorously evaluated with appropriate blood cultures, and therapy should be instituted as soon as possible. For the common organisms, therapy is the same as that outlined in Table 12-7. For the uncommon organisms, therapy should be dictated by appropriate sensitivity tests. Amphotericin B is the choice of treatment for fungal endocarditis, but it should be emphasized that successful therapy may be the exception rather than the rule. It should also be emphasized that the eradication of infection on a prosthetic valve is particularly difficult; replacement of the prosthesis is usually necessary and must be strongly considered unless there is an immediate and obvious response to antimicrobial therapy. It is imperative that blood cultures be obtained during and after therapy to ensure that treatment has been effective; persistent bacteremia or fungemia during or after appropriate therapy generally indicates that infection is persisting in or on the prosthesis and that surgical replacement is indicated.

MYOCARDITIS

Inflammatory lesions in the myocardium have been associated with almost every type of infectious agent, including bacteria, spirochetes, rickettsiae, viruses (especially the Coxsackie group), fungi, and parasites (Table 12-10). Although these lesions may be seen frequently at

Table 12-10   *Etiology of Myocarditis*

Infectious

Bacterial
  Diphtheria, *Staphylococcus aureus, Streptococcus pyogenes, H. influenzae,* Salmonella, *Nesseiria meningitidis, N. gonorrheae,* Brucella, TB

Rickettsial
  Epidemic typhus, Rocky Mountain spotted fever, scrub typhus

Viral
  ECHO, influenza, Coxsackie, rubeola, hepatitis, infectious mononucleosis, mumps, varicella, dengue, yellow fever

Fungal
  Blastomyces, Coccidioides, Histoplasma, Torula

Protozoan
  Chaga's disease, malaria, Toxoplasmosis

Metazoan
  Trichinosis, schistosomiasis, echinococcosis

Myocardial disease of obscure origin
Idopathic cardiomyopathies
Hemochromatosis
Sarcoidosis
Systemic lupus erythematosus
Scleroderma
Amyloidosis
Fiedler's myocarditis
Storage diseases
Drug-induced myocarditis
Hypersensitivity reactions
Endocardial fibroelastosis
Toxic myocarditis

---

careful postmortem examination, clinical myocarditis is uncommon. The frequency with which this diagnosis is made depends on the degree of suspicion of its presence and on the care given to interpretation of serial electrocardiograms. Myocarditis usually presents as cardiac arrhythmias but may present as cardiac arrest or sudden death. Congestive heart failure is uncommon. Myocarditis may be associated with pericarditis or endocarditis.

Myocardial abscesses generally are the result of bacteremia but may also develop by extension from valvular lesions of bacterial endocarditis. Rarely, an abscess will occur at the site of myocardial infarction. The majority of myocardial abscesses are small and of relatively little clinical significance. Their clinical manifestations usually are overshadowed by the associated infectious processes, but occasionally an abscess may cause or contribute to death.

The treatment of myocarditis depends upon the causative bacteria; the general principle of management is that of pericarditis.

THE HEART IN SEPTIC SHOCK

Although septic shock *per se* may involve the heart directly, as outlined in Table 12-11, any type of septic shock may directly or indirectly affect cardiac function simply by impairing the delivery of oxygenated blood to the myocardium. Therefore, it is appropriate that any type of septic shock be considered a cardiac emergency if adequate and effective cardiac function is to be maintained. The discussion below, therefore, applies to septic shock as a whole, but the implications with regard to the heart are obvious.

Septic shock is a dynamic syndrome induced by infections of varying types in which inadequate perfusion of tissues with blood develops. Although the microcirculation of the capillary loop is the final determinant of the events that occur in this condition, multiple factors are involved in the genesis and persistence of progressive decompensation of the capillary circulation and the cells that it supports. Effective therapy of septic shock requires knowledge of its pathogenesis, anticipation and recognition of the clinical picture, use of available bedside and laboratory techniques for assessing the nature and degree of the derangements, and rapid initiation of corrective measures.

Bacteremia is not a prerequisite for the development of septic shock, which may also be due to endotoxins, exotoxins, and direct bacterial invasion of, or obstruction of blood flow to, a vital organ. Although presence of gram-negative bacteria in the blood, with release of endotoxin, is the most common cause of this syndrome in hospitalized pa-

Table 12-11   *Cardiac Involvement in Septic Shock*

Mechanism	Cause
Impaired cardiac function	Myocarditis
	Cardiac tamponade
	Endocarditis, e.g., ruptured valve
	Myocardial infarction
	Mechanical outflow obstruction, e.g., Echinococcus cyst
Impaired venous return	
Reduced blood volume	Severe diarrhea
(loss of water and electrolytes)	Adrenal insufficiency, e.g., TB
	Salt-losing pyelonephritis
	Peritonitis
	Hemorrhage
Normal blood volume	Endotoxin shock
Disturbances of arteriolar tone	Destruction of vasomotor center, e.g., bulbar polio

tients and is second only to myocardial infarction as a cause of death on many large medical services, about one third of the cases of this type of shock follow invasion by staphylococci, streptococci, and clostridia; some cases may be associated with viral or rickettsial infections.

Shock due to the activity of endotoxin is most common in men over 40 years of age, but is fairly frequent in women with septic abortions and among neonates. Among the factors predisposing to the infections with which this syndrome is associated are urinary, intestinal, biliary-tract or gynecologic manipulation or surgery, transfusion of contaminated blood, hepatic cirrhosis, diabetes mellitus, burns, cancer (especially of the hematopoietic system), radiotherapy, and the use of antimetabolites, corticosteroids, and antibiotics. The organisms most frequently involved are *E. coli,* Proteus species, *Pseudomonas aeruginosa,* Klebsiella, Enterobacter, and Bacteroides. Hypotension is present in about 80% of patients who have bacteremia with gram-negative organisms. However, the complete syndrome of shock develops in only about 20% of patients; the mortality rate in this group may range from 40 to 80%.

The presence of any of the predisposing factors listed above should alert the physician to the possibility of endotoxic septic shock. If shaking chills, elevated temperature, and hypotension develop, or if high-grade fever appears in an elderly person (usually uncommon), a presumptive diagnosis of septic shock should be made. The early phase of the syndrome when it is produced by endotoxin is often marked by "warm shock," in which the skin is warm and dry, the pulse full, and the output of urine adequate despite the presence of hypotension. If not treated, this progresses to "cold shock," which is characterized by pallor, cold clammy skin, cyanosis of the nail beds, rapid thready pulse, collapse of veins, altered cerebral function, and reduction or total loss of urine flow. Also suggestive of endotoxic shock are tachypnea and respiratory alkalosis preceding acidosis and any alteration in the patient's clinical course (e.g., change in mental status, appetite, or sleeping habits; vomiting or diarrhea, unexplained urinary or gastric retention or ileus).

The development of shock in the course of infection is associated with three types of hemodynamic abnormalities (Table 12-11), any or all of which may be present at one time or another: Cardiac failure may occur as a result of myocarditis complicating diphtheria, influenza, Coxsackie-virus (Type B in very young children) and other virus infections and rickettsial disease or as a result of tamponade supervening during tuberculous, viral, or suppurative pericarditis; volume deficit may be the primary problem in severe infectious diarrhea, salt-losing pyelonephritis, adrenal insufficiency due to tuberculosis and infections associated with adrenal hemorrhage; and peripheral vascular failure may occur when autonomic ganglia or medullary centers are injured or destroyed, as in some cases of bulbar poliomyelitis and encephalitis.

The type of shock present can be measured in a variety of ways, which have been well described in the medical literature, but the ultimate goal should be to define the state of cardiac function and the adequacy of total and effective circulating blood volume. Once shock has been identified and the pathophysiologic basis defined, immediate therapy is indicated.

The present management of septic shock is based on several principles: (1) prevention and treatment of the situations known to be associated with its development; (2) anticipation of its occurrence when predisposing factors appear; and (3) therapy of the hemodynamic abnormalities and the infections with which it is associated. The most successful approach to the prophylaxis of septic shock is rapid and intensive therapy of the infection. Early and effective chemotherapy eliminates the risk of shock in most cases. Avoidance, if possible, of procedures that predispose to infection (such as the use of indwelling urinary-bladder catheters, unnecessary antimicrobial drugs, and venous catheters) is of obvious value. However, if these are necessary, patients subjected to them must be studied continually for clinical and microbiologic evidence of infection, which must be treated as soon as it is detected.

Paramount in the successful management of septic shock is rapid control of the responsible infectious process, but significant airway obstruction or blood loss must be ruled out as soon as the first evidence of shock becomes apparent. In many cases, a causative organism is not recovered, and the choice of treatment must be based on clinical grounds alone until the results of culture studies of blood, urine, sputum, and exudates or other body fluids are available. Since the recognition and identification of the shock state require the institution of antimicrobial therapy before culture results are available, it is helpful to know that certain gram-negative micro-organisms are statistically associated with diseases of particular anatomic areas (Table 12-12). The choice of antimicrobial agent(s) varies from physician to physician and clinic to clinic, but it is usually possible to make a rational choice based upon the available clinical data, gram stains of body fluids or exudates, and knowledge of the statistical likelihood that certain organisms are present. In many cases, a combination of two drugs is desirable until cultures are available: These combinations include cephalothin, 2.0 g IV every 4 hours, and gentamicin, 5 mg/kg per day in 3 divided doses IV; and clindamycin, 900 mg every 8 hours IV, and gentamicin. If the organism is known, then obviously the single most effective antimicrobial agent

Table 12-12   *Gram-Negative Sepsis:*
Etiologic Agent Suspected, by Anatomic Area

Site of Infection	Suspected Agent
Genitourinary tract	*Escherichia coli, Klebsiella pneumoniae, Proteus* spp., *Pseudomonas aeruginosa*
Gastrointestinal tract	*E. coli*, Bacteroides, Any coliform organism
Lower respiratory tract	*K. pneumoniae, Enterobacter* spp.
Ear–Mastoid	*Haemophilus influenzae, P. aeruginosa*
Skin	*P. aeruginosa, E. coli*

in the appropriate dose is indicated. In shock, it is always wise to use the intravenous route, since the absorption of intramuscularly administered drugs may be erratic. All antimicrobial agents excreted primarily by the kidneys must be given with extreme caution when shock is present because decreased renal perfusion results in accumulation of these agents in excessive and dangerous concentrations in the blood and in tissue fluids. Abscesses or other localized infections may not respond to chemotherapy alone and may require drainage. Careful control of acid–base balance is mandatory in patients with septic shock. Measurement of venous or arterial pH and serum lactate levels may prove of great help; the concentration of lactic acid in the blood is an important index of severe circulatory failure.

Vasopressor agents may be necessary in septic shock, but are *usually not indicated;* tissue perfusion must never be sacrificed for the sake of a rise in peripheral arterial pressure.

Because urine volume is somewhat proportional to renal blood flow, it is a good index of tissue perfusion. For this reason, an adequate output (at least 30 ml per hour) usually indicates effective blood supply to vital organs and reversal of the shock state much better than peripheral arterial pressure. Catheterization of the bladder should not be carried out, however, unless inability to void leads to significant distention of this organ.

The use of oxygen, although safe, is of questionable value since the anoxia in septic shock is of the static type. Hypothermia and antihistamines, aldosterone, heparin, and a number of other drugs have been employed in the management of experimental shock; their value in man remains to be proved.

The use of suprapharmacologic doses of corticosteroids is felt to be of value if they are given immediately and for a short period of time. The use of mannitol or other potent diuretics in the hope of maintaining urine output is also felt to be helpful but is not a mandatory part of the treatment regimen.

Whatever the etiology of shock, the basis of treatment remains prevention, if possible, and the immediate recognition, evaluation, and therapy of infection.

SUMMARY

Disease caused by virtually any of the known infectious agents may directly or indirectly involve the heart muscle or the membranes that line it. Diagnosis and treatment of infectious heart disease demand the same great care that is necessary in any other infectious or cardiac disease. Because cardiac involvement by infection can be life-threatening and can damage the heart permanently, every effort should be made to obtain the correct diagnosis and start proper therapy with a maximum of vigor and a minimum of delay. On the other hand, the urgency of the situation should never be allowed to cause panic in the physician, resulting in a decision to treat without being certain that treatable disease is present before sufficient information has been obtained to allow a rational choice of effective therapy.

SELECTED READING

Pericarditis

1. Benzing, G., III, and Kaplan, S.: Purulent pericarditis. Am. J. Dis. Child. 106:289, 1963.
2. Boyle, J. D. Pearce, M. L., and Guze, L. B.: Purulent pericarditis: Review of literature and report of 11 cases. Medicine 41:119, 1961.
3. Clark, E.: Pericarditis. Bull. N.Y. Acad. Med. 40:511, 1964.
4. Herrman, G. R., Marchand, E. J., Grur, G. H., et al.: Pericarditis: Clinical and laboratory data of 130 cases. Am. Heart J. 43:641, 1952.
5. Rooney, J. J., Crocco, J. A., and Lyons, H. A.: Tuberculous pericarditis. Ann. Intern. Med. 72:73, 1970.
6. Wolff, L., and Wolff, R.: Diseases of the pericardium. Ann. Rev. Med. 16:21, 1965.
7. Woodward, T. E., McCrumb, F. R., Carey, T. N., et al.: Viral and rickettsial causes of cardiac disease, including the Coxsackie virus etiology of pericarditis and myocarditis. Ann. Intern. Med. 53:1130, 1960.

Endocarditis

1. Amoury, R. A., Bowman, F. O., and Malm, J. F.: Endocarditis associated with intracardiac prostheses. J. Thorac. Cardiovasc. Surg. 51:36, 1966.
2. Andriole, V. T., Kravetz, H. M., Roberts, W. C., et al.: Candida endocarditis: Clinical and pathologic studies. Am. J. Med. 32:251, 1962.
3. Belli, J., and Waisbren, B. A.: Number of blood cultures necessary to diagnose most cases of bacterial endocarditis. Am. J. Med. Sci. 232:284, 1956.
4. Bennett, I. L., and Beeson, P. B.: Bacteremia: A consideration of some experimental and clinical aspects. Yale J. Biol. Med. 26:241, 1954.

5. Block, P. C., DeSanctis, R. W., Weinberg, A. N., et al.: Prosthetic valve endocarditis. J. Thorac. Cardiovasc. Surg. 60:54, 1970.
6. Blount, J. G.: Bacterial endocarditis. Am. J. Med. 38:909, 1965.
7. Braniff, B. A., Shumway, N. E., and Harrison, D. C.: Valve replacement in active bacterial endocarditis. N. Engl. J. Med. 276:1464, 1967.
8. Conway, N., Kothari, M. L., Lockey, E., et al.: *Candida* endocarditis after heart surgery. Thorax 23:353, 1968.
9. Davis, A., Binder, M. J., and Finegold, S. M.: Late infection in patients with Starr-Edwards prosthetic valves. Antimicrob. Agents Chemother. 5:97, 1965.
10. Denton, C., Pappas, E. G., Uricchio, J. F., et al.: Bacterial endocarditis following cardiac surgery. Circulation 15:525, 1957.
11. Derby, B. M., Coolidge, K., and Rogers, D. E.: *Histoplasma capsulatum* endocarditis with major arterial embolism. Arch. Intern. Med. 110:63, 1962.
12. Felner, J. M., and Dowell, V. R., Jr.: Anaerobic bacterial endocarditis. N. Engl. J. Med. 283:1188, 1970.
13. Goodman, J. S., Schaffner, W., Collins, H. A., et al.: Infection after cardiovascular surgery: Clinical study including examination of antimicrobial prophylaxis. N. Engl. J. Med. 278:117, 1968.
14. Hall, B., and Dowling, H. F.: Negative blood cultures in bacterial endocarditis: A decade's experience. Med. Clin. N. Am. 50:159, 1966.
15. Hancock, E. W., Shumway, N. E., and Remington, J. S.: Valve replacement in active bacterial endocarditis. (Editorial.) J. Infect. Dis. 123:106, 1971.
16. Hurley, E. J., Eldridge, F. C., and Hultgren, H. N.: Emergency replacement of valves in endocarditis. Am. Heart J. 73:798, 1967.
17. Kaplan, K., and Weinstein, L.: Diphtheroid infections of man. Ann. Intern. Med. 70:919, 1969.
18. Kaye, J. H., Bernstein, S., Frinstein, D., et al.: Surgical cure of *Candida albicans* endocarditis with open heart surgery. N. Engl. J. Med. 264:907, 1961.
19. Kaye, D., McCormack, R. C., and Hook, E. W.: Bacterial endocarditis: Changing pattern since introduction of penicillin therapy. Antimicrob. Agents Chemother. 37:46, 1961.
20. Kaye, J. H., Bernstein, S., Tsuji, H. K., et al.: Surgical treatment of Candida endocarditis. JAMA 203:621, 1968.
21. Kerr, A., Jr.: Clinical picture: Fever, murmur, evidence of bacteremia, p. 65. *In* Subacute Bacterial Endocarditis. Springfield, Ill., Charles C Thomas, 1955.
22. Lawrence, T., Shockman, A. T., and MacVaugh, H., III: *Aspergillus* infection of prosthetic aortic valves. Chest 60:406, 1971.
23. Lerner, P. I., and Weinstein, L.: Infective endocarditis in the antibiotic era. N. Engl. J. Med. 274:199, 259, 323, 388, 1966.
24. Mandell, G. L., Kaye, D., Levison, M. E., et al.: Enterococcal endocarditis. Arch. Intern. Med. 125:258, 1970.
25. Sande, M. A., Johnson, W. D., Jr., Hook, E. W., et al.: Sustained bacteremia in patients with prosthetic cardiac valves. N. Engl. J. Med. 286:1067, 1972.
26. Segal, C., Wheeler, C. G., and Tompsett, R.: Histoplasma endocarditis cured with amphotericin. N. Engl. J. Med. 280:206, 1969.
27. Shafer, R. B., and Hall, W. H.: Bacterial endocarditis following open heart surgery. Am. J. Cardiol. 25:602, 1970.
28. Walker, S. R., Shumway, N. W., and Merigan, T. C.: Management of infected cardiac valve prostheses. JAMA 208:531, 1969.
29. Weinstein, L.: Infected prosthetic valves: A diagnostic and therapeutic dilemma. (Editorial.) N. Engl. J. Med. 286:1108, 1972.
30. Weinstein, L., and Rubin, R. H.: Infective endocarditis—1973. Prog. Cardiovasc. Dis. 16:239, 1973.

31. Yeh, T. J., Anabtawi, I. N., Cornett, V. E., et al.: Bacterial endocarditis following open heart surgery. Ann. Thorac. Surg. 3:29, 1967.

Myocarditis

1. Abelmann, W. H.: Myocarditis. N. Engl. J. Med. 275:832, 1966.
2. Ryon, D. S., Pastor, B. H., and Myerson, R. M.: Abscess of the myocardium. Am. J. Med. Sci. 251:698, 1966.

Shock

1. Lillehei, R. C., Longerbeam, J. K., and Bloch, J. H.: Physiology and therapy of bacteremic shock: Experimental and clinical observations. Am. J. Cardiol. 13:599, 1963.
2. Lillehei, R. C., Longerbeam, J. K., Bloch, J. H., and Manax, W. G.: Modern treatment of shock based on physiologic principles. Clin. Pharmacol. Ther. 5:63, 1964.
3. MacLean, L. D., Duff, J. H., Scott, H. M., and Peretz, D. I.: Treatment of shock in man based on hemodynamic diagnosis. Surg. Gynecol. Obstet. 120:1, 1965.
4. McCabe, W. R., and Jackson, G. G.: Gram-negative bacteremia. I. Etiology and ecology. Arch. Intern. Med. 110:847, 1962.
5. McHenry, M. C., Martin, W. J., and Wellman, W. E.: Bacteremia due to gram-negative bacilli: Review of 113 cases encountered in five-year period 1955 through 1959. Ann. Intern. Med. 56:207, 1962.
6. Spink, W. W.: Endotoxin shock. Ann. Intern. Med. 57:538, 1962.
7. Udhoji, V. N., Weil, M. H., Sambhi, M. P., and Rosoff, L.: Hemodynamic studies on clinical shock associated with infection. Am. J. Med. 34:461, 1963.
8. Udhoji, V. N., and Weil, M. H.: Hemodynamic and metabolic studies on shock associated with bacteremia: Observations on 16 patients. Ann. Intern. Med. 62:966, 1965.
9. Weil, M. H., and Spink, W. W.: Comparison of shock due to endotoxin with anaphylactic shock. J. Lab. Clin. Med. 50:501, 1957.
10. Weil, M. H., Shubin, H., and Biddle, M.: Shock caused by gram-negative microorganisms: Analysis of 169 cases. Ann. Intern. Med. 60:384, 1964.
11. Weinstein, L., and Klainer, A. S.: Management of emergencies. IV. Septic shock—pathogenesis and treatment. N. Engl. J. Med. 274:950, 1966.

Chapter 13

PERICARDIAL TAMPONADE

DAVID H. SPODICK

Pericardial tamponade is the decompensated phase of cardiac compression resulting from an unchecked increase in intrapericardial pressure.[1] Rising pericardial pressure results from relentless accumulation within the pericardial sac of one or more fluids—inflammatory exudate, blood, pus, chyle, or gas—which initially fills and then stretches the parietal pericardium. When the elastic limit of this membrane is exceeded, intrapericardial pressure rises and the heart is compressed, causing progressive restriction of ventricular filling. Depending on the tempo of the inciting process, sooner or later cardiac compensation fails, producing signs of severe circulatory failure. A low-grade inflammation, for example, may slowly fill the sac with several hundred milliliters to one or two liters of fluid before this point is reached, because the pericardial fibrosa can yield considerably if distended slowly. By contrast, brisk intrapericardial hemorrhage from a heart wound or aortic dissection can cause lethal cardiac compression in seconds to minutes by as little as 150 ml of blood.

The course of events leading to pericardial tamponade is diagrammed in Figure 13-1. The normal potential pericardial space is filled by the first 80 to 120 ml,[1] after which the elastic tissue permits the parietal pericardium to "give" as fluid accumulates (Fig. 13-1*A*). During this period, arterial and ventricular systolic pressures are fairly well maintained in the face of rising ventricular diastolic, atrial, and venous pressures. This is possible because of compensatory mechanisms supporting

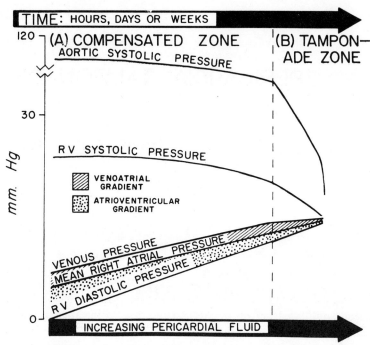

Figure 13-1. Schema of circulatory events during acute cardiac compression.
A, Period of effective compensation: Increasing pericardial fluid may cause increasing intrapericardial pressure but does not accumulate rapidly enough to overcome adjustments of the circulation; transvalvular gradients are maintained at some level, *B,* Pericardial tamponade: Either intrapericardial pressure rises too rapidly to permit compensation or compensatory mechanisms have been exhausted; pressure gradients—transvalvular and venoatrial—are rapidly liquidated. (Reprinted with permission from Spodick.[1])

atrial filling and ventricular minute output, principally tachycardia, arterial vasoconstriction, and expansion of venous blood volume with venous hypertension. The vertical broken line in Figure 13-1 indicates the point at which these mechanisms become inadequate and there is tamponade of the heart (Fig. 13-1*B*): rapid circulatory collapse marked by great venous hypertension and plunging arterial and ventricular systolic pressures. This may take hours, days, or weeks in most forms of pericarditis or pericardial neoplasia. An important exception is rapidly developing hemopericardium, particularly in cardiac wounds, aortic dissection, and ruptured myocardial infarction or aneurysm. Here, because of massive hemorrhage, the compensatory mechanisms rarely have a chance to operate. There is no time for intravenous blood volume expansion, and the heart is irretrievably compressed in seconds to minutes, with shock and no venous hypertension.

In all the above-mentioned circumstances, at some critical point (broken line in Fig. 13-1) during slow or rapid tamponade, quite small increments of intrapericardial contents cause disproportionate rises of pressure in the tight, low-compliance sac. The corollary to this, with crucial therapeutic implications, is that quite small decrements in intrapericardial contents can result in marked relief of cardiac compression. Thus, it is vital to recognize pericardial tamponade or impending tamponade in order to prevent or treat excessive cardiac compression with the expectation that appropriate treatment will usually give dramatic results. This is, in fact, usually the case, and relief of pericardial tamponade is often a most dramatic and rewarding experience.[1]

RECOGNITION OF PERICARDIAL TAMPONADE: DIAGNOSTIC OUTLINE

Accurate diagnosis of pericardial tamponade and its differentiation from other causes of circulatory embarrassment depend upon:

Awareness of appropriate clinical settings: systemic and local disorders associated with or capable of causing tamponade. These are listed in Table 13-1.

Recognition of any inflammatory or neoplastic pericardial disease as a potential source of tamponade.[1,3]

Anticipation of swift tamponade during diseases that, by penetrating the heart or aortic walls, may cause rapid exsanguination into the pericardial sac, notably dissecting aortic hematoma, acute myocardial infarction, and wounds of the chest or upper abdomen.

Detection of any pericardial effusion and its positive differentiation from cardiomegaly by echocardiography, cardioangiography, pneumoatriography, or radioisotope scanning.[2]

Detection of evidence that is more or less specific for pericardial tamponade if it occurs in appropriate clinical settings:

The picture of "shock" with venous distention.

Central venous pressure above 180 mm H_2O with absent y-descent in the venous pulse (except in patients with wounds of the heart or aorta who cannot elevate venous pressure but may have venous pulsations).

Marked pulsus paradoxus. Palpable inspiratory decline or absence of the pulse: inspiratory drop in systolic blood pressure exceed-

Table 13-1   *Etiologic Factors in Pericardial Tamponade*

Idiopathic pericarditis (syndrome)

Pericarditis due to living agents
Viral
Suppurative
Tuberculous
Other (e.g., parasites)

Trauma
Direct
  Penetrating chest or abdominal injury
  Surgical
  Cardiac catheterization
  Esophageal perforation
Indirect
  Nonpenetrating (blunt) chest injury
  Therapeutic irradiation of mediastinum or juxtacardiac structures
Postmyocardial/pericardial injury syndromes

Neoplasia
Secondary
  Pulmonary
  Breast
  Lymphoma
  Other
Primary (mesothelioma)

Diseases of contiguous or nearby structures
Myocardial infarction
  Pericardial effusion from "episteno-cardiac" pericarditis
  Myocardial rupture
  Hemopericardium associated (apparently) with anticoagulant administration

Hemopericardium of uncertain origin
Postmyocardial-infarction syndromes
Dissecting hematoma (aneurysm) of the aorta
Pleural and pulmonary diseases
  Pneumonia
  Pleuritis
  Neoplasia
Diseases of mediastinal structures
  Inflammations and infections
  Neoplasia

Disorders of metabolism
  Uremic pericarditis
  Hemorrhagic states
  Cholesterol pericarditis
  Others

Pericarditis with effusion in vasculitis-connective tissue disease group
Lupus erythematosus
Acute rheumatic fever
Rheumatoid arthritis
Others

Pericarditis in hypersensitivity states
Serum sickness syndrome
Others

Pericarditis of uncertain origin
Certain syndromes: Reiter's, Behcet's, Löffler's
Pericardial effusion associated with pancreatitis
Others

ing 15 mm Hg *or,* if the pulse pressure is less than this, equal to most or all of the pulse pressure.[2,4]

Absence of a third heart sound.

Marked electric alternation of the heart, particularly if this involves the P waves as well as the QRS.[4]

DEFINITIVE MANAGEMENT OF ACUTE TAMPONADE

Swift relief of acute or impending pericardial tamponade is mandatory. The pericardial contents must be evacuated as soon as possible. A few patients have overcome small degrees of cardiac compression, but this is unpredictable, and always hanging over the patient is the

Damoclean sword of a sudden increment in pericardial effusion or hemorrhage, which, even if small, would be catastrophic in an already tight system. The specific treatment of acute cardiac tamponade is *removal of pericardial fluid*—by needle paracentesis if possible, by surgical drainage if necessary. In the absence of significant complicating disorders (severe heart disease, true shock from exsanguination, overwhelming sepsis, constrictive epicarditis[5,6]), successful pericardial drainage produces truly dramatic subjective and objective changes in the patient: clearing of any mental confusion; a general feeling of relief; rise in arterial systolic and pulse pressure; decreased heart rate; diminution or disappearance of pulsus paradoxus, electric alternation, and venous distention; and disappearance of abnormal breathing patterns. Frequently, many of these changes occur upon removal of the first 50 to 150 ml of fluid[4]—the exact reverse of the "last straw" phenomenon, in which it is the last small increment of pericardial fluid that finally decompensates the cardiac response to even quite massive effusions. In other words, the patient's hemodynamics slide back along the pressure curves in Figure 13-1 from zone *B* to Zone *A*.

Indications for Pericardial Drainage

Absolute Indications.   The pericardium must be drained if there is frankly critical tamponade or when signs of early cardiac compression appear to be advancing. In particular, in the presence of adequate clinical or graphic evidence for pericardial effusion and acute cardiac compression,[2] pericardial drainage is often required if any of the following occur:

Cyanosis, tachypnea, a clear-cut shocklike syndrome, or impaired consciousness
Rising peripheral venous pressure above 130 mm H_2O
Pulsus paradoxus, measured by brachial sphygmomanometry to exceed 50% of the pulse pressure.

Relative Indications.   In the absence of florid tamponade, it may be desirable to drain large or increasing pericardial effusions for the following reasons:

To avert tamponade
To confirm the presence of effusion
To obtain fluid for etiologic diagnosis
To relieve intolerable chest discomfort
To instill certain therapeutic agents[1]

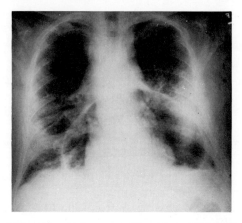

Figure 13-2. Induced pneumohydropericardium. Patient who had cardiac tamponade due to metastases from bronchogenic carcinoma (bilateral lung lesions evident). After relief of cardiac compression by pericardicentesis of tamponading effusion fluid, air has been insufflated into the pericardial sac through the needle used for the "tap." The heart is of normal size; the parietal pericardium is thin; there is residual fluid at the bottom of the sac.

To insufflate air (induced pneumohydropericardium) for demonstration of the state of the heart and pericardium[1,4,5] (Fig. 13-2)

Pericardial Paracentesis

Percutaneous needle aspiration of pericardial contents (pericardicentesis, pericardial tap) is the preferred method of drainage. In general, the distended pericardial sac can be tapped from any reasonably close location on the chest. In practice, certain "standard" points have been used (Fig. 13-3). The subxiphoid–subcostal approach (point 1, 2, or 3 in Fig. 13-3) seems to be the safest, and, in my experience, has nearly always been successful. The technique for this approach, which appears to minimize the risk of cardiac injury, is as follows:

Subxiphoid–Subcostal Pericardicentesis and Catheterization. Under strict aseptic technique, the needle is inserted in the left or right xiphocostal angle or beneath the xiphoid tip perpendicular to the skin and 3–4 mm below the costal margin. When the point of the needle penetrates to the level of the inner aspect of the rib cage, the hub of the needle is gently depressed so that the needle points towards the left shoulder ("northeast by north"). The needle now is cautiously advanced about 5 to 10 mm and its hub further depressed so that the point is only a few millimeters from the inner aspect of the rib cage (the hub

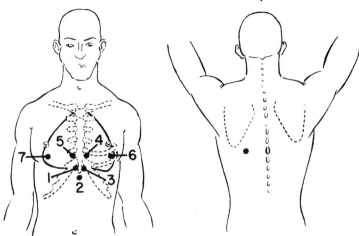

Figure 13-3. "Standard" locations for pericardicentesis approach. *Anterior view:* 1,2, and 3: Subxiphoid–subcostal approach points; 4 and 5: Fifth left and right intercostal spaces, respectively, 1 cm from sternal edge. 6: Apical. 7: Approach for major fluid accumulation on right side. *Posterior view:* Posterior approach. Details of subxiphoid–subcostal route are given in text. For details of other routes, see Spodick.[1] (Reprinted with permission from Spodick.[1])

at this point may have to be pressed into the abdominal wall in patients with protuberant abdomens). The needle is now cautiously advanced again by a worm-gear-type turning action of the fingers until fluid is reached. (N.B.: When the parietal pericardium is punctured, there is often but by no means always a distinct "give.") Should the epicardial surface of the heart be contacted, a definite "ticking" sensation is usually communicated to the fingers (and may even be audible inside a syringe attached to the needle hub); if this occurs, the needle is immediately withdrawn a few millimeters, the hub further depressed, and a new advance attempted in a parallel axis. If fluid is not encountered and the heart not contacted, the needle should likewise be withdrawn slightly and the hub elevated for another advance in another "northeast" axis. Once in place, the needle should be replaced by a plastic catheter, although quick removal of some fluid usually is desirable.

Equipment for Pericardicentesis and Pericardial Catheterization. Except in an immediate life-or-death crisis, a 20- or 21-gauge needle should first be used to anesthetize the skin and subcutaneous tissue with procaine or an equivalent anesthetic agent. Paracentesis is best performed with fairly large-bore needles and catheters, because proteinaceous inflammatory exudates, even those free of blood or pus, tend to congeal and because much more rapid evacuation is possible through wider lumens. A #16 Jelco- or Rochester-type needle can give good results and can be withdrawn, leaving its catheter inside the pericardial sac. For bloody or viscous fluids, a #14 thin-wall needle with obturator can be used with extreme care. Through it, a PE-190 plastic catheter can be passed and its external end attached to a syringe or suction apparatus via a Tuohey-type adapter. When using needles without attached catheters, soft-tip Amplatz-type "piano" wires can be passed through the needle, the needle withdrawn and an appropriate catheter threaded over the emplaced wire. It is desirable to use catheters that contain a radiopaque filament that will permit checking their location by fluoroscopy or radiography.

Safeguards. Pericardicentesis aims a sharp weapon at the heart. Certain protective measures are desirable:

• The usual "crash cart" items should be available, including pressor agents, intravenous fluids, oxygen, tracheal tubes, defibrillator–pacemaker, and ECG monitor.

• A slow intravenous drip of saline or glucose in water should be started to preserve a route for intravenous therapy.

• The shank of the paracentesis needle may be attached to the chest lead of an electrocardiograph or oscilloscope monitor by means of an insulated wire with an alligator clamp at each end. If the point of the needle contacts the ventricle, the S–T segment rises and there may be ventricular ectopic beats; when it touches the atrium, the P–R segment is elevated and atrial ectopic beats can be provoked. (Even with this safeguard, however, the needle should be advanced slowly, since there may be a delay in registering any change).

• A preliminary approach with a 20-gauge needle (which can be the needle used to deposit local anesthetic along the paracentesis route) sometimes will establish the adequacy of the route selected and the required depth of penetration and will occasionally suffice for removal of fluid.

• If bloody fluid is withdrawn, it is important to know quickly whether the needle has penetrated the heart. (In tamponade, removal of circulating blood from the heart or any vessel could be disastrous.) A microhematocrit apparatus should be available to compare the hematocrit of the first aliquot of fluid with that of the peripheral blood. Meanwhile, an agent used for circulation time estimation may be injected: If the patient tastes the sodium dehydrocholate, saccharin, or magnesium sulfate, the needle is surely in the heart or a blood vessel; the fluorescein–ultraviolet light technic may be used in patients unable to respond.

Failure of paracentesis to deliver fluid does not rule out pericardial effusion or hemorrhage. If the diagnostic criteria are strong, surgical intervention becomes mandatory.

Surgical Drainage of the Pericardium

When the diagnosis of pericardial effusion with tamponade is reasonably certain, failure to aspirate fluid or to successfully relieve tamponade by aspiration indicates surgical drainage (pericardiotomy). A small subcostal or intercostal incision may be adequate, although resection of a costal cartilage or even thoracotomy may be needed, especially in the case of loculated effusions. The individual situation will dictate the initial surgical approach and subsequent plan.

In tamponade due to penetrating wounds of the heart and great vessels, there is evidence favoring both routine surgical intervention, either following an initial tap or without delay, and surgery only if the patient becomes worse despite a successful pericardicentesis. The current trend in managing heart wounds is toward the more radical approach because paracentesis may not remove clots and because of late deaths and complications owing to repeated cardiac bleeding or progressive pericardial disease. Clotting is a serious problem in traumatic hemopericardium. In inflammatory and neoplastic effusions, intrapericardial blood obtained during pericardicentesis rarely tends to clot, owing to dilution and the defibrinating effect of being constantly agitated by cardiac motion. During pure pericardial bleeding, there is no dilution and tissue thromboplastic factors released by wounds will promote intrapericardial clotting, which tends to defeat pericardicentesis while permitting cardiac compression to proceed.

SUPPORTIVE MANAGEMENT

If there is difficulty in draining the pericardium or if there is delay in obtaining equipment, the heart and circulation can be maintained until either successful pericardicentesis or pericardiotomy is performed. Such supportive measures usually are unavoidable when tamponade is associated with significant blood loss. They include, particularly, use of intravenous fluids and adrenergic stimulants, which bolster physiologic compensatory mechanisms. Oxygen may be helpful, particularly in patients with marked dyspnea, cyanosis, or psychic disturbances, but it should not be delivered by positive-pressure breathing (which raises both intrapleural and intrapericardial pressures, thus reducing venous return to the heart). The place of digitalis and related substances is not clear; they may be of particular use in patients who also have heart disease.

Intravenously administered fluids maintain cardiac filling by expanding venous blood volume and maintaining the small venoatrial gradient. Glucose or saline may be used, but for traumatic bleeding and in patients with severe anemias, blood is preferable.

Pressor agents, particularly those with beta-adrenergic effects, produce increased myocardial stroke work per unit of effective filling pressure. They can thus support stroke volume despite pericardial tamponade. This is one of the few disorders in which the "ideal" beta-adrenergic stimulant, isoproterenol, can be truly effective. Norepinephrine, with both alpha- and beta-adrenergic stimulating properties, is also helpful.

SUMMARY

Pericardial tamponade, the decompensated phase of cardiac compression, occurs when relatively small increments in intrapericardial contents begin to cause disproportionate rises in intrapericardial pressure. Accurate diagnosis of tamponade depends on awareness of appropriate clinical settings, along with recognition of any inflammatory or neoplastic pericardial disease; detection of any pericardial effusion and its differentiation from cardiomegaly and congestive heart failure; anticipation of swift cardiac compression associated with diseases and wounds capable of producing intrapericardial hemorrhage. More or less specific evidence for tamponade includes "shock" with venous distention (in the absence of acute hemorrhage), increased venous pressure with absent y-descent in venous pulses, marked pulsus paradoxus, absence of third heart sound, and marked electric alternation on the electrocardiogram.

The specific management of tamponade is evacuation of pericardial contents by needle paracentesis if possible, or by surgical drainage if necessary. One of these is absolutely indicated if signs of cardiocirculatory embarrassment are either already marked or are moderate but detectably progressing. Relative indications include etiologic diagnosis of pericardial lesions, relief of symptoms (large effusions), intrapericardial administration of therapeutic agents, and production of an induced pneumohydropericardium. Utilizing appropriate safeguards, pericardial paracentesis can be performed using numerous approaches, but the subxiphoid–subcostal route is preferred. Insertion of an intrapericardial catheter should be routine to minimize trauma, permit continuous drainage, and obviate repeated needle punctures. Inability to remove fluid in this way mandates surgical drainage (which may be the definitive method for penetrating wounds of the heart and great vessels). While awaiting paracentesis or surgical equipment, temporary relief of tamponade can be obtained by intravenous administration of fluids and inotropic agents, particularly isoproterenol.

Infectious heart disease is described in detail in Chapter 12, and the surgical approach to cardiac emergency is treated in Chapter 17.

REFERENCES

1. Spodick, D. H.: Acute Pericarditis. New York, Grune & Stratton, 1959.
2. Spodick, D. H.: Acute cardiac tamponade: Pathophysiology, diagnosis and management. Prog. Cardiovasc. Dis. 10:64, 1967.
3. Spodick, D. H.: Differential diagnosis of acute pericarditis. Prog. Cardiovasc. Dis. 14:192, 1971.
4. Spodick, D. H.: Electric alternation of the heart: Its relation to the kinetics and physiology of the heart during cardiac tamponade. Am. J. Cardiol. 10:155, 1962.
5. Spodick, D. H.: Chronic and Constrictive Pericarditis. New York, Grune & Stratton, 1964.
6. Spodick, D. H., and Kumar, S.: Subacute constrictive pericarditis and cardiac tamponade. Dis. Chest 54:62, 1968.

Chapter 14
HYPERTENSIVE CRISIS

ALBERT N. BREST

Severe arterial blood pressure elevation may lead to a variety of clinical emergencies, including acute hypertensive encephalopathy, acute left ventricular failure, intracranial hemorrhage, acute coronary insufficiency, acute dissecting aneurysm of the aorta, and malignant hypertension. Such emergencies may occur during the course of either primary or secondary hypertension.

All of the various hypertensive crises demand rapid blood pressure reduction, although not necessarily to normotensive levels and not necessarily with the same urgency. Thus, hypertension associated with acute encephalopathy or aortic dissection requires immediate blood pressure reduction, i.e., within minutes or hours, whereas malignant or accelerated hypertension usually can be treated effectively by reduction of arterial pressure within days. Hypertensive crises associated with impaired renal or cerebral function should be treated initially by moderate blood pressure reduction, with careful observation of the patient's subsequent clinical status to determine whether further blood pressure reduction is feasible.

It is noteworthy that there is no single level of blood pressure elevation that augurs the development of a hypertensive emergency. Instead, a moderate arterial blood pressure elevation may in certain circumstances induce a hypertensive crisis, e.g., in patients whose hypertension develops rather suddenly (children and adolescents with acute renal disease or women with toxemia of pregnancy), whereas severe blood pressure elevation may at times occur without acute complications, e.g., in patients with long-standing hypertension.

CLINICAL ASPECTS

Acute Hypertensive Encephalopathy

This dramatic clinical syndrome is characterized by (1) sudden escalation of the blood pressure, i.e., an acute onset of hypertension or an acute exacerbation of previously existing hypertension, which is followed rapidly by (2) severe headache and altered consciousness. This disorder can eventuate in death within a few days if not promptly recognized and rapidly reversed.

Typically, diastolic blood pressure levels of 150 mm Hg or higher are encountered in this disorder. However, lesser levels may also be associated with hypertensive encephalopathy, especially in those patients with initial rather than long-standing hypertension. Accordingly, hypertensive encephalopathy may be encountered at times in patients whose diastolic blood pressure levels are no greater than 110 mm Hg, e.g., in youngsters with acute glomerulonephritis or in pregnant women with toxemia. In addition to the hypertension, the other typical physical abnormality in this disorder is found in the optic fundus, i.e., extreme retinal arterial narrowing. The severe arterial spasm is frequently, although not invariably, accompanied by papilledema. Less commonly, retinal hemorrhages and exudates are seen.

The encephalopathy is manifested predominantly by severe headache and altered consciousness, i.e., drowsiness, stupor, disorientation, and even coma. These manifestations may be accompanied by nausea, vomiting, visual blurring or blindness, and focal or generalized seizures. The clinical syndrome may be full-blown within a few hours, or it may take a day or two to develop.

The term "hypertensive encephalopathy" is sometimes used loosely to designate severe blood pressure elevation *per se,* without accompanying encephalopathy. However, this loose terminology is to be deplored, especially since the prognostic implications and therapeutic considerations for hypertensive encephalopathy are materially different than for severe hypertension by itself.

Pathologically, cerebral edema is the most commonly encountered abnormality. At times, the cerebral pathology will include petechial hemorrhages, tiny infarcts, and arteriolar necrosis; in some cases, herniation of the medulla into the foramen magnum may account for death.

The pathophysiologic sequence of hypertensive encephalopathy appears to derive from intense arterial spasm. The attendant cerebral ischemia is accompanied by increased capillary permeability, capillary wall ruptures, petechial hemorrhages, microinfarcts, and cerebral edema.

The clinical diagnosis can be recognized by the abrupt onset, the usually severe blood pressure elevation and the typical fundoscopic abnormalities, in combination with the rapidly progressive encephalopathy. The electroencephalogram generally reveals focal or generalized dysrhythmias, while the cerebrospinal fluid and protein content may be increased or normal. Skull x-rays, brain scan, and echoencephalogram are unremarkable in this disorder. Prompt clinical improvement (sometimes within an hour or two) following blood pressure reduction serves to confirm the clinical impression. Obviously, the more protracted the condition and the more severe the manifestations, the more prolonged and less complete the recovery.

The differential diagnosis of hypertensive encephalopathy includes various disorders in which blood pressure elevation and neurologic dysfunction coexist. Accordingly, this syndrome must be differentiated from certain cases of cerebral infarction and cerebral vascular insufficiency, intracerebral or subarachnoid hemorrhage, brain tumor, cerebral embolism, head injury, acute encephalitis, cerebral vasculitis, and epilepsy. The differentiation is aided if it can be shown that the blood pressure elevation had first occurred after the onset of cerebral symptoms or, in the case of antecedent chronic hypertension, if it can be demonstrated that the exacerbation of hypertension followed the onset of clinical symptoms. Unfortunately, in the clinical situation, such information may not be available. In this case, the overall clinical picture and, sometimes even more importantly, the favorable response (or lack of response) to emergency antihypertensive therapy may serve to confirm (or disprove) the clinical impression of hypertensive encephalopathy. If there is reasonable doubt about the diagnosis, prompt blood pressure reduction should be undertaken.

In addition to the aforementioned differential diagnostic considerations, clinical confusion sometimes arises in conditions such as acute pulmonary edema, acute coronary insufficiency, or acute anxiety, in which dramatic (albeit often transient) increases in blood pressure are sometimes encountered. However, in such instances, close examination of the total clinical picture generally serves to dispel the clinical diagnostic confusion.

As already indicated, the occurrence of hypertensive encephalopathy calls for prompt recognition and immediate blood pressure reduction to normal or near-normal levels. It is preferable to treat such patients in an intensive care unit, where changes in blood pressure, state of consciousness, convulsive activity, and airway obstruction can be monitored closely and treated expeditiously. Antihypertensive drug therapy should be administered parenterally in order to achieve blood pressure reduction without undue delay. The agents of choice in most instances are diazoxide, sodium nitroprusside, trimethaphan, or pentolinium. However, hydralazine may be particularly effective in controlling hypertensive encephalopathy associated with acute glomerulonephritis or toxemia of pregnancy. Reserpine and methyldopa should be used cautiously, especially because their sedative effects may lead to confusion in evaluating the patient's sensorium. Furthermore, the delayed antihypertensive response to both reserpine and methyldopa is an additional disadvantage in this emergency situation.

Acute Left Ventricular Failure

Blood pressure elevation increases the cardiac afterload, which may, in turn, result in sudden cardiac decompensation. Acute pulmonary edema is the usual clinical expression. In this situation, it is imperative to promptly reduce the workload of the incompetent left ventricle. Accordingly, prompt blood pressure reduction is generally more important therapeutically than digitalis administration, although the latter may be useful if the patient is not already taking the drug.

Reduction of blood pressure to normal levels is indicated in the management of acute heart failure associated with uncomplicated hypertensive heart disease. However, if the patient has accompanying symptomatic coronary disease, with or without acute myocardial infarction, less profound blood pressure reduction is indicated; otherwise, coronary insufficiency may be invoked.

The ganglioplegic drugs such as trimethaphan or pentolinium are particularly useful in the management of this hypertensive emergency because they reduce both the cardiac afterload and the preload, thereby decreasing systemic blood pressure and right ventricular pressure simultaneously. However, diazoxide or sodium nitroprusside also exert favorable antihypertensive effects in this situation. Potent diuretics, e.g., furosemide, should also be employed because they tend to enhance the blood pressure reduction and to exert favorable anticongestive effects as well. Ancillary therapeutic measures include bed rest, oxygen administration, morphine, and dietary salt restriction. Congestive heart failure and digitalization are discussed in detail in Chapters 1 and 7, respectively.

Intracranial Hemorrhage

Severe hypertension may be complicated by subarachnoid or intracranial hemorrhage. Blood pressure reduction is generally indicated in this situation. However, arterial spasm has been demonstrated angiographically in the area surrounding the bleeding site, and relief of the angiospasm by antihypertensive therapy may exacerbate this disorder. Accordingly, the blood pressure should be lowered cautiously, and the patient's neurologic status must be monitored carefully during attempted blood pressure reduction. If neurologic deterioration ensues, less aggressive blood pressure lowering is indicated. Conversely, if blood pressure reduction is well tolerated, it may be desirable to reduce the pressure to normotensive or even hypotensive levels. The antihypertensive agents of choice are trimethaphan, sodium nitroprusside, and pentolinium. Each has a rapid onset and short duration of action that makes dosage titration easier by intravenous infusion than when intramuscular or bolus intravenous injections are given; furthermore, none of these drugs produces somnolence that would interfere with neurologic evaluation. Neurologic consultation should also be obtained, especially in the case of subarachnoid hemorrhage, where surgical treatment may be more important than antihypertensive therapy.

The neurologic deficit associated with atherothrombotic stroke (cerebral infarct) is often aggravated by drastic reduction of the blood pressure. This complication results from decreased cerebral blood flow. Therefore, if aggravation of cerebral ischemia is to be avoided, blood pressure must be lowered cautiously. Again, the drugs of choice are trimethaphan, sodium nitroprusside, and pentolinium.

Acute Coronary Insufficiency

Blood pressure elevation usually increases myocardial oxygen requirement, and a sharp blood pressure rise may induce acute coronary insufficiency. This circumstance requires cautious blood pressure reduction. Drastic blood pressure fall must be avoided in order to prevent an undue fall in coronary blood flow and ensuing acute myocardial infarction. Reserpine is useful in this situation because of its gradual antihypertensive effect, as well as its sedative action.

Whereas acute hypertension may induce coronary insufficiency, it may also happen that coronary insufficiency initiates blood pressure elevation, so that hypertension actually follows rather than precedes the coronary attack. The blood pressure rise in this circumstance may be the result of extreme anxiety with reflexly induced blood pressure elevation; appropriate sedation will generally control the blood pressure rise.

Acute Dissecting Aortic Aneurysm

Hypertension is the most common precursor of acute aortic dissection. Although the aorta in these cases often shows evidence of cystic medial necrosis, the degree of this process frequently is comparatively minor. Therefore, the blood pressure elevation may be the more important factor in the pathogenesis of this disorder.

Until recent years, the general impression was that acute aortic dissection had a rapid devolutionary clinical course that invariably eventuated in death within a few hours, days, or weeks at the most, unless the lesion could be treated surgically. It is now evident, however, that acute aortic dissection can often be stabilized by hypotensive drug therapy.

Medical management consists essentially of intensive monitoring and the use of drugs that decrease cardiac impulse and lower the systolic blood pressure. A suitable response can generally be achieved with trimethaphan given intraveously, reserpine given intramuscularly, and guanethidine and propranolol given orally. The systolic blood pressure elevation should be maintained between 100 and 120 mm Hg. These drugs decrease myocardial contractility, thereby lessening the force that the cardiac impulse transmits to the dissecting aneurysm. Hydralazine and diazoxide should be avoided because they tend to greatly increase cardiac output and stroke volume, and such effects could aggravate the aortic dissection.

Malignant and Accelerated Hypertension

These conditions are associated with markedly elevated blood pressure and exudative retinopathy. In accelerated hypertension, the blood pressure elevation is accompanied by retinal hemorrhages and exudates, whereas papilledema is additionally present in malignant hypertension.

These disorders tend to be associated with rapid systemic deterioration. Typically, the pathology consists of diffuse necrotizing arteritis, which accounts for the attendant renal, cardiac, and cerebral dysfunction. In addition, acute renal ischemia usually induces marked renin production and secondary aldosteronism.

These conditions represent semi-emergencies, in that blood pressure reduction is required within days rather than within minutes or hours. Nonetheless, the rapid devolutionary course must not be underestimated.

Prompt blood pressure reduction may at times be achieved with oral antihypertensive therapy. However, to gain rapid control of hypertension, especially if oral medication is poorly tolerated because of nausea and vomiting, parenterally administered antihypertensive drugs may be valuable for several days. Diazoxide, reserpine, sodium nitroprusside, trimethaphan, or pentolinium may be useful in this circumstance.

Pheochromocytoma and Hypertensive Crises Associated with Monoamine Oxidase Inhibition

Pheochromocytoma should be suspected in patients with paroxysmal severe blood pressure elevation associated with headache, palpitation, excessive sweating, tachycardia, facial pallor, and tremor of the hands. Intravenous injection of 5 to 10 mg of phentolamine will serve both as a diagnostic test and a therapeutic measure for patients with pheochromocytoma. Intravenous infusion of sodium nitroprusside is also effective in controlling the blood pressure elevation associated with this disorder. Additionally, propranolol may be employed to control any cardiac dysrhythmias.

Acute hypertensive crises similar in signs and symptoms to those encountered in pheochromocytoma may occur also in some patients who receive monoamine oxidase (MAO) inhibitors and at the same time take catecholamine-releasing drugs (e.g., amphetamine or ephedrine) or ingest beverages or foods that contain much tyramine (e.g., chianti, some beers manufactured in countries other than the United States, unpasteurized cheeses, pickled herring, and chicken livers). This syndrome, as with pheochromocytoma, results from excess circulating catecholamines. The hypertensive emergency should be managed in the same way as pheochromocytoma.

ANTIHYPERTENSIVE DRUG THERAPY

Diazoxide

Diazoxide is a nondiuretic thiazide that exerts potent antihypertensive effects when administered intravenously. In contrast with the oral benzothiadiazine diuretics, the drug promotes sodium retention. Nonetheless, diazoxide is a potent and rapidly acting antihypertensive agent. It acts directly on the arterioles, with a resultant decrease in peripheral vascular resistance. Its antihypertensive effect is accompanied by an increase in heart rate and cardiac output. Furthermore, the fall in blood pressure produced by intravenous diazoxide is not ordinarily accompanied by a reduction in renal blood flow or glomerular filtration rate, and therefore the drug can usually be given safely to patients with renal insufficiency.

To be effective, diazoxide must be given rapidly (in 10 to 15 seconds) by intravenous push from a syringe without diluting the commercial preparation. The usual effective dosage is 300 mg. Blood pressure falls steeply, with a maximal effect achieved in 3 to 4 minutes, and the effect may persist for 12 hours or longer.

Diazoxide causes sodium and fluid retention, and therefore if the drug must be employed for more than 2 to 3 days, oral or parenterally administered diuretics should be used in addition. Because diazoxide induces hyperglycemia, the drug should be used with appropriate caution in diabetic patients. In addition, because diazoxide may cause abrupt cessation of labor, its use is limited in toxemia of pregnancy. Diazoxide should be avoided in the medical treatment of acute dissection of the aorta because its enhancement of cardiac output may provide additional stress at the site of intimal tear. Likewise, the abrupt decrease in blood pressure could be detrimental to patients with coronary or cerebrovascular insufficiency, and therefore the drug should not be given in these situations.

Sodium Nitroprusside

Sodium nitroprusside, like diazoxide and hydralazine, is a direct vasodilator, but it does not increase cardiac output and rate. The drug is instantaneously and consistently effective. A stock solution can be prepared by dissolving 50 mg of sodium nitroprusside USP in 25 ml of normal saline. Then 25 ml of the stock solution can be added to 1000 ml of normal saline or 5% glucose in water. The infusion of sodium nitroprusside is started at a rate of 5 or 10 drops per minute, and the rate is regulated according to the blood pressure response. The infusion of nitroprusside should be attended at all times, and the blood pressure should be checked every 10 minutes or less. Because of the precipitous fall in blood pressure that it causes, the infusion should be titrated with particular care in patients with coronary or cerebrovascular insufficiency.

The nitroprusside ion is converted to thiocyanate, so serum levels of thiocyanate should be determined every other day if the infusion must be continued for longer than 72 hours. The infusion should be discontinued if the serum concentration of thiocyanate exceeds 12 mg/100 ml to avoid an acute toxic reaction manifested by psychosis and confusion.

Ganglion-Blocking Agents

The ganglioplegic drugs are potent antihypertensive agents, but their usefulness in the treatment of hypertensive emergencies is necessarily limited by the fact that their greatest effect is exerted when the patient is in the upright position. These compounds are particularly indicated in those instances of severe congestive heart failure in which blood pressure elevation is sudden. As therapeutic blockade is established, venous tone is reduced, with a resultant decrease in venous pressure, decrease in right atrial pressure, and increase in cardiac output. Consequently, relief of pulmonary edema is often dramatic. To obtain maximum benefit from ganglion-blocking agents, the patient should be semireclining and the head of the bed should be elevated 10 to 12 inches on blocks.

When pentolinium (Ansolysen) is given by continuous intravenous infusion for hypertensive emergencies, 50 to 200 mg is placed in 1000 cc of 5% glucose in water. The drug is infused at a moderate rate until the blood pressure begins to fall, and then the rate of infusion is adjusted so as to maintain an adequate blood pressure reduction. For intramuscular injection, an initial dose of 5 mg is used and subsequent doses can be progressively increased, at 1–2-hour intervals, until reduction is adequate or a maximum dose of 50 mg is being given. Response is rarely greater with larger doses. A similarly useful ganglioplegic drug is trimethaphan camphorsulfonate (Arfonad), which may be given intravenously in a concentration of 1000 mg per liter of 5% glucose in water.

Continuous parenteral use of the ganglion-blocking agents frequently leads to the development of ileus and urinary retention. Foley catheters are nearly always required for elderly men who receive ganglion-blocking compounds for any significant period. Cathartics should be used freely for relief of constipation, and cholinergic agents are sometimes even more effective.

Reserpine

Parenteral reserpine is a potent antihypertensive agent that is effective in most hypertensive emergencies. Equally important is the fact that its antihypertensive effect is manifested in the recumbent as well as the upright position, an attribute of particular importance in the acutely ill, bedfast patient. However, there is a latent period of 1 to 2 hours before the blood pressure decreases, following either intravenous or intramuscular administration of the drug. If immediate reduction of blood pressure is desirable, a more rapidly acting drug must be administered.

The initial recommended dosage of parenteral reserpine is 1 to 2.5 mg. Thereafter, the dosage may be increased by 2.5-mg increments until an adequate blood pressure reduction is achieved; however, at least 2 hours must be allowed between doses in order to observe the maximum response to any single administration. If necessary, subsequent doses of 5 or even 10 mg may be given, but individual doses should rarely exceed 10 mg and the total dose should not exceed 20 mg per day.

After the proper dosage has been established, the patient can be placed on a regular schedule, which usually consists of 2.5 to 5 mg of reserpine given every 6 to 12 hours. The dosage and the interval between doses depend on the blood pressure response and are adjusted so as to maintain the desired blood pressure level.

The side effects associated with reserpine tend to become more prominent as the dosage or the frequency of administration is increased. Prolonged daily administration of more than 10 mg depresses cerebration and may cause a Parkinsonlike syndrome. The latter manifestations are temporary, however, and tend to disappear several days after discontinuation of the drug. Reserpine may also activate peptic ulcers, leading to acute gastrointestinal bleeding. However, the major disadvantage of the drug is its tendency to cause profound somnolence. This soporific effect is particularly troublesome in cerebral hemorrhage or hypertensive encephalopathy, because it interferes with the clinical evaluation of the sensorium, which is so important in assessing the progress of these patients.

Hydralazine

This drug is especially effective in the management of hypertensive encephalopathy complicating acute or chronic glomerulonephritis or eclampsia. The onset of blood pressure reduction (15 to 20 minutes) after administration of hydralazine is more rapid than after administration of reserpine. However, the best results are often obtained when the two drugs are used in combination, hydralazine producing the more rapid action and reserpine allowing a more sustained effect.

When hydralazine is administered, an initial dose of 10 to 20 mg should be given intravenously as a single injection over a 5-minute period, or a dose of 10 to 50 mg may be given intramuscularly. Then 100 mg may be placed in 1000 cc of 10% glucose in water and administered by continuous intravenous injection. The rate of infusion should be adjusted according to the blood pressure. In other instances, blood pressure reduction may be maintained by giving hydralazine intramuscularly in doses ranging from 10 to 50 mg as often as every 4 hours.

Phentolamine

Phentolamine is an alpha-adrenergic blocking agent. Its use in hypertensive crises is recommended only for patients with increased levels of circulating catecholamines, i.e., those with pheochromocytoma or hypertensive emergencies associated with MAO inhibition. The drug is ineffective in managing hypertensive crises arising from other causes. The effect of phentolamine is short-lived, usually lasting less than 15 minutes. It may be desirable to administer phentolamine by constant intravenous infusion after the blood pressure has been controlled initially by rapid intravenous injection of 5 to 15 mg from a syringe.

Methyldopa

Intravenously administered methyldopa has a delayed onset of action (4 to 6 hours), and this limits its effectiveness in hypertensive emergencies. The drug is less consistently effective than is reserpine. Furthermore, like reserpine, methyldopa may also cause sedation, thereby inter-fering with evaluation of the patient's sensorium. Methyldopa should be administered intravenously by intermittent infusion over a 30–60-minute interval; the usual dosage is 250 to 500 mg/100 ml.

Diuretics

The antihypertensive action of all the aforementioned antihyperten-sive drugs is enhanced by the concomitant administration of a diuretic. The diuretic drugs of choice are furosemide or ethacrynic acid because (1) they can be given intravenously, (2) they are rapidly effective, and (3) they do not cause an acute decline in glomerular filtration rate (in contrast with the thiazide diuretics). The usual dosage of furosemide is 40 to 80 mg, while ethacrynic acid is given in a dosage of 50 to 100 mg. Larger doses may be required in patients with renal function impairment. Both furosemide and ethacrynic acid may cause nerve deaf-ness when rapidly infused intravenously in large doses in azotemic patients.

Overall Therapeutic Approach

An outline for the drug treatment of hypertensive emergencies is given in Table 14-1. Quick appraisal of the state of renal compensation is extremely important in these patients, as is evaluation of their cardiac and cerebral status. Renal function evaluation can best be done by mea-surement of serum creatinine. When the creatinine is elevated, serial values should be measured every 2 to 3 days while the blood pressure is being regulated. When evidence of rising creatinine is observed, the blood pressure should be allowed to increase slowly by decreasing the dose of antihypertensive agent until the creatinine again decreases to pretreatment levels.

Should undue blood pressure reduction occur during treatment, a direct pressor agent such as levarterenol bitartrate (4 mg/liter) may be employed to treat the drug-induced hypotension. However, discon-tinuation of the infusion will usually suffice when short-acting depressor agents such as sodium nitroprusside or trimethaphan are employed. Re-plenishment of plasma volume by infusions of saline, whole blood, or low-molecular-weight dextran is important when diuretic drug therapy has induced oligemia.

After the hypertensive emergency is over and the blood pressure and general status of the patient have been stabilized for 3 to 7 days, oral antihypertensive drug treatment should be substituted for the parenteral medication.

Table 14-1   *Outline for Parenteral Drug Treatment of Hypertensive Emergencies*

Emergency	Preferred Drugs	Drugs to Avoid or Use with Caution
Acute hypertensive encephalopathy	Diazoxide Sodium nitroprusside Trimethaphan Pentolinium	Reserpine Methyldopa
Acute left ventricular failure	Trimethaphan Pentolinium Diazoxide Sodium nitroprusside	Hydralazine
Intracranial hemorrhage	Sodium nitroprusside Trimethaphan Pentolinium	Reserpine Methyldopa
Acute coronary insufficiency	Reserpine	Hydralazine
Acute dissecting aortic aneurysm	Trimethaphan and reserpine	Hydralazine Diazoxide
Malignant and accelerated hypertension	Diazoxide Reserpine Sodium nitroprusside Trimethaphan Pentolinium	
Pheochromocytoma and hypertensive crises associated with MAO inhibition	Phentolamine Sodium nitroprusside	All others

SUMMARY

A variety of hypertensive emergencies may be encountered during the course of primary or secondary hypertension. These emergencies include acute hypertensive encephalopathy, acute left ventricular failure, intracranial hemorrhage, acute coronary insufficiency, acute dissecting aortic aneurysm, and malignant hypertension. Each of these requires prompt recognition and rapid blood pressure reduction, although not necessarily to normotensive levels and not necessarily with the same urgency. Preferably, such patients are treated initially in an intensive care unit, where changes in blood pressure, state of consciousness, convulsive activity, and airway obstruction can be monitored closely and treated expeditiously. Antihypertensive drug therapy is administered parenterally, and the individual drug selection is determined by the specific emergency and by the patient's overall clinical condition (especially the cardiac, renal, and cerebral status). After the hypertensive emergency is controlled and the blood pressure and general status of the patient have been stabilized for 3 to 7 days, oral antihypertensive drug treatment should be substituted for the parenteral medication.

SELECTED REFERENCES

1. AMA Committee on Hypertension: The treatment of malignant hypertension and hypertensive emergencies. JAMA 228:1673, 1974.
2. Bhatia, S. K., and Frohlich, E. D.: Hemodynamic comparison of agents useful in hypertensive emergencies. Am. Heart J. 85:367, 1973.
3. Finnerty, F. A., Jr.: Hypertensive encephalopathy. Am. J. Med. 52:672, 1972.
4. Freis, E. D.: Hypertensive crisis. JAMA 208:338, 1969.
5. Gifford, R. W., Jr., and Richards, N. G.: Hypertensive encephalopathy. Stroke 5:43, 1970.
6. Hypertension Study Group: Resources for the management of emergencies in hypertension. Circulation 43:A157, 1971.
7. Koch Weser, J.: Current concepts: Hypertensive emergencies. N. Engl. J. Med. 290:211, 1974.
8. Mroczek, W. J., Davidov, M., Gavrilovich, L., et al.: The value of aggressive therapy in the hypertensive patient with azotemia. Circulation 40:893, 1969.
9. Vaamonde, C. A., David, N. J., and Palmer, R. F.: Hypertensive emergencies. Med. Clin. N. Am. 55:325, 1971.
10. Woods, J. W., and Blythe, W. B.: Management of malignant hypertension complicated by renal insufficiency. N. Engl. J. Med. 277:57, 1967.

Chapter 15
DIGITALIS INTOXICATION

EDWARD K. CHUNG

Cardiac glycoside has probably been the most valuable drug available for treatment of heart disease from the time digitalis was introduced by the British physician William Withering in 1785.[1] It is well documented that cardiac glycoside is an essential drug in the management of congestive heart failure regardless of underlying heart disease and of various supraventricular tachyarrhythmias, particularly atrial fibrillation with rapid ventricular response.[2]

In recent years, however, the incidence of digitalis toxicity has increased because of the frequent use of potent purified cardiac glycosides in conjunction with potent diuretics, which predisposes to the development of hypokalemia. The incidence of digitalis intoxication in general hospitals has been estimated to be approximately 20%.[2] Digitalis intoxication is often unavoidable, because the margin between therapeutic and toxic doses is relatively narrow. This margin is further reduced in elderly and seriously ill patients and those with various modifying factors, such as hypokalemia, myxedema, electrolyte imbalance, hypoxia, and pulmonary disease. It has been shown that the therapeutic dose is approximately 60% of the toxic dose.

Although cardiac glycoside is indispensable in the treatment of heart failure and various supraventricular tachyarrhythmias, the drug is no longer beneficial to a patient who has developed manifestations of digitalis toxicity. Frequently, digitalis intoxication may develop in a patient after a relatively small dose that is either therapeutic or inadequate for other patients. This is especially true when there are various modifying factors such as those listed above. Consequently, the digitalis requirement varies from patient to patient and within the same patient from time to time. Use of the standard dosage for digitalization without adjusting to the individual response is a common cause of digitalis toxicity. It is not uncommon for digitalis to reach intoxicating levels without having the desired therapeutic effect, especially in patients with intractable congestive heart failure. In retrospect, apparently inexplicable death in patients with refractory congestive heart failure can often be attributed to digitalis intoxication.

Although digitalis is certainly one of the oldest and most commonly used drugs, it is not possible for physicians to determine precisely the optimal therapeutic dosage. The determination of serum digoxin or digitoxin value is widely utilized at many institutions in order to assess the therapeutic and toxic doses of digitalis.[3,4] A markedly increased serum digitalis level usually indicates digitalis toxicity, whereas very low levels of digitalis in the serum often indicate underdigitalization. Serum digitalis determination is extremely valuable in patients suffering from intractable congestive heart failure or complex cardiac arrhythmias when little or no information regarding previous digitalization is available. Determination of serum digitalis level will be discussed in detail later in this chapter.

The most common manifestations of digitalis intoxication are gastrointestinal disturbances, various cardiac arrhythmias, aggravation of preexisting congestive heart failure or the development of new congestive heart failure, neurologic disturbances, and visual disturbances.[2] Common and uncommon manifestations of digitalis intoxication are listed in Table 15-1.

GASTROINTESTINAL SYMPTOMS

Anorexia is often the earliest sign of digitalis toxicity, and it is usually followed by nausea and vomiting within 2 to 3 days if digitalization is continued. Nausea and vomiting are considered to be central rather than gastric in origin.

Diarrhea is a rather uncommon manifestation of digitalis toxicity, and constipation and abdominal pain have also been reported rarely. Gastrointestinal symptoms are often not clearly evident in elderly patients, probably being masked by the severity of the congestive heart failure and cerebral insufficiency. It is well documented that most of the purified glycosides produce nausea and vomiting much less frequently than digitalis leaf. Thus, digitalis-induced arrhythmias are frequently the earliest manifestation of digitalis toxicity with these preparations. When nausea

Table 15-1   *Manifestations of Digitalis Toxicity*

Symptoms	Common	Uncommon
Gastro-intestinal	Anorexia, nausea, vomiting	Abdominal pain, constipation, diarrhea, hemorrhage
Cardiac	Worsening of congestive heart failure, ventricular premature contraction, paroxysmal atrial tachycardia with block, nonparoxysmal AV nodal tachycardia, AV block, sinus bradycardia	Atrial fibrillation, atrial flutter, ventricular tachycardia, ventricular flutter, sinus arrest, SA block, atrial premature contraction, AV nodal premature contraction
Visual	Color vision (green or yellow) with halos	Blurring or shimmering vision, scotoma, micropsia or macropsia, amblyopia
Neurologic	Fatigue, headache, insomnia, malaise, confusion, vertigo, depression	Neuralgia, convulsions, paresthesia, delirium, psychosis
Nonspecific	—	Allergic reaction, idiosyncrasy, thrombocytopenia, gynecomastia

and vomiting develop, and the possibilities of overdigitalization and underdigitalization are almost equal, digitalis should be discontinued immediately and the patient should be re-evaluated.

VISUAL AND NEUROLOGIC MANIFESTATIONS

Green or yellow color vision with colored halos has been considered to be a pathognomonic feature of digitalis toxicity for many years.[2] Other visual disturbances may include scotoma, blurring, shimmering vision, and, less commonly, micropsia and temporary or permanent amblyopia.[2] These visual manifestations may easily go unrecognized unless the physician inquires specifically about them.

Cardiac glycosides may produce various neurologic symptoms, including headache, fatigue, lassitude, insomnia, malaise, depression, confusion, delirium, and vertigo and, less commonly, convulsions, neuralgias, especially trigeminal nerve and paresthesia. Visual and neurologic manifestations usually develop later than gastrointestinal symptoms or cardiac arrhythmias, and most of the above-mentioned symptoms are less specific for digitalis toxicity than gastrointestinal manifestations or arrhythmias, except for the color vision. Furthermore, neurologic symptoms are often difficult to evaluate in elderly individuals because these manifestations may be due to many other conditions, such as cerebrovascular accidents and chronic brain syndrome.

RARE MANIFESTATIONS

Allergic manifestations, such as urticaria and eosinophilia, and idiosyncrasy are *not* true manifestations of digitalis intoxication.[2,5] Similarly, unilateral or bilateral gynecomastia that develops during digitalis therapy does not seem to be a manifestation of digitalis toxicity, although some investigators consider it to be so. This author has seen several patients who have shown no other toxic manifestations after the development of gynecomastia in spite of continued digitalis therapy.[2] Therefore, gynecomastia due to an estrogenlike activity of digitalis is most likely not a toxic manifestation.[6] Furthermore, digitalis-induced gynecomastia seems to be duration-dependent rather than dosage-dependent because it usually develops when patients receive cardiac glycosides for more than 2 years.

A rare occurrence of digitoxin-induced thrombocytopenia has been reported, and it was considered to be a specific sensitivity reaction to digitoxin bound to the gamma globulin fraction of the serum.[7]

CARDIAC MANIFESTATIONS

There are two major cardiac manifestations induced by digitalis—alteration in contractility and digitalis-induced arrhythmias—and they often occur simultaneously.[2]

Alteration of Contractility

A worsening of pre-existing congestive heart failure or the development of new heart failure during digitalization is a not uncommon manifestation of digitalis toxicity.[2,5] Indeed, intractable or refractory congestive heart failure is frequently due to digitalis intoxication, and this relationship may be much more common than is recognized. Regardless of the fundamental mechanism involved, all patients with intractable congestive heart failure should be carefully re-evaluated for possible digitalis toxicity.

Digitalis-Induced Cardiac Arrhythmias

Although cardiac glycoside is often essential in the treatment of most supraventricular tachyarrhythmias, the drug may produce almost every known type of cardiac arrhythmia by altering impulse formation, conduction, or both.[2] Recognition of digitalis-induced arrhythmias is extremely important because various cardiac arrhythmias may be not only the earliest but also the only sign of digitalis intoxication. Use of purified glycosides in recent years has led to an increase in incidence of cardiac arrhythmias without other symptoms of toxicity. Furthermore, hypo-kalemia induced by frequent use of potent diuretics predisposes to the development of digitalis-induced cardiac arrhythmias.[2]

It has been estimated that some form of cardiac arrhythmia occurs in 80% to 90% of patients with digitalis intoxication.[2,8] Various combi-nations of cardiac arrhythmias are commonly observed in patients with advanced digitalis toxicity; it is not uncommon for cardiac arrhythmias to change from one type to another in the same electrocardiographic tracing.[2]

It should be emphasized that the classical digitalis effect (S–T and T-wave changes) in the electrocardiogram during digitalis therapy is completely unrelated to digitalis toxicity.[2,8] The digitalis effect in the electrocardiogram may be absent in about two thirds of the cases with digitalis toxicity, and, by the same token, striking S–T and T-wave changes are frequently observed in the absence of any evidence of digi-talis toxicity. Other electrocardiographic findings during digitalis ther-apy, such as a shortening of the Q–T interval, increased amplitude of the U waves, and peaking of the terminal portion of the T waves, also are not indicative of digitalis toxicity.[2]

Ventricular bigeminy or trigeminy is probably the most common digi-talis-induced cardiac arrhythmia. Almost equally common are A–V nodal (junctional) arrhythmias, especially in the presence of pre-existing atrial fibrillation.[2]

Almost all types of cardiac arrhythmias may be induced by digitalis, but there are some arrhythmias that do not seem to be related to cardiac glycosides. Non-digitalis-induced cardiac arrhythmias include Mobitz type II AV block, parasystole, bilateral bundle branch block of varying degree, sinus tachycardia, and paroxysmal AV nodal (junctional) tachycardia.

Disturbances of Sinus Impulse Formation and Conduction. Minor toxic effects of digitalis may induce sinus bradycardia (Fig. 15-1), which may lead to more serious arrhythmias, such as sinus arrest and sinoatrial block, if digitalization continues. A sudden reduction of the heart rate to below 50 per minute in an adult patient during digitalization should raise the suspicion of digitalis intoxication (Fig. 15-1). A pulse rate below 100 per minute in infancy has the same clinical significance. Sino-atrial block with or without Wenckebach phenomenon is not uncommon in digitalis intoxication, especially in children.[2] Indeed, digitalis may be the most common cause of SA block. Sinus tachycardia does not seem to be induced by digitalis. However, it should be noted that some patients with congestive heart failure may have persisting sinus tachycar-dia even after full digitalization. This is observed when the congestive

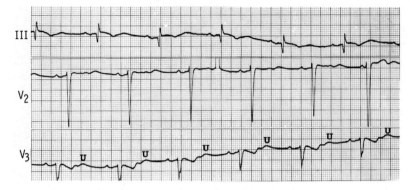

Figure 15-1. Sinus bradycardia with a rate of 49 beats per minute. Note prominent U waves due to hypokalemia.

heart failure is associated with other diseases, such as chronic pulmonary diseases, hyperthyroidism, obesity, and anemia.

Atrial Arrhythmias. It is well documented that various atrial tachyarrhythmias may be produced by digitalis, even though digitalis is the drug of choice in the treatment of most atrial tachyarrhythmias. Atrial tachycardia is the commonest digitalis-induced atrial arrhythmia, and it is frequently associated with varying-degree AV block[2,9] (Fig. 15-2). This condition is called paroxysmal atrial tachycardia (PAT) with block. Although the frequent occurrence of digitalis-induced PAT with block is often emphasized, is actually accounts for only about 10% of digitalis-induced cardiac arrhythmias.[2]

It has been said that carotid sinus stimulation frequently terminates PAT with block not due to digitalis toxicity and is ineffective when digi-

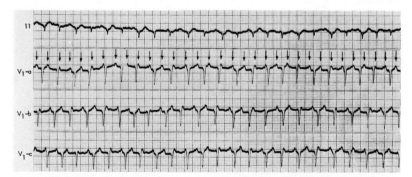

Figure 15-2. Leads V₁-a,b, and c are continuous. Arrows indicate P waves. The rhythm is atrial tachycardia (atrial rate: 210 beats per minute) with varying-degree Wenckebach AV block (ventricular rate: 145–165 beats per minute).

talis is the etiologic factor.[8] However, the danger of applying carotid sinus stimulation to patients with suspected digitalis intoxication cannot be overemphasized. It has been shown that some patients have died from ventricular fibrillation during or after carotid sinus stimulation.[10,11] All of these patients had been critically ill and had received cardiac glycosides. Based on these observations, carotid sinus stimulation should be avoided if at all possible in patients who are taking even small amounts of digitalis.

As for the fundamental mechanism responsible for the production of atrial tachycardia, the refractory period of the atrial musculature is markedly shortened by an indirect vagal stimulating action of digitalis. Thus, increased conductivity within the atrial muscle can produce various atrial tachyarrhythmias. A combination of the depressive effect on the AV conduction and the shortening effect on the atrial refractory period results in atrial tachycardia with varying-degree AV block.[2]

Atrial fibrillation or flutter may be produced by digitalis, but its occurrence is very rare indeed. It is unclear why digitalis-induced atrial fibrillation or flutter is so rare, in comparison with atrial tachycardia. Although atrial premature contractions are not as common as ventricular ones, if they do occur, the ectopic P waves are frequently not conducted to the ventricles (nonconducted or blocked atrial premature contractions) in spite of relatively long coupling intervals. The combination of impaired AV conduction and the increased excitability in the atria results in frequent nonconducted atrial premature contractions.

AV Nodal (Junctional) Arrhythmias. As mentioned earlier in this chapter, the incidence of various AV nodal (junctional) arrhythmias in digitalis toxicity is probably as high as that of ventricular premature contractions.[2] Digitalis induces various AV nodal (junctional) arrhythmias, due either to passive impulse formation resulting in AV nodal escape rhythm (Fig. 15-3) or to enhancement of AV nodal impulse

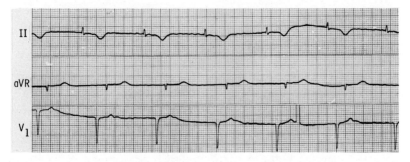

Figure 15-3. Atrial fibrillation with AV nodal (junctional) escape rhythm (rate: 46 beats per minute) due to complete AV block.

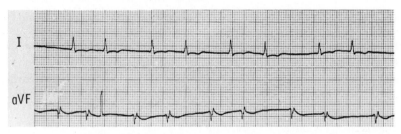

Figure 15-4. Nonparoxysmal AV nodal (junctional) tachycardia (rate: 68 beats per minute) in the presence of atrial fibrillation producing complete AV dissociation.

formation resulting in nonparoxysmal AV nodal (junctional) tachycardia (Fig. 15-4).

In advanced digitalis intoxication, exit block of varying degree may develop around the AV nodal (junctional) pacemaker, and the ventricular cycle may become slower and/or irregular. When the exit block is Wenckebach type, the ventricular cycle may show regular irregularity (Fig. 15-5). Ventricular tachycardia may be closely simulated by AV nodal (junctional) tachycardia with aberrant ventricular conduction, especially in the presence of pre-existing atrial fibrillation. In rare occasions, double AV nodal (junctional) rhythm or tachycardia may be produced by digitalis; this is a rare form of AV dissociation (Fig. 15-6). It should be emphasized that the basic rhythm is frequently atrial fibrillation when digitalis-induced AV junctional arrhythmias develop (Fig. 15-3 through 15-5). At times, the atrial mechanism may be atrial flutter or tachycardia in the presence of AV junctional tachycardia (Fig. 15-7), leading to double supraventricular tachycardia.

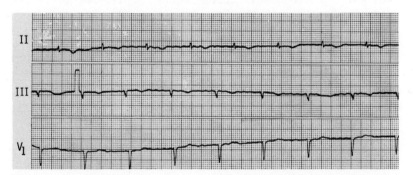

Figure 15-5. Nonparoxysmal AV nodal (junctional) tachycardia with 3:2 Wenckebach exit block in the presence of atrial fibrillation, producing complete AV dissociation.

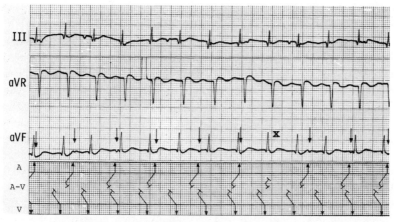

Figure 15-6. Double AV nodal (junctional) tachycardia. The rate of the AV junctional tachycardia (75 beats per minute) controls the atria in a retrograde fashion (indicated by arrows), whereas another AV junctional tachycardia activating the ventricles produces a faster rate (rate: 100 beats per minute). Retrograde block is most likely responsible for the absence of a P wave in lead aVF (marked *X*).

AV Conduction Disturbances. Digitalis may produce various degrees of AV block resulting from both the direct and indirect actions of the drug.[2] These actions are, needless to say, essential in the management of various supraventricular tachyarrhythmias, especially atrial fibrillation. The degree of AV block in digitalis intoxication depends largely

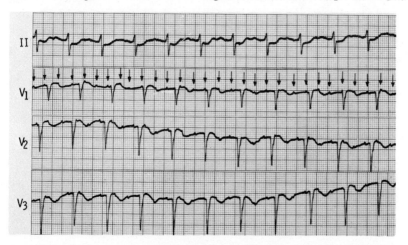

Figure 15-7. Arrows indicate atrial activity. The rhythm is atrial tachycardia (atrial rate: 220–240 beats per minute) with nonparoxysmal AV junctional tachycardia (rate: 94 beats per minute), producing complete AV dissociation (double supraventricular tachycardia).

upon the dosage of the drug, underlying heart disease, pre-existing AV conduction disturbances, and electrolyte imbalance.

Although first-degree AV block is one of the earliest manifestations of digitalis toxicity, some investigators do not include it among the toxic manifestations of the drug. However, digitalis-induced second-degree or higher AV block is often followed by first-degree AV block when digitalis is stopped. Therefore, first-degree AV block during digitalization should definitely be considered a manifestation of digitalis toxicity.

The average incidence of second-degree AV block in different series is estimated to be 11%.[2,8] Among second-degree AV blocks, Wenckebach (Mobitz type I) AV block is more common than 2:1 AV block. On the other hand, Mobitz type II AV block has not been reported as a manifestation of digitalis toxicity. It is common to observe that Wenckebach AV block and 2:1 AV block often coexist in the same electrocardiographic tracing (Fig. 15-8).

High-degree (advanced) or complete AV block is very common in digitalis intoxication when the underlying rhythm is atrial fibrillation (Fig. 15-3). It has been said that digitalis intoxication is the second most common cause of complete AV block.[2]

Ventricular Arrhythmias. Ventricular premature contractions are the most common and often the earliest manifestation of digitalis toxicity in the adult population. The incidence has been reported to be approximately 50% of all digitalis-induced arrhythmias. It has been known for many years that ventricular bigeminy (Fig. 15-9) is a hallmark of digitalis-induced arrhythmia.[2,8] Diagnostic probability of digitalis intoxication is 100% when ventricular bigeminy coexists with nonparoxysmal AV nodal (junctional) tachycardia or AV block, especially in the presence of atrial fibrillation (Fig. 15-9).

In children and healthy adults, supraventricular arrhythmias and AV conduction disturbances are a more common occurrence than ventricular

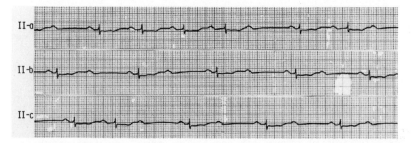

Figure 15-8. Leads II-a,b, and c are not continuous. The tracing shows sinus rhythm (atrial rate: 66 beats per minute) with 2:1 AV block and intermittent Wenckebach (varying-degree) AV block.

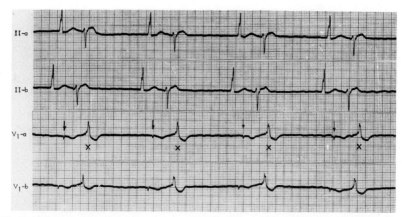

Figure 15-9. Leads II-*a* and *b* are continuous, as are leads V₁-*a* and *b*. The rhythm is atrial fibrillation with AV nodal (junctional) escape rhythm (indicated by arrows) due to complete AV block and ventricular bigeminy (marked *X*).

premature contractions.[2,8] Ventricular bigeminy or trigeminy induced by digitalis occurs frequently in the presence of a diseased myocardium, particularly in the aged. Ventricular premature contractions may originate from a single focus or may be multifocal. Multifocal ventricular premature contractions are more pathognomonic for digitalis intoxication than unifocal ones.

When ventricular premature contractions are frequent, particularly multifocal or bidirectional ones, ventricular tachycardia may develop, producing unidirectional or bidirectional tachycardia or even ventricular fibrillation. The average incidence of ventricular tachycardia has been estimated to be 10% of all digitalis-induced arrhythmias.[2,8] If ventricular tachycardia persists, there is always the possibility of the development of ventricular fibrillation and sudden death. The mortality of patients with digitalis-induced ventricular tachycardia is extremely high (68–100%).

Bidirectional ventricular tachycardia (Fig. 15-10) is considered to be a more pathognomonic feature of digitalis toxicity than the unidirectional entity.[2] This tachycardia is more common in advanced heart disease, and frequently the basic atrial mechanism is atrial fibrillation, flutter, or tachycardia (Fig. 15-10).

Except for idioventricular rhythm, the mechanism of ventricular tachycardia or fibrillation is most likely similar to that responsible for the production of ventricular premature contractions. Enhancement of automaticity is probably responsible for most digitalis-induced ventricular arrhythmias.

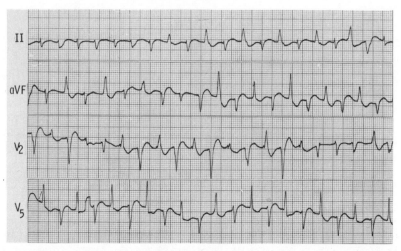

Figure 15-10. Tracing taken from a 70-year-old man with cor pulmonale and thyrotoxicosis who died soon after this ECG was recorded. The serum digoxin level was more than 10 ng/ml. The rhythm is atrial fibrillation with bidirectional ventricular tachycardia (rate: 176 beats per minute) producing complete AV dissociation.

DETERMINATION OF SERUM DIGITALIS LEVEL BY RADIOIMMUNOASSAY

In the past 10 years, various methods of determining serum cardiac glycosides in order to assess an optimal therapeutic dosage and to diagnose digitalis toxicity with accuracy[3,4] have been proposed. The radioimmunoassay method most commonly used at present was first employed by Oliver and co-workers[12] to determine serum digitoxin level. Later, Smith and associates[3] developed a radioimmunoassay method for measuring serum digoxin level.

The clinical importance of serum cardiac glycoside levels rests in the reasonably close correlation between blood content and tissue content of digitalis: The blood levels reflect total body and myocardial concentrations.[4] This relationship was first noted by Doherty and associates, who observed a relatively constant ratio between blood and myocardial levels of digoxin in animals as well as in man.[4]

At present, it is generally agreed that patients with unequivocal digitalis intoxication have significantly higher serum or plasma levels of digoxin or digitoxin than nontoxic patients. Nevertheless, there is substantial overlap between toxic and nontoxic serum or plasma cardiac glycoside levels. This is particularly true with patients suffering from intractable congestive heart failure or various complex arrhythmias. As has been emphasized repeatedly, the dosage of digitalis varies not only from patient to patient, but also from time to time in the same patient. Similarly, toxic and nontoxic serum or plasma digitalis levels may differ from patient to patient because of various modifying factors, including electrolyte imbalance, thyroid disease, renal disease, acute or chronic lung disease, and, particularly, the nature and severity of the underlying heart disease.

According to a prospective study on 931 consecutive patients with digitalis intoxication by Beller and associates,[13] serum concentrations of digoxin and digitoxin in toxic patients were 2.3 ± 1.6 ng/ml and 34 ± 18 ng/ml, respectively. On the other hand, serum digoxin and digitoxin levels in nontoxic patients were 1.0 ± 0.5 ng/ml and 20 ± 11 ng/ml, respectively, in the same study. Clearly, there is significant overlap between values for the two groups.

In general, serum digoxin levels of 2.0 ng/ml or below and serum digitoxin levels of 20 ng/ml or below are considered to be nontoxic, even though toxic patients may have serum levels below these values.[3,4,12,13] Very low serum cardiac glycoside concentrations (digoxin levels below 0.4 ng/ml or digitoxin levels below 10 ng/ml) usually indicate underdigitalization.[3,4,12,13] Values this low are, as a rule, not observed among toxic patients.

The radioimmunoassay methods are extremely valuable when the serum cardiac glycoside levels are used in conjunction with the total clinical picture and electrocardiographic findings. Serum digitalis level determination is useful when little or no information is available about previous digitalization. Once the serum digitalis level in such a patient is known, additional digitalis dosage may be determined much more accurately. Serum digitalis levels are also valuable in patients in whom various modifying factors dictate daily regulation of digitalis dosage. Another role of serum digitalis level determination is to assess underdigitalization, which may be difficult or even impossible to ascertain clinically or electrocardiographically, especially in the presence of sinus rhythm.

The most important role of the determination of serum digoxin or digitoxin levels by radioimmunoassay methods will be in establishing optimal dosage for a given patient. It is to be hoped that these methods will enable many physicians to prescribe cardiac glycosides more effectively and more appropriately, so that the risk of digitalis intoxication can be minimized or even eliminated.

DETERMINATION OF SALIVA ELECTROLYTES

Recently, it has been shown that the electrolyte content of the saliva has a close relationship with digitalis intoxication. Wotman and associ-

ates[14] demonstrated that patients with digitalis intoxication have dispro-
portionately high concentrations of potassium and calcium. This test
also shows some overlap between toxic and nontoxic groups, although
mean values of saliva potassium and calcium were significantly higher
in the group with digitalis toxicity. Further clinical evaluation will be
needed to assess the value of the saliva test.

It must be remembered that the evaluation of the total clinical picture
of each patient during digitalis therapy is essential, and that the results
of any single laboratory test must not be used as the basis for treatment
or diagnosis.

MANAGEMENT OF DIGITALIS INTOXICATION
(TABLE 15-2)

Unfortunately, there is no known drug that is an antagonist to digitalis. Various agents have been tried in the treatment of digitalis intoxication with varying success; diphenylhydantoin (Dilantin) and potassium have proved to be the most effective in terminating various
digitalis-induced tachyarrhythmias.

The most important treatment for digitalis toxicity is, needless to say,
the immediate withdrawal of the drug, not merely a reduction in dosage.[2]
Most patients with mild digitalis intoxication, such as sinus bradycardia,
first-degree AV block, and occasional ventricular premature contractions, can recover from digitalis toxicity if the drug is discontinued for
several days. Generally, in patients with digitalis toxicity, emotional
stress and physical activity should be restricted, and all factors that may
aggravate the toxicity should be eliminated. Any patient with advanced
digitalis intoxication, particularly serious cardiac arrhythmias, should
be treated in a cardiac care unit or a room with similar facilities. Various
agents can be given orally, intramuscularly, or intravenously, depending
upon the clinical situations.

Potassium

Potassium is one of the most effective agents for abolishing various
atrial and ventricular tachyarrhythmias in digitalis intoxication.[2,15] The
amount of potassium to be administered depends upon the severity of
the toxicity, the degree of suspected potassium deficiency in the myocardium, and the response to potassium therapy. Potassium is definitely
contraindicated in the presence of renal failure and hyperkalemia. Potassium is also relatively contraindicated in the presence of second-degree
or complete AV block unless the serum potassium is very low. Potassium in the form of potassium chloride may be administered orally in
doses of 20 to 80 mEq/liter daily or by a slow intravenous infusion

Table 15-2   *Treatment of Digitalis Intoxication*

Drugs and Other Methods	Mild Toxicity	Severe Toxicity	Contraindications
IMMEDIATE WITHDRAWAL OF DIGITALIS!			
Potassium	1–2 g KCl q̄ 4 hr	40–60 mEq/liter KCl in 500 ml 5% D/W IV injection (2–3 hr period) under ECG monitor and periodic serum K^+ determination	Hyperkalemia, uremia, 2nd and 3rd-degree AV block, SA block
Dilantin (diphenylhydantoin)	100 mg tid or qid by mouth	125–250 mg IV injection (2–3-min period) under ECG monitor. Same dosage may be repeated q̄ 5–10 min	2nd- and 3rd-degree AV block, SA block, marked sinus bradycardia
Xylocaine (lidocaine)		1 mg/kg body wt IV injection q̄ 20 min Maximum dose: 750 mg	Similar to Dilantin (see above)
Inderal (propranolol)	10–30 mg tid or qid before meals and at bedtime	1–3 mg slow IV injection (not to exceed 1 mg/min) under ECG monitor. Second dose may be repeated after 2 min. Additional medication should be withheld for at least 4 hr	Bronchial asthma, allergic rhinitis, marked sinus-bradycardia, SA block, 2nd- and 3rd-degree AV block, cardiogenic shock, heart failure, pulmonary hypertension
Pronestyl (procaine amide)	250–500 mg q 3–4 hr by mouth	50–100 mg q̄ 2–4 min slow IV injection or 1 g in 200 ml 5% D/W IV drip (30–60-min period) under ECG monitor. Maximum dose: 2.0 g	Similar to Dilantin (see above)
Quinidine		0.6 g in 200 ml 5% D/W IV drip (30–60 min-period) under ECG monitor	Similar to Dilantin (see above)
Magnesium sulfate	Slow (1 cc/min) IV infusion (20 cc of 20% solution) under continuous electrocardiographic monitoring		
Sodium EDTA	Not recommended for clinical use		
DC countershock	Not recommended except as a last resort after all available measures have been exhausted		
Artificial pacemaker	Temporary demand pacemaker is indicated for 3rd-degree AV block and occasionally for 2nd-degree AV block or SA block		

in doses of 40 to 60 mEq/liter over a 2–3-hour period initially. Intravenous administration is preferred because the exact amount received by the patient can be controlled and the drug may be discontinued at any time.[2] Oral administration is widely used for milder cases with digitalis toxicity when hypokalemia is suspected or present. During intravenous administration of potassium, continuous electrocardiographic monitoring is essential in order to prevent toxic signs of hyperkalemia or any cardiac arrhythmia. Frequent determination of serum potassium is also indicated. Needless to say, the efficacy of potassium is most pronounced when a significant hypokalemia is present (Fig. 15-1).

Diphenylhydantoin (Dilantin)

Clinical investigations have demonstrated that Dilantin is effective in treating digitalis-induced arrhythmias, including paroxysmal atrial tachycardia, AV nodal (junctional) rhythm, wandering atrial pacemaker, ventricular bigeminy, multifocal ventricular premature contractions, and AV nodal (junctional) or ventricular tachycardia[2,15–17] (Fig. 15-11). Most patients respond within 3 seconds to 5 minutes with intravenous administration. The duration of response varies from 5 minutes to 4–6 hours. The initial intravenous dose is between 125 and 250 mg for 1 to 3 minutes under electrocardiographic monitoring. The same dose may be repeated every 5 to 10 minutes until the effect is established. Toxic manifestations or side effects of Dilantin include respiratory arrest, skin

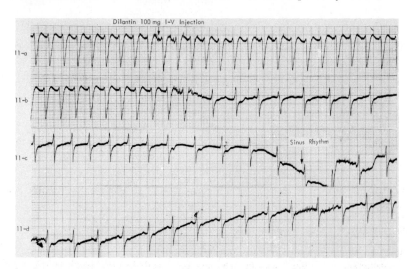

Figure 15-11. Leads II-*a,b,c*, and *d* are continuous. Ventricular tachycardia (rate: 155 beats per minute) has been converted to sinus rhythm by Dilantin, 100 mg, injected intravenously.

reaction (urticaria, purpura), drowsiness, depression, nervousness, arthralgia, gingival hyperplasia, transient eosinophilia, and transient hypotension, but these manifestations are rare and usually not serious. After conversion to sinus rhythm or the disappearance of digitalis-induced arrhythmias, oral maintenance dosage (200–400 mg) in divided doses is sufficient.

It has recently been shown that Dilantin is of prophylactic value before direct current shock in a digitalized patient. The drug is capable of preventing arrhythmias induced by cardioversion[2] by increasing the threshold of the excitability of the heart by counteracting the electrophysiologic actions of digitalis. Dilantin is probably the safest and most effective drug in the treatment of all types of digitalis-induced tachyarrhythmias.

Beta-Adrenergic Blocking Agents

Propranolol is the most commonly used beta-adrenergic blocking agent.[18,19] The usual intravenous dose of propranolol is between 1 and 3 mg under continuous electrocardiographic monitoring. The drug should be administered slowly, at a rate not exceeding 1 mg (1 cc) per minute. Sufficient time should be allowed to enable a slow circulation to carry the drug to its site of action. A second dose, if needed, may be repeated after 2 minutes. Additional medication should be withheld for at least 4 hours. Propanolol may be given orally as soon as cardiac arrhythmias are abolished or are markedly improved.[18,19] Intravenous atropine (0.5–1.0 mg) may be needed if marked bradycardia occurs. In nonurgent situations, propanolol may be given orally in doses ranging between 10 and 30 mg three to four times daily, before meals and at bedtime. The same dosage schedule is also recommended for long-term use or for prophylaxis.

Propranolol is probably contraindicated for patients with bronchial asthma and allergic rhinitis (especially during the pollen season), marked sinus bradycardia, second- or third-degree AV block, SA block, sinus arrest, cardiogenic shock, and significant congestive heart failure.[18,19] The drug is also contraindicated when patients are receiving any anesthetics that produce myocardial depression, such as chloroform and ether. Patients receiving adrenergic-augmenting psychotropic drugs (including MAO inhibitors) also should not receive the drug. Propranolol may be given with caution after the 2-week withdrawal period from such drugs. It should be emphasized that electrocardiographic monitoring is mandatory during the intravenous administration of propranolol. In this author's experience, propranolol is not as effective as potassium or Dilantin for the treatment of digitalis toxicity.

Procaine Amide (Pronestyl) and Quinidine

Procaine amide and quinidine may be effective in abolishing supraventricular and ventricular tachyarrhythmias induced by digitalis.[2] Procaine amide may be used if potassium, Dilantin, and propranolol are ineffective or contraindicated. The drug may be given intravenously in a slow drip not exceeding 50–100 mg every 2–4 minutes, or orally in a dose of 250–500 mg every 3 to 4 hours. Quinidine has been less widely used because of the frequent occurrence of hypotension during parenteral administration. Its effect is unpredictable and often hazardous. During parenteral administration of either procaine amide or quinidine, electrocardiographic monitoring and frequent blood pressure determinations are indicated. A vasopressor agent should be readily available.

The therapeutic effects of quinidine and procaine amide include prolongation of the Q–T interval, widening and notching of the P waves, flattening or inversion of the T waves, and depression of S–T segments. If patients develop toxic manifestations from these drugs, the electrocardiogram will show varying degrees of AV block, progressive intraatrial and intraventricular block, and atrial standstill. In severe cases, ventricular fibrillation or tachycardia may develop. Both procaine amide and quinidine are contraindicated in the presence of AV or intraventricular block.

Xylocaine (Lidocaine)

Like procaine amide, the antiarrhythmic mechanism of Xylocaine is related to the drug's ability to raise the diastolic stimulation threshold of the ventricles.[20,21] Xylocaine penetrates the tissue more rapidly than procaine or procaine amide, but its action is often transient. Xylocaine may be effective for the treatment of digitalis-induced ventricular arrhythmias.[20,21]

Xylocaine may be given in doses of 1 to 2 mg per kilogram body weight intravenously over 1 to 2 minutes. The same dose may be repeated at 20-minute intervals if needed. A constant intravenous drip is often necessary following a direct intravenous bolus of Xylocaine since the duration of the antiarrhythmic effect is relatively brief (10 to 20 minutes). Although most adult patients require 75 to 150 mg of the drug, as much as 750 mg of Xylocaine has been safely used in anesthetized patients during the first hour of administration.

Side effects include hypotension, depression of the central nervous system, and convulsions.[20,21] Xylocaine is contraindicated in the presence of AV block, SA block, intraventricular block, and hypotension.

Chelating Agent

Sodium EDTA (ethylenediaminetetraacetic acid) is occasionally of value in the treatment of digitalis-induced ventricular arrhythmias and AV block.[22,23] The chief advantage of this drug is its rapid onset of action, while its disadvantages include transient effect and occasional hypotension and renal damage following large doses. Chelating agents may be used when potassium and Dilantin are contraindicated or ineffective. In general, chelating agents are not recommended for clinical use because of the many superior agents now available.

Magnesium Sulfate

Recent clinical and experimental investigations have shown that hypomagnesemia predisposes to digitalis intoxication. Therefore, magnesium sulfate should be administered when digitalis toxicity is associated with hypomagnesemia.[24,25] The drug may be given by slow (1 cc per minute) intravenous infusion (20 cc of 20% solution) under continuous electrocardiographic monitoring.

Direct Current Shock

Cardioversion should not be attempted on patients with suspected or proven digitalis-induced arrhythmias because the procedure frequently induces more serious and irreversible arrhythmias, such as ventricular tachycardia or fibrillation.[2,26] If cardioversion is definitely needed, prophylactic administration of Dilantin or potassium may prevent the occurrence of serious arrhythmias. It is essential to discontinue cardiac glycosides before cardioversion. If a short-acting preparation has been given, the procedure should be postponed for at least 24–48 hours; if long-acting preparations have been used, the procedure should be delayed for at least 3–5 days.

In general, when treating the digitalis-induced tachyarrhythmias, cardioversion should be attempted only as a last resort, after all other available measures have failed.[2]

Artificial Pacemakers

The primary indication for an artificial pacemaker is AV block associated with the Adams-Stokes syndrome. Although digitalis intoxication is reported to be the second most common cause of complete AV block, the Adams-Stokes syndrome as a manifestation of digitalis overdose has been found to be rare, since the ventricular rate in digitalis-induced complete AV block tends to be faster than that in complete AV block due

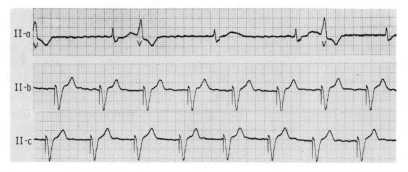

Figure 15-12. Leads II-*b* and *c* are continuous. A temporary demand pacemaker was inserted (leads II-*b* and *c*) for the treatment of symptomatic high-degree AV block in the presence of atrial fibrillation and frequent ventricular premature contractions (marked *V*) shown in lead II-*a*.

to other causes.[2] Therefore, a withdrawal of digitalis alone is often sufficient treatment. However, if the underlying rhythm is atrial fibrillation, the incidence of Adams-Stokes seizures increases. When Adams-Stokes syndrome develops as a result of digitalis intoxication, a temporary demand pacemaker is quite suitable because the AV block induced by digitalis is often transient and intermittent (Fig. 15-12). The use of an artificial pacemaker with a fixed rate is not recommended, because of the danger of provoking a pacemaker-induced parasystolic rhythm that competes with the patient's own basic rhythm or ectopic rhythm, resulting in ventricular tachycardia or fibrillation. Permanent pacemaker implantation for the treatment of digitalis-induced AV block is rarely called for unless there are other coexisting causes of AV block.

SUMMARY

Once a patient develops digitalis toxicity, digitalis is no longer beneficial even in the presence of congestive heart failure. Therefore, the most important therapeutic approach to digitalis intoxication is an immediate discontinuation of the drug, rather than a mere reduction of the dosage. Almost every known type of cardiac arrhythmia may be induced by digitalis. The most common digitalis-induced arrhythmias include ventricular premature contractions and nonparoxysmal AV junctional tachycardia, particularly in the presence of atrial fibrillation.

Mild forms of digitalis-induced arrhythmias usually disappear after discontinuation of digitalis. However, advanced and more serious tachyarrhythmias require the use of pharmacologic agents in addition to the discontinuation of digitalis. The most effective agents are diphenylhydantoin (Dilantin) and potassium. Digitalis-induced bradyarrhythmias usually improve after withdrawal of digitalis. In rare cases of high-degree or complete AV block, especially when the underlying rhythm is atrial fibrillation, a temporary demand pacemaker may be required. A permanent pacemaker is almost never indicated.

It should be re-emphasized that the dosage of digitalis not only varies from patient to patient but that it also may vary from time to time in the same individual, depending upon various modifying factors, such as the status of underlying heart disease, the presence or absence of hypokalemia and hypoxia, and the status of renal and thyroid function.

The serum digitalis level determination is extremely useful, but the value should be interpreted carefully in conjunction with clinical background and the electrocardiographic findings.

It should be remembered that cardiac glycoside is the most useful and essential drug in treatment of heart disease, but it may produce serious untoward effects and even death from digitalis intoxication. Serious manifestations of digitalis intoxication can be avoided if all physicians thoroughly familiarize themselves with this most valuable drug, particularly with regard to digitalis toxicity.

REFERENCES

1. Withering, W.: An Account of the Foxglove and Some of Its Medical Uses with Practical Remarks on Dropsy and Other Diseases. London, M. Swinney, 1785. (Reproduced in Med. Classics 2:30, 1937).
2. Chung, E. K.: Digitalis Intoxication. Baltimore, Williams & Wilkins, 1969.
3. Smith, T. W., and Haber, E.: Current techniques for serum or plasma digitalis assay and their potential clinical application. Am. J. Med. Sci. 259:301, 1970.
4. Doherty, J. E., Perkins, W. H., and Flanigan, W. J.: The distribution and concentration of tritiated digoxin in human tissues. Ann. Intern. Med. 66:116, 1967.
5. Somylo, A. P.: The toxicology of digitalis. Am. J. Cardiol. 5:523, 1960.
6. Navab, A., Koss, L. G., and LaDue, J. S.: Estrogen-like activity of digitalis. JAMA 194:30, 1965.
7. Young, R. C., Nachman, R. L., and Horowitz, H. I.: Thrombocytopenia due to digitoxin. Am. J. Med. 41:605, 1966.
8. Irons, G. V., Jr., and Orgain, E. S.: Digitalis-induced arrhythmias and their management. Prog. Cardiovas. Dis. 8:539, 1966.
9. Lown, B., Wyatt, N. F., and Levine, H. D.: Paroxysmal atrial tachycardia with block. Circulation 21:129, 1960.
10. Alexander, S., and Ping, W. C.: Fatal ventricular fibrillation during carotid stimulation. Am. J. Cardiol. 18:289, 1966.
11. Hilal, H., and Massumi, R.: Fatal ventricular fibrillation after carotid-sinus stimulation. N. Engl. J. Med. 275:157, 1966.
12. Oliver, G. C., Jr., Parker, B. M., and Brasfield, D. L. et al.: The measure of digitoxin in human serum by radioimmunoassay. J. Clin. Invest. 47:1035, 1968.
13. Beller, G. A., Smith, T. W., Abelmann, W. H., Haber, E., and Hood, W. B., Jr.: Digitalis intoxication. A prospective clinical study with serum level correlations. N. Engl. J. Med. 284:989, 1971.

14. Wotman, S., Bigger, J. T., Mandel, I. D., and Bartelstone, H. J.: Cardiologists hear about rapid saliva test for digitalis toxicity. JAMA 215:1068, 1971.
15. Lyon, A. F., and DeGraff, A. C.: Reappraisal of digitalis. X. Treatment of digitalis toxicity. Am. Heart J. 73:835, 1968.
16. Ruthen, G. C.: Antiarrhythmic drugs. IV. Diphenylhydantoin in cardiac arrhythmias. Am. Heart J. 70:275, 1965.
17. Conn, R. D.: Diphenylhydantoin sodium in cardiac arrhythmias. N. Engl. J. Med. 272:277, 1965.
18. Irons, G. V., Jr., Ginn, W. N., and Orgain, E. S.: Use of a beta adrenergic receptor blocking agent (propranolol) in the treatment of cardiac arrhythmias. Am. J. Med. 43:161, 1967.
19. Stock, J. P. P.: Beta adrenergic blocking drugs in the clinical management of cardiac arrhythmias. Am. J. Cardiol. 18:444, 1966.
20. Jewitt, D. E., Kishon, Y., and Thomas, M.: Lignocaine in the management of arrhythmias after acute myocardial infarction. Lancet i:266, 1968.
21. Harrison, D. C., Sprouse, J. H., and Morrow, A. G.: Antiarrhythmic properties of lidocaine and procaine amide: Clinical and physiologic studies of their cardiovascular effects in man. Circulation 28:486, 1963.
22. Rosenbaum, J. L., Mason, D., and Sever, M. J.: The effect of disodium EDTA on digitalis intoxication. Am. J. Med. Sci. 240:111, 1960.
23. Cohen, B. D., Spritz, N., Lubash, G. D., and Rubin, A. L.: Use of a calcium chelating agent (Na EDTA) in cardiac arrhythmias. Circulation 19:918, 1959.
24. Seller, R. H., and Moyer, J. H.: Magnesium and digitalis toxicity. Heart Bull. 18:32, 1969.
25. Kim, Y. W., Andrews, C. E., and Ruth, W. E.: Serum magnesium and cardiac arrhythmias with special reference to digitalis intoxication. Am. J. Med. Sci. 242:87, 1961.
26. Kleiger, R., and Lown, B.: Cardioversion and digitalis. II. Clinical studies. Circulation 33:878, 1966.

Chapter 16

CARDIOPULMONARY EMERGENCY CARE IN CHILDREN

GEORGE H. KHOURY

The basic pathophysiology of cardiopulmonary emergencies is similar in the adult and child. However, the incidence, causes, clinical manifestations, and management differ according to the specific age group in children. The immediate recognition and treatment of various emergencies in children, particularly in early infancy, are essential in achieving a successful outcome and improving the morbidity rate. In this chapter, congestive heart failure, cyanotic spells, cardiac arrhythmias, respiratory failure, and cardiac arrest will be discussed in detail.

CONGESTIVE HEART FAILURE

The incidence of congestive heart failure due to congenital heart disease is high during the first 6 months of life and is usually associated with a high morbidity rate.[1-8] The causes of heart failure can be classified into three main categories: (1) pressure-overloading lesions, such as obstruction of either the aortic or pulmonary valve and complete transposition of the great vessels; (2) volume-overloading lesions, such as large ventricular septal defect, patent ductus arteriosus, valvular insufficiency, and severe anemia; and (3) diffuse myocardial disease, such as endocardial fibroelastosis and myocarditis.

Several studies have demonstrated that there is a correlation between type of cardiac defect and age at onset of heart failure (Fig. 16-1).

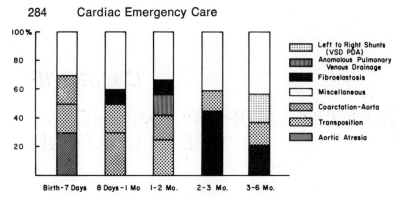

Figure 16-1. Causes of heart failure from birth to 6 months as found in a study of 161 infants. (VSD PDA, ventricular septal defect patent ductus arteriosus.)

This correlation is helpful to clinicians in making an exact diagnosis of the underlying cardiac lesion. During the first week of life, the most common cause of heart failure is hypoplastic left heart syndrome, for which the outlook is bleak. From 8 days to 1 month of age, coarctation of the aorta and complete transposition of the great vessels are leading causes. The prognosis for these lesions is improving with continuing advances in surgical treatment. In infants older than 1 month of age, a frequent cause of heart failure is large ventricular septal defect. In each age range, there is a group of miscellaneous causes, including atrioventricular canal defect, pulmonary atresia, cerebral arteriovenous fistula, and paroxysmal atrial tachycardia.

The clinical presentation of heart failure in infancy is more subtle than in older children. The cardinal clinical features indicating the presence of heart failure include dyspnea, tachycardia, hepatomegaly, and venous congestion. These occur in various degrees, depending on the severity of the lesion. In the newborn, one has to rely more on the presence of dyspnea and hepatomegaly than the degree of tachycardia because the heart rate in the healthy newborn infant is rapid, with a wide range of normal variation. Other common symptoms of heart failure in early infancy are poor feeding, vomiting, cough, irritability, and excessive perspiration over the forehead.

The diagnosis of heart failure is usually not difficult when a typical clinical picture is present. However, the condition has frequently been either overlooked or overdiagnosed.

When the only manifestation is increased respiratory activity—that is, tachypnea—the differential diagnosis should include primary pulmonary disorders, such as respiratory distress syndrome, pneumonia, and bronchiolitis. A chest roentgenogram is very helpful in differentiating between these conditions and congenital heart disease (Figs. 16-2 and

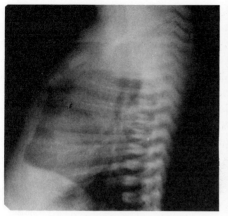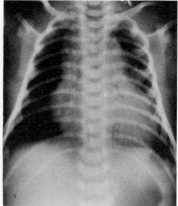

Figure 16-2. Chest roentgenogram of a 3-day-old baby who, at autopsy, was found to have "hypoplastic left-heart complex." Notice the gross cardiomegaly with bilateral venous congestion. In the lateral view, the posterior cardiac border is straight.

16-3). On the other hand, overdiagnosis of heart failure is often made in patients with cyanotic congenital heart diseases in which the patient is subject to anoxic, blue, or paroxysmal dyspneic spells.

In older children, the most common cause of heart failure is myocarditis of either viral or rheumatic etiology, but there may be other causes,

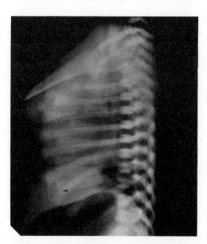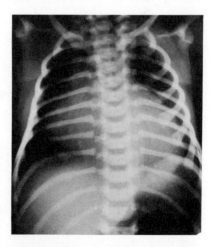

Figure 16-3. Chest roentgenogram of a 2-day-old baby with "hypoplastic right-heart complex," which consists of pulmonary atresia, tricuspid stenosis, and right ventricular hypoplasia. Notice the large right atrial shadow. The pulmonary vascular markings are decreased. In the lateral view, the lower retrosternal space is clear.

such as acute glomerulonephritis, chronic lung disease, and anemia. The onset is usually sudden, and the manifestation is usually that of pulmonary edema. The diagnosis is made on the basis of sudden dyspnea and tachypnea with air hunger. The chest roentgenogram is usually classical in this situation (Fig. 16-4). It shows bilateral venous congestion, which is denser in the hilar area. Immediate recognition of the problem is mandatory if the child is to be saved.

Therapy for heart failure has three main components: digitalis, diuretics, and oxygen. There are guidelines for digitalis therapy that must be followed (see Chapter 7). It is improper to digitalize acutely ill patients without careful clinical and electrocardiographic monitoring. There are many preparations of digitalis available, but the physician should become accustomed to one type; for children, digoxin (Lanoxin) is considered to be the safest preparation. Digoxin may be administered either orally or parenterally[a] (see Chapter 7). The parenteral route is usually preferred if the infant or child has severe congestive heart failure or if there is a history of vomiting. Dosage may be prescribed in different ways, as shown in Table 16-1, but, in any case, the order must be clearly and precisely written. Every physician should be familiar with the usual digitalizing methods (see Chapter 7). Digitalis toxicity is manifested by vomiting and diarrhea followed by various cardiac arrhythmias, mainly ventricular ectopic beats, supraventricular tachycardia, and varying degrees of AV block (see Chapter 15).

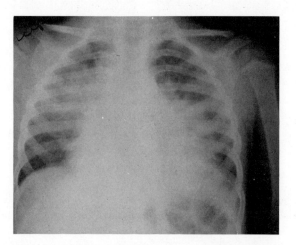

Figure 16-4. Chest roentgenogram of a 2-year-old boy who was admitted in severe pulmonary edema. The heart is enlarged. Note the bilateral hilar pulmonary infiltrate with venous congestion.

Table 16-1   *Digoxin Dosages*

Digitalizing Dose	Age of Child (yr)	
	<2	>2
Oral	0.07 mg/kg	0.04 mg/kg
IM or IV	0.05 mg/kg	0.03 mg/kg
Oral	0.03 mg/lb	0.02 mg/lb
IM or IV	0.02 mg/lb	0.015 mg/lb
Oral	1.6 mg/m²	1.0 mg/m²
IV	0.9 mg/m²	—

Maintenance dose: $\frac{1}{3}$ to $\frac{1}{5}$ of the digitalizing dose.

The diuretics most commonly used in acute congestive heart failure are Lasix and ethacrynic acid. Ethacrynic acid should only be given intravenously. The dose is 1 mg/kg body weight.[10] When using diuretics, one should be alert to the possibility of hypochloremia and hyponatremia, which make the patient less responsive to digitalis and predispose to digitalis toxicity.

Surgical therapy is sometimes indicated when there is no respone to the decongestive measures. A notable example is in coarctation of the aorta or transposition of the great vessels. One can only stress that severe congestive heart failure in infants should be considered an emergency, because a delay in either medical or surgical treatment may result in death.

CYANOTIC SPELLS

Cyanosis is an alarming symptom, particularly when it is associated with respiratory distress and when it manifests itself in the first few days of life. First, it must be determined whether the cause of cyanosis is cardiac or noncardiac. This determination is made with the aid of careful history taking and physical examination, in conjunction with a chest roentgenogram, electrocardiogram, and blood gas analysis. When a cyanotic congenital heart disease is suspected, an aggressive approach should be adopted, since a delay in diagnosis and treatment may be disastrous.

Patients with cyanotic heart diseases and decreased pulmonary blood flow, such as tetralogy of Fallot, are susceptible to cyanotic spells. These spells are also known as "paroxysmal dyspneic spells," "blue spells," or "anoxic spells." The cyanotic spells are characterized by a sudden hyperpnea, marked cyanosis, generalized limpness, and fainting. Occasionally, the patient may develop severe convulsion, resulting in death.

The incidence of these spells in those suffering from cyanotic heart disease varies from 20% to 40%.[11,12] The spells are usually triggered by crying or tachycardia, which results in an increase in right-to-left shunt, producing a sudden alteration in arterial oxygen and carbon dioxide tension and hydrogen ion concentration. These manifestations in turn stimulate the respiratory center and cause the hyperpnea, which perpetuates the cycle.

Treatment consists of immediate administration of oxygen and sedation in the form of morphine 0.1 mg/pound. Propranolol has been used at a dosage of 1 to 2 mg/kg orally in cases of tetralogy of Fallot with infundibular stenosis. Frequent spells will dictate an early surgical correction of the lesion.

In addition to cyanotic spells, one must be aware of other complications in cyanotic heart diseases, such as acidosis, hypocalcemia, and hypoglycemia.

In order to improve the salvage rate of patients with cyanotic heart diseases, one should refer them to a fully equipped medical center where an accurate diagnosis can be established and proper management can be instituted before complications develop.

CARDIAC ARRHYTHMIAS

Cardiac arrhythmias are encountered less frequently in the pediatric age group than in the adult population. Causes of the cardiac arrhythmias seen in childhood are listed below:

Idiopathic
Congenital heart disease
Familial
Autonomic immaturity
Hypoxia
Infections: Myocarditis
Cardiac tumors
Iatrogenic   (cardiac   surgery,   cardiac   catheterization,   drugs,
anesthesia)

Serious arrhythmias commonly seen in children are those that will produce clinical symptoms, including supraventricular tachycardia, atrial flutter, congenital AV block, and postsurgical arrhythmias.

Supraventricular Tachycardia

Supraventricular tachycardia is the most common serious arrhythmia occurring between 2 weeks and 6 months of age. The true incidence is unknown, but an estimate of 1:25,000 was given by Keith, Rowe, and Vlad.[13] The onset of the arrhythmia is usually sudden and is precipitated by infection, commonly pneumonia. The baby may be asymptomatic in the early stages, in which case the only abnormal finding will be the tachycardia itself. However, if the tachycardia persists, the baby usually develops congestive heart failure and presents with peripheral vascular collapse. The patient is usually ashen gray or cyanotic, clammy, and cold. Respiration is rapid and labored. The heart rate may vary from 180 to 300 beats per minute (Fig. 16-5). Peripheral pulses are usually weak and thready. In 15% to 20% of the cases, the electrocardiogram during sinus rhythm exhibits Wolff-Parkinson-White syndrome.

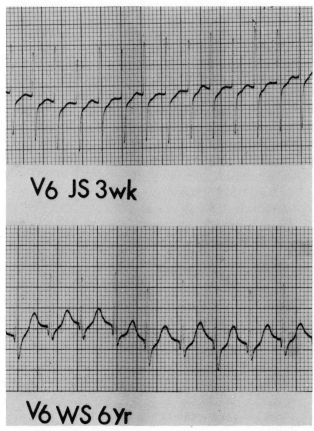

V6 JS 3wk

V6 WS 6Yr

Figure 16-5. The top tracing shows supraventricular tachycardia with a ventricular rate of 280/minute in a 3-week-old baby. The bottom tracing shows a paroxysmal supraventricular tachycardia with a ventricular rate of 180/minute in a 6-year-old boy.

The paroxysms occurring before 6 months of age are more common in males than in females, and the recurrence rate is very low. In older children, supraventricular tachycardia usually has less effect on cardiovascular hemodynamics, and the main symptom is usually palpitation.

The treatment usually consists of rapid intravenous or intramuscular digitalization (see Chapter 7). However, in severe heart failure, immediate termination of the tachycardia is desirable, and in this situation, DC cardioversion is the treatment of choice (see Chapter 9). The longer the duration of tachycardia, the higher the incidence of heart failure. Propranolol, in combination with digoxin, provides effective prophylaxis against recurrent supraventricular tachycardia (see Chapter 7). Several antiarrhythmic drugs have been used in adults but are of little value in children.

Congenital Atrioventricular Block

The clinical picture in congenital AV block differs from that of AV block in adults.[14] The cardiac output is usually normal; this is accomplished by increased stroke volume. The majority of patients are asymptomatic except for easy fatigability and subnormal exercise tolerance. When symptoms do occur, the prognosis is usually less favorable. The two most common symptoms of congenital AV block are congestive heart failure and Adams-Stokes attacks in the form of fainting spells or convulsions or both. These symptoms are likely to occur in patients with a slow ventricular rate, usually below 30–40 beats/minute, and wide QRS complex, which indicates the block is in the lower part of the bundle of His. When the ventricular rate is faster than 60 beats/minute, the diagnosis may be missed, especially when the electrocardiogram is not taken (Figure 16-6). On auscultation, a systolic ejection murmur in an infant with a heart rate of 60 beats or less is a clinical sign strongly suggesting complete AV block.

The indications for cardiac pacing in congenital AV block are (1) persistent heart failure in spite of therapy with digitalis and diuretics; (2) occurrence of Adams-Stokes syndrome; and (3) ventricular rate below 40 beats/minute with symptoms on exercise. His bundle recording are of value in delineating the level of the block and in clarifying the prognosis in individual cases. The use of artificial pacemakers is discussed in detail in Chapter 10.

Atrial Flutter

Atrial flutter in infancy is very rare. It may occur in a congenital form, which can usually be predicted prenatally.[15] The presenting symptoms of atrial flutter with 1:1 AV response are heart failure and/or

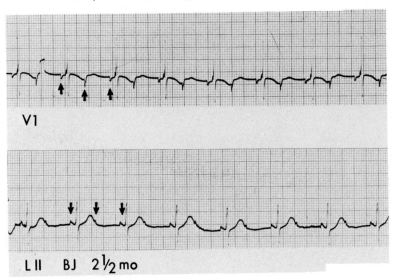

Figure 16-6. The electrocardiogram shows 2:1 AV block with atrial rate of 160 per minute and ventricular rate of 80 per minute.

repeated bouts of vomiting (Fig. 16-7). Therapy consists of cardioversion (see Chapter 9) or the use of antiarrhythmic drugs, particularly diphenylhydantoin (Dilantin) and quinidine (see Chapter 7).

Postsurgical Arrhythmias

Postsurgical arrhythmias in the pediatric age group commonly occur following open-heart surgery, but they can occur during anesthesia. The common arrhythmias include AV junctional tachycardia, atrial flutter, complete AV block, premature ectopic beats, and ventricular tachycardia. In dealing with postsurgical arrhythmias, one must consider the following questions: (1) Is the patient symptomatic or asymptomatic? (2) What is the status of the cardiovascular hemodynamics? (3) Does

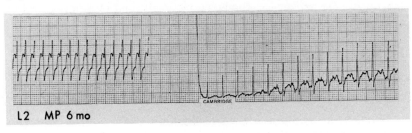

Figure 16-7. Atrial flutter with 1:1 AV response (ventricular rate, 360 per minute). Restoration of sinus rhythm with a rate of 150 per minute by DC cardioversion.

Table 16-3   *Dosages of Antiarrhythmic Drugs*

Quinidine gluconate:
IM: 2 mg/kg as initial test dose; then 5 to 10 mg/kg every 6 hours as needed
IV: 0.5 mg/kg given slowly over 10 to 15 minutes with electrocardiographic monitoring; stop if bradycardia develops
PO: 10 to 30 mg/kg/day
Propranolol (Inderal):
PO: 1 to 2 mg/kg
Diphenylhydantoin (Dilantin):
PO: 2 to 5 mg/kg/day in two or three doses
IV: 3 to 5 mg/kg injected slowly over 5 to 10 minutes
Lidocaine (Xylocaine):
IV: 0.15 to 1.0 mg/kg every 20 to 60 minutes as needed

---

the patient have hypotension? (4) Is he in congestive heart failure? In other words, one must determine the urgency of termination of the arrhythmia. Antiarrhythmic drugs (Table 16-3) should be used judiciously, with constant electrocardiographic monitoring. Detailed description of antiarrhythmic therapy may be found in Chapter 7.

RESPIRATORY FAILURE

Acute respiratory distress is an emergency that requires immediate recognition and a prompt multidisciplinary approach in its management. Respiratory failure may occur in any patient who has a severe pulmonary, cardiac, or central nervous system disorder.[16] In the pediatric age group, the causes, clinical presentation and management of respiratory failure vary with age (Table 16-4).

The symptoms and signs that should alert the physician to the possibility of impending respiratory failure are tachypnea, dyspnea, erratic breathing, chest wall retraction, cyanosis, generalized hypotonia with depressed reflexes and systemic hypotension or hypertension. These findings should be corroborated by evaluation of arterial blood gases at room air and after breathing 100% oxygen for 10–15 minutes. Biochemically, the patient has combined metabolic and respiratory acidosis in this situation.

The blood gas indices that indicate the presence of respiratory failure and signal the need for assisted ventilation also vary according to its cause. However, in general, hypoxemia (PO_2 50 mm Hg or less for newborns after breathing 100% oxygen and less than 100 mm Hg in older children) and hypercarbia (PCO_2 75 mm Hg or over) should alert the physician to the need for assisted ventilation.

In the newborn period, hyaline membrane disease (HMD) is the leading cause of respiratory failure, and hence it merits some discussion.

Table 16-4   *Common Causes of Acute Respiratory Failure*

Age	Cause

Newborns	Respiratory distress syndrome due to:
	  Hyaline membrane disease
	  Pneumonia
	  Atelectasis
	  Pleural effusion, bilateral
	  Diaphragmatic hernia
	  Congestive heart failure, severe
	  Central nervous system disorders

Infants and children	Acute bronchiolitis Epiglottitis Status asthmaticus Bronchopneumonia with tenacious secretions Cardiac surgery Infectious polyneuritis Drowning Septic shock

It is primarily a disease of premature infants, but it can occur in full-term infants born by caesarean section or to diabetic mothers. The principal cause of HMD is a deficiency of pulmonary surfactant, a lipoprotein complex consisting of two molecules, lecithin and sphingomyelin. The lack of pulmonary surfactant leads to collapse of alveolar sacs and ducts, with deposition of an eosinophilic membrane along the inner lining of the terminal bronchioles and alveolar sacs and ducts.

Suspected HMD can be confirmed prenatally by examining the amniotic fluid for the lecithin/sphingomyelin (L/S) ratio.[17] The clinical diagnosis of HMD depends on the presence of characteristic findings, which consist of tachypnea, expiratory grunting, subcostal and intercostal retractions, nasal flaring, cyanosis, and poor muscle tone. However, these signs could be indicative of other causes of respiratory distress, including pneumonia, pneumothorax, pleural effusion, pulmonary hemorrhage, atelectasis, diaphragmatic hernia, and ascites. The diagnosis of HMD is usually confirmed by radiographic demonstration of a reticulogranular pattern usually described as a ground-glass appearance of both lungs and an air bronchogram extending beyond the cardiac shadow.

In the management of respiratory failure in infants, adequate caloric intake should be maintained. Body temperature should be regulated to prevent hypothermia. Complications, such as sepsis, bleeding, vascular problems due to vessel catheterization, and oxygen toxicity, should be prevented.

CARDIAC ARREST

Cardiac arrest means an abrupt cessation of circulation of blood due to either ventricular asystole or ventricular fibrillation. In association with cardiac arrest, the respiratory efforts are ineffective and hence pulmonary ventilation is poor. Cardiac arrest may occur in any age group, and it is often unexpected. Its cause is any condition leading to hypoxia, myocardial depression, or arrhythmia; drug poisoning; anesthesia; electrolyte imbalances; and any condition leading to shock.

The success of cardiopulmonary resuscitation depends on many factors, including primary causative disease, adequacy and timing of emergency treatment, and adequacy of drug therapy in conjunction with the use of defibrillator as needed.

In cardiopulmonary resuscitation, certain principles must be kept in mind: (1) Cardiac output must be maintained by closed cardiac massage. (2) The most efficient type of artificial ventilation is expired ventilation using the mouth-to-mouth method or a mask and bag tightly applied to the mouth. (3) Acidosis often develops rapidly after cardiac arrest, and prompt treatment is absolutely necessary.

Phase 1.   The exact time of the arrest should be recorded, if possible. Apply a sharp blow to the precordium, and call for help. In order for the mouth-to-mouth breathing to be effective, the airway should be opened by tilting the head backward, and a tight seal should be applied over the nose and mouth. Tracheal intubation should be performed only by skilled personnel. Closed cardiac massage should follow ventilation; the pressure point in infants and small children is on the lower half of the breast plate just above its soft lower end. In infants, the chest should be held with both hands and the thumbs held exactly over the lower breast plate. In older children, the heel of one hand should be placed over the lower sternum. Compression should be in the form of rhythmic pressure of $1-1\frac{1}{2}$ inches at a rate of 100–120 per minute. The effectiveness of the cardiac massage should be evaluated by noting the patient's color, size of pupils, pulse, and cardiac action.

Phase 2.   This is the period during which an electrocardiogram should be recorded to determine the type of electrical activity, which may be asystole—that is, a total absence of electrical activity—or ventricular fibrillation. Intravenous infusion should be started immediately; the drugs and dosage frequently used in cardiopulmonary resuscitation are summarized in Table 16-5.

Phase 3.   This phase is the aftercare of the patient after cardiac action has been restored and an adequate cardiac output established, with or without adrenergic drugs. The patient should then be moved

Table 16-5   *Drugs Used for Cardiopulmonary Resuscitation*

Drug	Dosage
Sodium bicarbonate	2 mEq/kg every 10 minutes (monitor pH)
Epinephrine	0.1–0.5 mg IC or IV
Calcium gluconate (10 %)	3–5 cc IV
Isoproterenol (Isuprel)	Initial dose 0.5 mg diluted in 10 ml 5 % D/W IV or IC. Then slow IV drip 1 mg in 250 ml 5 % D/W (discontinue if tachycardia or arrhythmias occur)
Metaraminol bitartrate (Aramine)	IV drip 0.3 mg/kg in 250 ml 5 % D/W

to the intensive care unit, where he is carefully monitored, since cardiac arrest may recur. Every effort should be made to eliminate the possible causes of arrest. The success of cardiopulmonary resuscitation depends on a well-disciplined and organized team effort. Cardiopulmonary resuscitation is described in detail in Chapter 11.

SUMMARY

The incidence, causes, clinical manifestations, and management of cardiopulmonary emergencies in children are different from those in the adult population. The immediate recognition and treatment of various emergencies, particularly in early infancy, are essential in achieving a successful outcome and improving the salvage rate. In this chapter, congestive heart failure, cyanotic spells, cardiac arrhythmias, acute respiratory failure, and cardiac arrest have been discussed.

The incidence of heart failure due to congenital heart disease is high during the first 6 months of life and is usually associated with a high morbidity rate. The cardinal clinical features indicating the presence of heart failures are dyspnea, tachycardia, hepatomegaly, and venous congestion. Other common symptoms include poor feeding, vomiting, cough, irritability, and excessive perspiration over the forehead. The initial therapy of heart failure is medical, but surgical therapy is indicated in such instances such as coarctation of the aorta and transposition of the great vessels when there is no response to decongestive measures.

Cyanotic spells, known also as paroxysmal dyspneic spells, are characterized by a sudden hyperpnea, marked cyanosis, generalized limpness, and fainting. The incidence of these spells varies from 20% to 40% in patients with cyanotic heart diseases associated with decreased pulmonary blood flow. The treatment consists of immediate administration of oxygen and sedation in the form of morphine or phenobarbital.

Frequent spells will dictate an early surgical correction of the cardiac lesion.

Cardiac arrhythmias are encountered less frequently in the pediatric age group than in the adult population. The most common arrhythmias are supraventricular tachycardia and postsurgical arrhythmias. The use of antiarrhythmic drugs varies according to the specific type of rhythm disturbance. They should be used judiciously and with constant electro-cardiographic monitoring.

Acute respiratory distress is an emergency that requires immediate recognition and prompt multidisciplinary approach in management. The causes, clinical presentation, and management of respiratory failure vary with age and with specific cause. In the newborn, hyaline membrane disease is the leading cause of respiratory failure, and its diagnosis is usually confirmed by the radiographic demonstration of a reticulogranu-lar pattern described as a ground-glass appearance of both lungs and an air bronchogram that extends beyond the cardiac shadow.

Cardiac arrest, from whatever cause, requires prompt cardiopulmo-nary resuscitation. The principles of cardiopulmonary resuscitation in children are the same as in adults (see Chapter 11), but the technique differs somewhat. The success of cardiopulmonary resuscitation depends on a disciplined and organized team approach.

REFERENCES

1. Keith, J. D.: Congestive heart failure. Pediatrics 18:491, 1956.
2. Nadas, A. S., and Hauck, A. J.: Pediatric aspects of congestive heart failure. Circulation 21:424, 1960.
3. Neill, C. A.: Recognition and treatment of congestive heart failure in infancy: I. Diagnosis. Mod. Concepts Cardiovasc. Dis. 28:499, 1959.
4. Neill, C. A.: Recognition and treatment of congestive heart failure in infancy: II. Treatment. Mod. Concepts Cardiovasc. Dis. 28:507, 1959.
5. McCue, C. M., and Young, R. B.: Cardiac failure in infancy. J. Pediatr. 58:330, 1961.
6. Engle, M. A.: Cardiac failure in infancy: Recognition and management. Mod. Concepts Cardiovasc. Dis. 32:825, 1963.
7. Lambert, E. C., Canent, R. V., and Hohn, A. R.: Congenital cardiac anoma-lies in the newborn. A review of conditions causing death or severe distress in the first month of life. Pediatrics 37:343, 1966.
8. Khoury, G. H., and Hawes, C. R.: Congestive heart failure in infancy: Pitfalls in diagnosis and management. Med. Times 97:142, 1969.
9. Hauck, A. J., Ongley, P. A., and Nadas, A. S.: The use of digoxin in infants and children. Am. Heart J. 56:443, 1958.
10. Sparrow, A. W., Friedberg, D. Z., and Nadas, A. S.: The use of ethacrynic acid in infants and children with congestive heart failure. Pediatrics 42:291, 1968.
11. Morgan, B. C., Guntheroth, W. G., Bloom, R. S., and Fyler, D. C.: A clinical profile of paroxysmal hyperpnea in cyanotic congenital heart disease. Circula-tion 31:66, 1965.
12. Guntheroth, W. G., Morgan, B. C., and Mullins, G.: Physiologic studies of

paroxysmal hyperpnea in cyanotic congenital heart disease. Circulation 31:70, 1965.

13. Keith, J. D., Rowe, R. D., and Vlad, P.: Heart Disease in Infancy and Childhood. 2nd ed. New York, The MacMillan Co., 1967.

14. Paul, M., Rudolph, A., and Nadas, A. S.: Congenital complete atrioventricular block: Problems of clinical assessment. Circulation 18:183, 1958.

15. Landtman, B., and Kassila, E.: Auricular flutter in infancy. Acta Paediatr. Scand. 44:272, 1955.

16. Downes, J. J., Fulgencio, T., and Raphaely, R. C.: Acute respiratory failure in infants and children. Pediatr. Clin. N. Am. 19:423, 1972.

17. Gluck, L., Kulvoich, M. V., Borer, R. C., et al.: Diagnosis of the respiratory distress syndrome by amniocentesis. Am. J. Obstet. Gynecol. 109:440, 1971.

Chapter 17

SURGICAL APPROACH TO CARDIAC EMERGENCY

STANLEY K. BROCKMAN

The emergency operative approach to cardiac disease or injury requires that the surgeon and team be totally familiar not only with standard methods but also with the techniques of extracorporeal circulation and circulatory assist devices. The team must also be familiar with appropriate monitoring devices and have available an emergency room, an operating room, and a postoperative care unit with personnel trained in the care of complicated cardiac problems.

No effort has been made here to present an exhaustive review of the literature, since the subject material may change and even become outdated. Emphasis has been placed on practices and techniques currently in use at our institution and elsewhere.

CARDIAC TRAUMA

Cardiac trauma is a growing source of mortality and morbidity, paralleling advances in our mechanized society and an increasing incidence of man raising weapons against his fellows. When death results from an automobile accident, approximately two thirds of those killed have some cardiac trauma. Stab wounds of the heart continue to present themselves with unabating regularity. Gunshot wounds of the heart are increasing at an alarming rate in some localities. In many instances, cardiac trauma is not isolated, but is associated with massive chest trauma or trauma that involves multiple organ systems. Trauma to the heart has classically been divided into penetrating and nonpenetrating wounds. Most penetrating wounds are produced by sharp instruments, such as knives or ice picks, or by gunshot wounds. Penetrating cardiac trauma compromises circulation and may cause death by producing cardiac tamponade, hemorrhage, or an ineffective heartbeat.

Penetrating Cardiac Trauma

The first successful suture closure of an actively bleeding wound of the human heart was by Rehn in 1897.[1] The first successful suture closure of such a wound in the United States was performed by Hill in 1902.[2] In 1920, Tuffier[3] reviewed 305 cases of cardiac trauma and reported a recovery rate of approximately 50%, which confirmed the use of cardiorrhaphy as the treatment of choice for penetrating wounds of the heart. In 1943, Blalock and Ravitch[4] suggested pericardial aspiration as an alternative method of treatment of tamponade associated with penetrating wounds of the heart. These authors indicated that open operation should be reserved for those wounds that were not immediately fatal and in which pericardiocentesis alone would not suffice. The conservative approach utilizing pericardiocentesis has been employed with claims of goods results. However, during the last 15 years, many inadequacies of pericardiocentesis have been recognized. The comparison of early thoracotomy with pericardiocentesis has been somewhat misleading since patients treated by pericardiocentesis are carefully selected and those with massive hemorrhage and severe wounds have been omitted from most studies. Although unanimity is still lacking, most authors now clearly prefer early thoracotomy with pericardiotomy and cardiorrhaphy as the most effective method in the definitive treatment of patients with penetrating wounds of the heart. Early operation with cardiorrhaphy has again emerged as the treatment of choice for penetrating wounds of the heart. (See Chapter 13 for a detailed discussion of cardiac tamponade.)

Over half the patients with penetrating cardiac trauma do not reach the hospital alive. This depends largely upon the severity of the wound, so that patients with massive injuries, particularly gunshot wounds, are least likely to reach the hospital alive. Approximately 70% of penetrating injuries to the heart occur in the ventricles, and the right ventricle is involved more frequently than the left. Ten per cent of the wounds are in the atrium, and 20% involve the pulmonary artery, vena cava, coronary vessels, intrapericardial aorta, or the pericardium alone.[5-8] In an excellent study, Sugg and his co-workers[8] demonstrated that wounds of the left ventricle have the highest mortality rate: Only 8% of patients with isolated left ventricle wounds reached the hospital alive.

The pathophysiology is essentially the production of acute hemopericardium with cardiac tamponade. Were it not for the unyielding presence of the tough, fibrous pericardium, most patients would suffer hopeless hemorrhage and immediate death. The restraining force of the pericardium, with its consequent pericardial tamponade, enables the patient to survive long enough to reach the hospital and the operating table. In surviving patients, there is a balance between the lifesaving effect of the pericardial tamponade and its lethal effects. The limitation of diastolic expansion of the ventricle caused by the pericardial tamponade decreases cardiac filling. Cardiac output and blood pressure fall, venous pressure rises, and the clinical picture of shock evolves. In acute hemopericardium, 150–200 ml of blood can cause severe shock and death as a result of the tamponade. At these levels, pericardial aspiration of only 10–20 ml of blood may spell the difference between life and death.

Most patients are admitted to the emergency room with a history of trauma, and in most instances the nature of the weapon is known. The most important factor in the diagnosis of penetrating wounds of the heart is the high index of suspicion. When a high index of suspicion is present, it should be assumed that there is a penetrating wound of the heart until proven otherwise. The majority of patients are in shock that is frequently out of proportion to the severity of the wound or the obvious loss of blood. Almost half of the patients have no detectable blood pressure when they are first seen in the emergency room. Approximately 23% of the patients have a systolic blood pressure that is not above 40 mm Hg, and approximately 31% of the patients have a systolic blood pressure that is 70 mm Hg or above.[8] The other clinical signs of shock, such as a dull sensorium, agitation, disorientation, rapid thready pulse, and cold clammy skin, are frequently present. The neck veins may be distended, the heart sounds muffled and difficult to hear, and a falling or absent blood pressure with a rising or elevated venous pressure confirm the diagnosis of pericardial tamponade. As soon as the diagnosis is suspected, a pericardiocentesis should be performed immediately for diagnostic and therapeutic purposes. If blood is removed from the pericardium, the diagnosis is certain. However, even when blood is not aspirated, at least 15% of the patients will still have hemopericardium.

In patients with massive trauma without pericardial tamponade who survive to reach the hospital, the clinical manifestations will be predominantly those of shock due to massive blood loss. In addition, these patients will have signs and symptoms resulting from associated trauma, such as pneumothorax, hemothorax, or tension pneumothorax, adding to the picture of shock. Chest roentgenograms may help by showing enlargement of the cardiac shadow or an associated hemothorax or pneumothorax. The roentgenogram may show the location of a bullet and aid in plotting its course and determining what organ structures may have been affected. In many patients, however, the time necessary for obtaining a chest roentgenogram might be better utilized in direct route to the operating room. The electrocardiogram usually shows S–T and T-wave changes,[6] but is not of great help in the diagnosis of severity of a penetrating wound of the heart. If a patient's condition is relatively stable, the electrocardiogram can be obtained, but if his condition is unstable, operation should not be delayed. Within a few days after injury, most patients will demonstrate elevation of the S–T segments, which may be followed by inversion of the S–T segments in some of the leads. These changes may be temporary or permanent; if permanent, they should not be mistaken later for ischemic heart disease.

Before 1965, most penetrating wounds of the heart were treated by pericardiocentesis and observation, reserving the operating room for those instances in which this type of treatment was unsuccessful. Since 1965, pericardiocentesis has been used more sparingly and only to substantiate the diagnosis and to decompress the tamponade while the patient is being prepared for surgery. The results of pericardiocentesis have been enigmatic, and the reports have been misleading, since massive injuries with exsanguinating hemorrhage have not been included. In patients with large pericardial lacerations and penetrating injuries of the heart, brisk hemorrhage occurs, requiring prompt cardiorrhaphy. Pericardiocentesis alone has the following disadvantages: (1) Tamponade may persist or recur; (2) the patient may deteriorate rapidly during an observation period; (3) clots may be present that cannot be removed; (4) secondary hemorrhage may occur days or weeks later; (5) constrictive pericarditis may result from trapped clotted blood; (6) rarely, a traumatic ventricular aneurysm may result; and, finally, (7) damage may be done to the heart by the probing needle.[5–8] Current practice requires that any patient strongly suspected of having penetrating cardiac injury with tamponade be moved to the operating room as rapidly as possible for thoracotomy, pericardiotomy, and direct repair of the wound. Time is spent in the emergency room and en route to the operating room only for typing and cross-matching of blood, beginning infusions, maintenance of airway, insertion of Foley catheter, and diagnostic and therapeutic pericardiocentesis. (See Chapter 13 for a full discussion of pericardial tamponade.)

Diagnostic studies such as roentgenograms, venous pressure, and electrocardiogram may be performed when it is clear that the additional time will not jeopardize the patient. Patients with shock and anoxia may be prone to cardiac arrest during induction of anesthesia, and in this instance rapid thoracotomy is required. Penetrating wounds of the heart are best handled through a left anterolateral thoracotomy through the fourth or fifth intercostal space. This may be extended across the sternum for additional exposure of the right side of the heart. When the wound of entrance is on the right side of the heart, a right-sided thoracotomy may be carried out. In some instances, a median sternotomy may be a preferable incision, particularly when cardiopulmonary bypass would likely be used.

The pericardium is widely incised, blood and clots are rapidly evacuated, and the point of bleeding is controlled by direct digital pressure. Release of the cardiac tamponade and control of hemorrhage is the most crucial point of the operation. When digital control of bleeding under direct vision has been achieved, blood and fluid replacement is given to establish normal circulation before definitive repair of the wound is accomplished. If the heart is asystolic, it is advantageous to close the wound quickly prior to cardiac massage and resuscitation. Circulation must be restored as soon as possible to prevent cerebral damage.

The wound is closed by suture repair beneath the occluding finger, and each suture is tied before the next suture is placed, until the wound is completely closed. In some instances, small pledgets of Teflon or Dacron felt may be helpful. When a wound is adjacent to a coronary vessel, the suture may be passed beneath the coronary vessel in a mattress fashion to avoid obstruction of coronary flow.

When there are extensive cardiac wounds or when there are posterior wounds that are difficult to expose, emergency cardiopulmonary bypass may be lifesaving. In some cases with massive hemorrhage, an autotransfusion device may be helpful or lifesaving. Finally, a circulatory assist device such as a balloon counterpulsation device may aid the patient through a period of depressed circulation that would otherwise have been fatal. Wounds of the atrium may be best handled by the use of noncrushing vascular clamps rather than digital pressure because of the thin and yielding nature of the atrial wall.

It should be stressed that careful examination of the heart in the operating room is required, and a wound of exit, as well as a wound of entrance, should be sought after. Cases have been reported in which a wound of exit has been missed, with tragic results.

The complications of penetrating wounds of the heart that may require further therapy are constrictive pericarditis, the postpericardiotomy syndrome, congestive heart failure from valvular damage, ventricular septal defects, aortic–ventricular fistula, and ventricular and coronary artery aneurysms. The early operative management of penetrating wounds of the heart should prevent the occurrence of late constrictive pericarditis by removal of all blood and clots from the pericardium and establishment of good postoperative drainage. There may be an occasional instance in which continued small leaks in the immediate postoperative period could produce constrictive pericarditis. The development of a ventricular coronary artery aneurysm also should largely be prevented by adequate initial repair, but it theoretically could develop with a lead through a ventricular suture line or a missed coronary artery wound. The postpericardiotomy syndrome will occur in a small percentage of the patients with or without operation; if therapy is required, salicylates or steroids are used. When valvular insufficiency, ventricular septal defect, or other intracardiac defects are produced, they are rarely, if ever, corrected at the time of initial operation. Corrective operation is usually performed electively weeks after the original injury and after cardiac catheterization and angiography have precisely defined the nature and severity of the defect.[17,18]

The results of surgery, in general, reflect the severity of the injury. Most of the deaths are in patients who enter the emergency room with irreversible shock and severe injuries. The mortality rate for penetrating wounds of the heart with cardiac tamponade treated by pericardial aspiration alone has ranged from 0 to 25%.[9-15] As already noted, these figures may be somewhat misleading, since they did not include severe injuries with massive hemorrhage. Beall and his co-workers[9] reported a mortality rate of 5.5% in 78 patients treated by pericardiocentesis. In 23 patients who did not respond to pericardiocentesis, the mortality rate was 26.7% if thoracotomy and cardiorrhaphy were carried out almost immediately, but this figure more than doubled if significant delays were permitted. In a more recent report, the same group now advocates the aggressive operative management of penetrating chest trauma.[13]

Mortality figures similar to those for pericardiocentesis have been reported for early thoracotomy: 0–36%.[5-8,29-31] It is significant that mortality has been reduced since 1965 by early thoracotomy. This approach was championed by Naclerio in an important paper in 1964.[6] In 1968, Sugg and his associates[8] reported a mortality rate of 36% in patients treated prior to 1966. Of 18 deaths, 10 were due to secondary recurrent tamponade, and the authors felt that these wounds could have been repaired by thoracotomy. The same group reported a mortality rate of only 5% after 1966, when early thoracotomy was adopted.

In 1970, Borja and his associates[7] reported a mortality rate of 16.6% in 54 cases of stab wounds of the heart treated by early thoracotomy from 1951 through 1968. Of the deaths in this group, two patients died from transfusion reaction of unmatched blood, three patients from cardiac arrest in the recovery room, and one from a myocardial infarction in the left anterior descending coronary artery caused by an inappropriately placed suture. One patient was clinically dead on arrival in the operating room, and one patient died from exsanguination with irreversible brain damage. Thus, the deaths could not be ascribed to the use of thoracotomy as compared with pericardiocentesis.

In 1971, Hutchinson and his associates[19] reported 34 patients with penetrating cardiac wounds from 1967 to 1970 of whom 31 were in severe shock at the time of admission. There were only 8 deaths in this series. Three deaths were the result of severe gunshot wounds, and seven of the eight patients who died had no obtainable blood pressure when admitted to the operating room. The excellent results of Hutchinson are attributed to early thoracotomy.

Balanowski and associates[16] reported a mortality rate of 15% in 34 patients with cardiac stab wounds and a mortality of 60% in those with cardiac gunshot wounds; all of these patients were treated with immediate thoracotomy.

In 1972, Carrasquilla and his associates[21] reported a series of patients having penetrating wounds of the heart, almost 50% (27) of which were caused by gunshot. Twenty of the twenty-seven patients survived, and this survival is largely attributed to early thoracotomy. In this group the protective effect of tamponade is strikingly demonstrated by the fact that all deaths occurred in patients without tamponade. Until this report, survival after gunshot wounds of the heart was thought to be uncommon, and one of the better survival rates (64.5%) was reported by Ricks and his associates.[20] Thirteen of the patients had no obtainable blood pressure upon admission and five of these died. Of 14 patients with a systolic pressure exceeding 50 mm Hg, only 2 died. Of the 14 patients who had tamponade, only 2 died; in contrast, of 13 patients who did not have tamponade, 5 died.

In all of these reports, postoperative morbidity was mainly that of pulmonary dysfunction, including atelectasis and pleural effusion. There was an occasional occurrence of pericarditis and the postpericardiotomy syndrome, as well as the morbidity of intercardiac defects mentioned above, which would be handled by elective cardiopulmonary bypass at a later date.

Nonpenetrating Cardiac Trauma

Nonpenetrating cardiac trauma most frequently produces contusion of the heart in surviving patients; this can be treated by bed rest and medications designed to relieve pain. Sometimes, however, patients with massive nonpenetrating cardiac trauma, particularly rupture of the myocardial chamber or disruption of a cardiac valve, will survive a long enough time to allow emergency correction of the defect.

In 1958, Parmley and his associates[22] presented a review of 546 autopsy cases of nonpenetrating traumatic injuries to the heart. Cardiac contusion and laceration were the two most common lesions of nonpenetrating traumatic injury in this series. Ventricular rupture was most common and was usually associated with immediate death except for one patient who lived for 4 hours until massive exsanguination caused death. Thirteen patients with atrial rupture, 19% of the atrial ruptures, survived the initial injury and might have been saved by emergency operation. In the series of nonpenetrating cardiac injuries reported by Bright and Beck,[23] 14 of 66 patients with rupture of the atrium survived long enough to allow operation. In a review by Kohn and his associates,[24] there were 79 cases of atrial rupture, and 19 of these survived long enough to permit operation. It is clear, therefore, that approximately 20% of atrial ruptures secondary to nontraumatic injury of the heart allow survival long enough for emergency operation. It is assumed that those who die of exsanguination have an associated large pericardial tear that produces early exsanguination and death rather than cardiac tamponade, which would allow longer survival.

Rupture of the ventricular septum was found in 30 patients in Parmley's series[22] and in 5 of these the septal rupture was the sole cardiac lesion. Both immediate and delayed rupture of the intraventricular septum following nonpenetrating cardiac trauma has been documented. The defects usually occur in the muscular septum near the apex, but they may occur at any site. Delayed septal defects are presumably due to necrosis of previously contused muscle. Some of these patients may survive long enough for operative correction.

Disruption of the atrioventricular valves was the most frequent of the valvular injuries in Parmley's series, but there was usually enough associated myocardial injury that the patient did not survive long enough for operative correction. Of greater interest to the surgeon are the four cases of aortic valvular rupture in Parmley's series, since there have been a number of reports of successful operative correction of these lesions. Nonpenetrating trauma can produce almost any type of cardiac injury, some of which may be surgically remediable; cardiac catheterization and angiography are in order when such conditions are suspected.

The principles of treatment described for penetrating cardiac trauma apply to nonpenetrating cardiac trauma, particularly when there is a rupture of the atrium. There have been at least nine successful repairs of atrial rupture reported.[24,25] Most of these were repaired by direct suture without need for extracorporeal circulation.

Traumatic disruption of the aortic valve results when nonpenetrating trauma to the chest occurs during the diastolic phase of the cardiac cycle. The left and/or noncoronary aortic leaflets are the most commonly perforated or detached. The diagnosis is usually suggested by the typical high-pitched musical aortic diastolic murmur and may be confirmed by aortography. The physician must be extremely sensitive to the lethal nature of this lesion, and if it is suspected, immediate operation with cardiopulmonary bypass and aortic valve replacement must be performed. The classical description of traumatic rupture of the aortic valve, including a review of 113 cases, is that of Howard in 1928.[26] In 1955, Leonard and his associates[27] reported the first operative correction, which was achieved by inserting a Hufnagle plastic valve into the descending aorta. The first successful total correction followed insertion of a ball valve by Beall and Shirkey[28] in 1964. At least seven instances of survival following operative correction have been reported.[26-29]

There have been two successful valve replacements for traumatic insufficiency of the tricuspid valve.[30,31] I have successfully corrected one instance of traumatic disruption of the mitral valve by valve replacement. Lesions of the tricuspid and mitral valve were not of an emergency nature and were repaired under extracorporeal circulation electively. Ventricular septal defect secondary to nonpenetrating trauma of the heart rarely requires emergency operation if it is the sole lesion. These lesions are usually identified by cardiac catheterization and angiography and operated on electively at a later date. Patch closure of the defect in the muscular septum is recommended.

DISSECTING HEMATOMA (ANEURYSM) OF THE AORTA

Dissecting hematoma of the ascending aorta is a true cardiac emergency that will tax the judgment of cardiac surgeon and cardiologist. Cystic medionecrosis is the most common pathologic finding in the ascending aorta in patients with dissecting hematoma. Most patients with this condition have hypertension. Approximately one third of the cases will occur in association with Marfan's syndrome. In some instances, atherosclerosis alone may be an etiologic factor. There are a number of other conditions, including coarctation of the aorta, patent ductus arteriosus, pheochromocytosis, and Cushing's disease, that may be associated with dissecting hematoma of the aorta.

There are three types of dissecting hematoma of the ascending aorta.[32] Type I accounts for at least two thirds of the dissecting hematomas;

it begins in the ascending aorta and propagates distally for varying distances. Type II is rare and may be found in Marfan's syndrome; it remains confined to the ascending aorta. Type III originates at or just beyond the origin of the left subclavian artery and will progress distally for varying lengths. Approximately one fifth to one third of the patients seen will have Type III dissecting hematoma. It is unusual for Type III to extend proximally, although this has been observed.

In untreated acute aortic dissecting hematoma, death will occur in approximately 20% of the patients within 24 hours, two thirds within 2 weeks, and 90% within 3 months due to rupture of the aorta with hemorrhage and/or cardiac tamponade. So-called healed dissecting hematoma of the aorta has been reported as an incidental autopsy finding in later life, so survival without treatment is possible.

The diagnosis of dissecting hematoma of the aorta is usually made or suspected on the basis of typical clinical symptoms of severe tearing chest pain, which may be associated with hypertension, and weak or absent pulse in one or more of the extremities. Once there is a high index of suspicion and a presumptive diagnosis has been made, it must be confirmed by thoracic and abdominal aortography within a few hours to precisely define the site of the intimal tear as well as the extent of the dissecting hematoma and the involvement of the aortic branches.

There is still controversy about treatment, particularly concerning emergency operation. At present, this author agrees with the concepts that have been set down by Wheat and his associates,[33,34] in which drug therapy is the treatment of choice in the immediate management of patients with acute dissecting hematoma of the aorta, except in special circumstances. If drug treatment is chosen, the systolic blood pressure is reduced to 100–120 mm Hg with trimethaphan given intravenously and reserpine intramuscularly. When trimethaphan is no longer effective because of tachyphylaxis 24–48 hours after initiation of treatment, reserpine and guanethidine will usually suffice for control of blood pressure. In many instances, propranolol may be helpful. The patient's urine output, pulses, ECG, blood pressure, blood urea nitrogen, and sensorium are carefully followed in the intensive care unit.

This approach should be abandoned when (1) pain is not alleviated, indicating progression and extension of the dissecting hematoma of the aorta; (2) the blood pressure cannot be brought under control, while the urine output, blood urea nitrogen, and sensorium of the patient remain adequate; (3) the aortic valve is insufficient; (4) there is roentgenographic evidence of enlargement of the aneurysm; (5) there is suspicion that the dissecting hematoma is leaking or that rupture is imminent; (6) patients who respond well to hypotensive drug therapy enter a chronic stage, developing an acute sacular aneurysm or aortic insufficiency. Approximately 20–30% of patients in this last group will require operation.

When there is obstruction of a major branch of the aorta, a local operative procedure, such as segmental replacement, may suffice. Thus, the combination of hypotensive drug therapy with operative intervention, when required, will best serve the overall interests of the patient with a dissecting hematoma of the aorta. In general, Type I and Type II dissecting hematomas of the aorta are associated with valvular insufficiency and are usually treated by emergency operative intervention with results that are excellent.[35–37]

From a technical point of view, the operative approach has gone through a metamorphosis, beginning with the palliative "fenestration" operation together with segmental excision with end-to-end anastomosis. In 1961, DeBakey reported 72 cases of dissecting aneurysm of the aorta treated operatively with good results.[38] Many of DeBakey's patients had some type of graft replacement for aneurysm, and it was difficult to ascertain which procedures were done on an emergency basis and which were done in a chronic stage.

In a Type I dissecting hematoma, current technique utilizes total extracorporeal circulation. The ascending aorta is transected just above the aortic valve, and the proximal and distal double-barreled lumen are oversewn and reapproximated with or without a prosthetic tubular graft. This procedure will resuspend the aortic valve leaflets and abolish the insufficiency in most instances. In those cases in which the aortic leaflets are still insufficient, a prosthetic valve may be required. The operative approach for Type II aneurysm is similar to that for Type I. Most Type III aneurysms are successfully treated by hypotensive drug therapy. When this type of therapy fails, operation is undertaken with partial extracorporeal circulation by a femorofemoral bypass or by left atrium to femoral artery bypass. The aneurysm is isolated by means of vascular clamps placed proximally and distally, and then it is excised. The double-barreled lumens are oversewn both proximally and distally and the two ends of the aorta connected by a Dacron prosthesis.

The complications of the operative approach are mainly postoperative hemorrhage, along with congestive heart failure, arrhythmias, and myocardial infarction. There has been a reported operative mortality rate of 10–25% with a primary operative approach for Type I and Type II aneurysms.[35–37] There is a late mortality rate of 10–20% in patients who survive operation. Hypotensive drug therapy also has untoward effects, largely due to poor tissue perfusion; these effects include tubular necrosis of the kidney, duodenal ulcer associated with reserpine therapy,

depressed sensorium with confusion and lethargy due to postural hypotension, and occasionally, drug-induced jaundice.[33,34]

CARDIAC TUMORS

Seventy to eighty per cent of cardiac neoplasms are benign. Myxoma
accounts for approximately 50% of all neoplasms and is of great interest
to the surgeon. Myxomas arise in the left atrium in 70–80% of instances, with most of the remainder arising in the right atrium. A number of myxomas have been removed from the right and left ventricles.
Myxomas vary in size and configuration and are usually attached by
a narrow pedicle to the atrial septum in the area of the fossa ovalis.
The tumor may have a ball valve effect, passing back and forth from
atrium to ventricle, when the pedicle is long enough, to intermittently
obstruct the mitral valve. In other instances, the tumor may produce
no clinical symptoms and may be an incidental finding.

The clinical symptoms of myxoma are due to embolization, obstruction to blood flow at the level of the atrioventricular valve with congestive heart failure, and certain constitutional effects, including arthralgia,
weight loss, anemia, fever, and hyperglobulinemia. The constitutional
effects are poorly understood at present. The diagnosis is confirmed by
catheterization and angiography.

The clinical course of myxoma may be quite uncertain, with severe
disabling features due to peripheral emboli, progressive deterioration
of valvular function, and severe congestive heart failure. In some instances, sudden death may occur; thus, the presence of a myxoma is
considered an indication for emergency operation as soon as possible
after the diagnosis is made. Under extracorporeal circulation, the
myxoma is removed, along with a small portion of the adjacent atrial
septum. Although many operations have been done without removing
a portion of the atrial septum, there have been reports of recurrence.[39,40]

The mortality rate has been low following excision of the atrial
myxoma. Patients who survive operation for removal of atrial myxoma
are usually asymptomatic and can lead normal lives.

VALVULAR HEART DISEASE

Aortic valve replacement is usually performed on an elective basis
in patients with significant symptoms of congestive heart failure, syncope, or angina. There may be an occasional instance in which the clinical symptoms indicate that the patient is at extreme risk of sudden death
and the operation is performed on an urgent basis. When acute severe
aortic valve insufficiency occurs, the hemodynamic derangement may
be so severe as to rapidly lead to heart failure and death. Acute valve

insufficiency may follow acute dissecting hematoma of the aorta, trauma, or infective endocarditis.

The emergency operative approach to aortic insufficiency resulting from dissecting hematoma of the aorta and from trauma have already been covered (p. 307). Emergency operation may be required for patients with infective endocarditis. Because of the success of anti-biotics, aortic valve perforation with severe cardiac failure has become the leading cause of death in patients treated for infective endocarditis. When cardiac failure is present, it may be extremely difficult to "steril-ize" patients with bacterial endocarditis. When progressive and intract-able cardiac failure occurs with aortic valve insufficiency, there is no alternative to emergency replacement of the aortic valve even when anti-biotic therapy has just been begun. There have been a great number of reports of surgery for bacterial endocarditis with cardiac valve in-volvement and cardiac failure in which aortic valve replacement has been performed under emergency conditions even without definite anti-bacterial measures, with excellent results. (See Chapter 12 for a full dis-cussion of infectious heart disease.)

Operations upon the mitral valve are almost always performed on an elective basis. When papillary muscle rupture occurs as a complica-tion of myocardial infarction, emergency operative correction should be undertaken, since death may result rapidly secondary to the acute hemodynamic derangement. This is covered below in the section on complications of myocardial infarction (p. 313).

ISCHEMIC HEART DISEASE

Aortocoronary saphenous vein bypass has emerged as the operative procedure of choice in patients with ischemic heart disease. Chronic, intractable angina pectoris constitutes the main indication for aortocoro-nary bypass on an elective basis. Urgent or emergency operative treat-ment of ischemic heart disease has been advocated in unstable angina pectoris and acute evolving myocardial infarction and when the ana-tomic lesion constitutes a severe threat to life. Unstable angina pectoris (crescendo angina, acute coronary insufficiency, preinfarction angina, im-pending myocardial infarction) is indicated by angina occurring for the first time, increasing severity of stable pre-existing angina, angina ex-tending for prolonged periods, and angina not relieved by rest or nitrates; formerly asymptomatic patients with a history of myocardial infarction who suddenly begin to have angina again also have unstable angina. There are no changes in the electrocardiogram or in the serum enzymes diagnostic of myocardial infarction. Although the natural his-tory of these patients is still somewhat enigmatic, it has been reported that up to 40% may experience myocardial infarction within 3 months, with relatively high mortality rates.[41-43]

Because of the high incidence of myocardial infarction, most centers performing aortocoronary saphenous bypass operations have developed an aggressive attitude with urgent or emergency operative correction of patients with impending myocardial infarction. These patients have arteriographic lesions which are essentially the same as patients with stable angina pectoris. This approach is based on the theory that immediate surgical intervention carries a risk essentially the same as patients undergoing an operation for stable angina, and avoids the higher risk of infarction and death. In 1973, a review of 420 patients operated on for impending myocardial infarction showed an operative mortality of 4.3%.[44] A review of 1500 patients in 1974 operated on for unstable angina showed an operative mortality rate of 7.7%.[45] Emergency operation for unstable angina is still controversial, and there is a passing need for controlled prospective double-blind analysis of therapy in this condition. In view of the excellent results of the emergency operative approach in these patients, however, it has become more difficult for major centers to carry out such a prospective study for fear of depriving patients of the benefit of operation. (The variant of coronary insufficiency described by Prinzmetal and his associates[46,47] is a form of angina pectoris associated with elevation of S–T segments in a specific area of the myocardium; patients suffering from this disorder should be classified with unstable angina patients when operation is considered.)

Emergency aortocoronary bypass grafts for acute myocardial infarction are even more controversial, but they may have application in selected instances. The justification for emergency operation in these patients is based on the improvement of oxygen delivery to the area of myocardium adjacent to the area of necrotic infarction, the "twilight zone" of ischemic tissue. Salvage of the potentially reversible ischemic myocardium would reduce the size of the infarct. This ischemic tissue may be reversible for up to 48 hours.

Experience with emergency operation for acute myocardial infarction is limited, and the operative mortality is higher than in patients with stable angina or impending myocardial infarction. Patients who suffer myocardial infarction during coronary angiography are a separate group in whom emergency operation is undoubtedly justified, and the results in this group have been gratifying.[48] Several centers have reported relatively small numbers of emergency operations for acute myocardial infarction with satisfactory results,[48-52] while other groups with similarly small numbers of patients have reported extremely discouraging results.[53-55] These contradictory results emphasize the controversial nature of emergency operation for acute myocardial infarction. The operative results have been more gratifying when patients did not have significant impairment of the left ventricular function or cardiogenic shock.

Case selection is most important when considering emergency operation for impending or proven myocardial infarction. Wiener and his associates[49,56] have attempted to improve selection by adding the use of metabolic evaluation of coronary sinus efflux to determine operability. Patients were considered to be candidates for surgery if abnormalities in lactate metabolism (increased lactate production) were present despite the efflux of creatinine phosphokinase (CPK) in coronary sinus blood. These authors reason that this was a determinant of ischemic, but still viable, myocardium and that the optimal time for operation was during the early CPK efflux in the coronary sinus blood, before systemic CPK elevation occurred. Utilizing this approach, these authors reported 2 deaths among 24 patients, 10 with impending myocardial infarction and 14 with evolving myocardial infarction, a mortality rate of 8.3%. Such an approach may help to define those individuals who are candidates for emergency operation following acute myocardial infarction.

Patients with critical stenosis (72% or greater) of the left main coronary artery have a potentially lethal lesion. Cohen and his associates[57] have reported a 50% mortality rate at the end of a 2-year period in a small group of patients who were not treated surgically. The operative mortality among patients with left main coronary artery stenosis—reported to be 12–35%[58,60]—is higher than among patients with stable angina or impending myocardial infarction without left main coronary artery stenosis. The condition of the survivors was considerably improved. Thus, at present emergency surgery for patients with left main coronary artery stenosis seems justified.

COMPLICATIONS OF MYOCARDIAL INFARCTION

Ventricular Aneurysm

Left ventricular aneurysm following myocardial infarction has been reported to occur in between 5% and 35% of patients. From the surgeon's point of view, a ventricular aneurysm is often a thick scar replacing a portion of the left ventricular wall usually adherent to the pericardium and usually containing thrombus on the endocardial surface. Differences in interpretation of angiograms may account for the varying reports of the incidence of this condition.

Most left ventricular aneurysms are in the anterior or apical portion of the heart, and the rest are in the posterior portion. Most posterior aneurysms involve the mitral valve mechanism, causing death from severe mitral insufficiency. Among patients with myocardial infarction who also develop left ventricular aneurysm, the survival rate is approximately one third of that of those who do not develop an aneurysm.[61] Most of the deaths are accounted for by congestive heart failure that follows the mechanical dysfunction produced by the mechanical effects of the aneurysm.[61,62] A significant percentage of the deaths result from arrhythmias; peripheral emboli may be troublesome in 5–10% of the cases.

Most operations for left ventricular aneurysm are performed on an elective basis because of the presence of refractory congestive heart failure. In some instances, the presence of emboli may constitute the indication for operation. In a small percentage of cases, the presence of difficult-to-treat cardiac arrhythmias is an indication for operation, and it is in these instances that emergency operation may be required. Cardiac arrhythmias have ranged from supraventricular to ventricular tachycardias and have included conduction disturbances such as intraventricular block, right bundle-branch block, left bundle-branch block, and frequent ventricular extrasystoles. There have been a number of instances in which emergency operation has been performed for intractable arrhythmias, particularly ventricular tachycardia, with success. There have also been instances of successful emergency operation performed for severe, life-threatening congestive heart failure.[62–64] The patients who survive usually have an excellent postoperative course, with greatly improved ventricular performance and, usually, disappearance of the arrhythmia once the mechanical deficits and ventricular irritability secondary to the aneurysm have been removed.

Postinfarction Ventricular Septal Defect

This condition is not common: 1–2% of patients dying of acute myocardial infarction will have experienced ventricular septal defect. In two thirds of these patients, the defect is in the apical portion of the septum, and in a few it is in the posterior, middle, or superior portion of the septum. In an occasional instance, multiple perforations may be found. Perforation of the ventricular septum frequently occurs between 5 and 15 days after the myocardial infarction and coincides with the time of maximal degeneration of the muscular tissue. One third of the patients have an associated left ventricular aneurysm, so this condition should always be suspected in the presence of an acquired ventricular septal defect.

Once a perforation of the ventricular septum occurs, one fourth of the patients will die within 24 hours and two thirds of them will die within 2 weeks. At the end of 1 year, less than 10% of the patients will be alive. The resulting congestive heart failure is usually refractory to conservative management because of the burden of the left-to-right shunt superimposed on the already damaged myocardium. Operation is performed in patients whose condition is deteriorating despite intensive medical management; over 100 operations have been reported. In many instances, operation will be an emergency lifesaving procedure. In those instances in which the diagnosis is uncertain and mitral insufficiency is suspected, the Swans-Gantz catheter may be used for confirmatory diagnosis at the bedside.[65]

The result will be best if operation can be delayed from 3 to 6 weeks after the occurrence of the ventricular septal defect to allow fibrous edges to develop so that a secure repair can be performed. Nevertheless, emergency operation may be undertaken because of rapid degeneration of the patient. In 26 patients operated on within 2 weeks of the infarction, the operative mortality was 56%.[66] Of patients operated on considerably under 6 weeks following the occurrence of the infarction, only 9% were alive at the end of 1 year, whereas when operation was undertaken 6 weeks or more after the occurrence of a ventricular septal defect, at least 35% of the patients were alive at the end of 1 year. In a recent report from the Mayo Clinic[66] there was a 54% survival rate at the end of 1 year or longer when the operation was undertaken 3 weeks or more after the occurrence of ventricular defect. In selected patients with a rapid downhill course that may be ascribed to a postinfarction ventricular septal defect, the balloon assist device may be of aid in tiding the patient over the initial critical period till operation can be performed.

Postinfarction Mitral Regurgitation

Rupture of the papillary muscle accounts for approximately 1% of deaths following myocardial infarction. The posterior papillary muscle is usually involved, and the infarction is located in the diaphragmatic surface of the heart.

Most of these patients have widespread diffuse coronary vessel disease. Intractable left ventricular failure follows papillary muscle rupture. Over two thirds of these patients will die within 24 hours, and almost 90% of them will die within 2 weeks. Operative intervention for this lesion is almost always undertaken as an emergency measure in the acute postinfarction period. There are only a few reports of successful mitral valve replacement in mitral insufficiency due to postinfarction rupture of the papillary muscle. The most important prognostic criteria are the extent of the infarct and the quality of the remaining muscle. Concomitant aortocoronary saphenous vein bypass will improve results in most instances. In some instances, the balloon assist device may arrest the patient's initial downhill course, permitting cardiac catheterization and emergency operative intervention. The first successful operative correction with valve replacement was performed in 1965.[67] When patients have enough viable myocardium to sustain life following mitral valve replacement, the results are satisfactory.

Cardiogenic Shock

Cardiogenic shock still has a high mortality rate despite all modalities of therapy. Diastolic augmentation with balloon counterpulsation may allow the patient to survive for hours or days, but will not itself alter the outcome. It will permit cardiac catheterization and an emergency operation to be performed. Emergency bypass surgery in this desperate situation is highly controversial, but, in selected instances where survival is theoretically possible, it may be the only alternative to certain death. In 10 reports of a total of 80 operations, there was a 39% survival following emergency operation.[68] In general, the surviving patients were those who had adequate amounts of viable myocardium. Surviving patients were usually those who received prompt treatment and who experienced cardiogenic shock for no longer than 12 hours. In one excellent study, of 42 patients who had intra-aortic balloon assist for 36 hours to 14 days, 5 patients are reported to have survived on a long-term basis. Emergency operative intervention was performed on 16 of these patients. Fourteen patients had aortocoronary bypass grafts, 8 had infarctectomy and bypass graft, 2 had infarctectomy alone, and 2 patients had mitral valve replacement. At the end of 1 month to 1 year, 7 of these patients were alive. The treatment of cardiogenic shock following acute myocardial infarction is still controversial, and further changes in therapy are expected in the immediate future. Cardiogenic shock is described in detail in Chapter 3.

PERICARDITIS

Surgery for pericarditis, including chronic pericardial effusion, acute inflammation of the pericardium, and chronic constrictive pericarditis, is usually performed on an elective basis when it becomes clear that the impairment has produced an increase in venous volume and pressure proximal to the ventricles in both systemic and pulmonary circulation, causing low cardiac output. There are a few instances in which emergency operation may be appropriate, particularly in purulent pericarditis and uremic pericarditis. Open drainage of the pericardium, pericardiotomy, or pericardiostomy may be required in purulent pericarditis, particularly when repeated needle aspirations are unsatisfactory. This procedure is merely the classical surgical principle of incision and drainage of an abscess in a closed space and under pressure. The type of technical operative approach would be selected in each instance. Tube pericardiostomy would be the treatment of choice in many cases while the more radical procedure of open drainage or pericardiotomy can be performed when required. Emergency operation may also be required in patients with uremic pericarditis, particularly those who may later have renal transplantation. Almost half the patients on chronic dialysis will experience pericarditis with effusion, usually bloody, with or without tamponade. This can usually be treated by pericardiocentesis or by tube pericardiostomy. If these procedures fail, urgent pericardiotomy may be required. Infectious heart disease and pericardial tamponade are discussed in detail in Chapters 12 and 13, respectively.

ARRHYTHMIAS

Certain arrhythmias may benefit from urgent or emergency operative treatment. The operative approach to severely symptomatic Wolff-Parkinson-White (WPW) syndrome is becoming established.[69,70] The indication for operation is disabling and life-threatening supraventricular and ventricular tachycardia.

Sealy and his associates[69] have described an excellent technique that requires electronic mapping and an incision, which is later sutured, around the mitral or tricuspid valve and carried through the annulus fibrosus. In this manner the accessory bundle of Kent may be located and divided, whether the WPW syndrome is Type A or Type B. Sealy and his co-workers[69] have reported 20 operative cases with 1 death, 2 failures, 3 partial successes; the remainder enjoyed good to excellent results. Good results have been achieved in the Type B. In the Type A variety of WPW, excellent results have been achieved when the accessory bundle of Kent was located laterally; the results were not as good when the accessory bundle of Kent was not located posteriorly. When the accessory bundle of Kent travels close to the bundle of His, close to the membranous septum, the results have not been entirely satisfactory; this type has been referred to by Sealy as septal Type A.[70]

Ventricular aneurysmectomy may be an effective means of controlling refractory ventricular and supraventricular tachyarrhythmias when aneurysm is present, and, as already noted, operation may be required on emergency basis. Ventricular arrhythmias probably have their origin in the marginal zone of the aneurysm separating the aneurysmal scar from the surrounding viable myocardium. This area is subject to continuous mechanical stress. The presence of uncontrolled supraventricular tachycardia is difficult to explain, but it may be related to the increased pressure and volume load in the atrium or it may be a consequence of the generalized ischemic process.

There have been occasional reports of intractable ventricular tachycardia for which no etiology was found. A few bilateral cervicothoracic sympathectomies with some success have been reported in such patients.[71] It is difficult to understand how bilateral thoracic sympathectomy is of benefit to patients with ventricular tachycardia refractory to the usual medical treatment, but it may be a method deserving of some consideration under unusual circumstances.

Medical management of cardiac arrhythmias is discussed in detail in Chapters 7 through 10.

CONGENITAL HEART DISEASE IN INFANTS

The mortality from congenital heart disease is highest in the first 6 months of life, accounting for approximately 80–85% of all deaths in this period. Refinements in pediatric cardiology and cardiac catheterization, along with the refinements in the performance of operations, have provided the cardiac surgeon with an increasing number of candidates in the first few months of life for emergency palliative and, in some instances, corrective procedures.

In a few cases, infants under 4 weeks of age and even premature infants may have severe congestive failure secondary to a large patent ductus arteriosus. Emergency closure of the patent ductus through a thoracotomy in the usual manner has been performed in this group with a mortality rate of approximately 15%.

Coarctation of the aorta producing severe congestive heart failure in the first year of life constitutes an emergency. Over two thirds of these infants have associated lesions, such as patent ductus arteriosus, ventricular septal defect, or an area of tubular hypoplasia (the so-called infantile type of coarctation). The operative mortality in these patients is higher than when this procedure is performed electively at a later age, largely because of the associated anomalies, which may not be amenable to correction at the time of operation. There is usually concomitant pulmonary vascular disease. Nevertheless, emergency operative intervention is required in these patients, since it is far more successful than conservative medical management alone. The best results will be obtained in infants with classic coarctation of the aorta without associated significant cardiac defects and in severe congestive heart failure not responding to medical therapy. In infants operated on during the first year of life, the mortality rate has ranged from 20–55%.

Congenital valvular aortic stenosis producing intractable congestive heart failure in the first year of life is uncommon, and it may require emergency operative intervention. Associated conditions such as endo-cardial fibroelastosis or coarctation should be watched for; they will in-crease the mortality rate. The infant with critical aortic stenosis should undergo urgent cardiac catheterization and operative correction. Incision of the fused commissure is required to relieve the stenosis. The operative mortality in the first year of life may be as high as 50%, but the emer-gency surgical management of such a critically ill child is imperative, since conservative treatment with medical management will result in death in almost every instance.

The prognosis for individuals with pulmonary stenosis or pulmonary atresia with an intact septum depends on the severity of the obstruction. In infants with moderate to severe obstruction, the disease is essentially lethal. Sudden death may follow the severe congestive heart failure de-spite all therapeutic efforts. Most infants with severe obstruction have some degree of cyanosis and usually a patent foramen ovale; death oc-curs within the first 3 to 6 months of life following congestive heart failure with attacks of hypoxemia. Emergency operation is indicated when congestive heart failure with dyspnea and fatigue are present along with hypoxic attacks. When infants have cyanosis due to reversed shunt through a patent foramen ovale, emergency operation is indicated. In patients with pulmonary valve stenosis, the basic principles of the opera-tion are incision of the fused commissures of the stenotic pulmonary valve. In patients with pulmonary atresia and an intact septum, a patent ductus arteriosus and atrial septal defect are usually present and re-quired for survival. Emergency operative creation of an aortopulmonary shunt of the Waterston or Blalock type is performed. In some instances, closed pulmonary valvulotomy may also be performed.

Congenital tricuspid atresia is an uncommon complex anomaly found in approximately 5% of the patients with cyanotic congenital heart dis-ease. Two thirds of these patients will be dead by 1 year of age. Death is due to congestive heart failure, along with anoxic attacks. The pres-ence of cardiac failure and hypoxic attacks is indication for emergency operative intervention. When the pulmonary flow is adequate, a pallia-tive systemic pulmonary artery shunt should be created by the method of Waterston or Blalock. In all instances, operation should be preceded by cardiac catheterization with balloon atrioseptotomy to ensure ade-quate emptying of the right atrium.[72] When there is an associated trans-position of the great vessels, there may be large blood flows into the lungs, so balloon atrioseptotomy should be followed by emergency oper-ative banding of the pulmonary artery. The operative risk is high, and development of congestive heart failure in the postoperative period is frequent.

In desperately ill infants with transposition of the great vessels, emergency cardiac catheterization with balloon atrioseptotomy is always performed. If, after this procedure, arterial oxygen saturation is found to be over 60%, corrective operation can be deferred to the second or third year of life. In infants who are incapacitated by associated pulmonary stenosis and inadequate blood flow, palliation can be achieved by emergency systemic pulmonary artery shunt of the Blalock or Waterston type. Corrective operation can then be deferred until the child is 2 to 4 years old. Over 50% of infants with transposition of the great vessels will die during the first month of life because of mixing between the two circuits. In many instances there are few, if any, associated cardiac lesions, so these patients are candidates for total correction by the Mustard procedure even at this early date. Rather than subject the patient to repeated balloon septostomy or accept the mortality of operative septectomy, early corrective operation is being performed when initial balloon atrial septostomy yields unsatisfactory palliation. In a series of 15 corrections, 10 in patients under 21 months of age and 4 in patients under 6 months of age, only two operative deaths were reported.[73] These data indicate that total correction by the Mustard procedure can be performed successfully in children under 6 months of age. Increasing numbers of successful total correction of transposition of the great vessels in infants under 1 year of age are being reported.

Without treatment, approximately three quarters of the patients with total anomalous venous return will die within the first year of life. Early diagnosis and operation are required if death is to be prevented. The natural history and survival of patients with this condition is determined by the degree of pulmonary hypertension and obstruction of the pulmonary venous return by constriction of the anomalous venous trunk. When severe pulmonary hypertension associated with pulmonary vascular disease is present, prognosis is poor and patients are usually dead within 6 to 12 months. When there is a good shunt at the atrial level without pulmonary hypertension, cyanosis, or cardiac failure, and symptoms are not severe, the patient will attain adulthood, and total operative correction at a later date is possible. The mortality rate following emergency correction of total anomalous venous return is related to age, pulmonary vascular resistance, and the severity of the cyanosis. The mortality rate in patients under 1 year of age as reported in the literature ranges from 47% to 70%. Operative management requires early diagnosis with cardiac catheterization, followed by operation. Corrective operation includes connection of pulmonary venous return to the left atrium, closure of the atrial septal defect, and closure of the abnormal venous return to the right atrium. Little or no attempt is made to manage the patient medically. Ventilatory support is maintained postoperatively, and acid–base balance is carefully regulated. Other groups have utilized extracorporeal circulation with or without surface hypothermia. It is difficult to be certain whether the differences in technique are important since satisfactory results have been obtained both with extracorporeal circulation alone and with surface cooling in addition to extracorporeal circulation.

Occasionally, infants with tetralogy of Fallot may require urgent operation because of severe cyanotic or apneic spells. Usually, anastomosis of ascending aorta to right pulmonary artery, as described by Waterston, is performed in babies under 6 months of age.

Emergency operations in infants with ventricular septal defects or atrial septal defects and refractory congestive heart failure are rarely required.

The emergency treatment of infants with congenital cardiac anomalies is a great challenge that must be met largely through surgical intervention. Most infants with cardiac defects become symptomatic during the first month of life and do not survive without operative intervention. Despite the high risk involved, curative or palliative operations are available and must be performed. Results obtained with this approach have been gratifying and encouraging, and the list of long-term survivors is growing rapidly.

Cardiopulmonary emergency care in infancy and childhood is described in detail in Chapter 16.

SUMMARY

It is generally agreed that the heart is amenable to emergency operative repair, provided the facilities are adequate and a knowledgeable team is available. The emergencies that confront the cardiac surgeon include cardiac trauma and a wide variety of acquired and congenital cardiac lesions. The surgeon must be thoroughly familiar with all basic aspects of traumatic surgery as well as with the highly specialized use of extracorporeal circulation and circulatory assist devices. Proper use of appropriate techniques in emergency situations yields excellent overall results.

REFERENCES

1. Rehn, L.: Uber penetrirende herzwanden und herznaht. Arch. Klin. Chir. 55:315, 1897.
2. Hill, L. L.: Report of a case of successful suturing of heart, and table of 37 other cases of suturing by different operators with various terminations and conclusions drawn. Med. Rec. (November 29), p. 846 1902.
3. Tuffier, T.: La chirurgie du coeur. Cinquième Congrès de la Société Internationale de Chirurgie, Paris (July 19–23) 1920. Extrait, Brussels, Hayez, 1920.
4. Blalock, A., and Ravitch, M. M.: Consideration of nonoperative treatment of cardiac tamponade resulting from wounds of heart. Surgery 11:157, 1943.

5. Maynard, A. D. L., Brooks, H. A., and Froix, C. J. L.: Penetrating wound of the heart. Report on a new series. Arch. Surg. 90:680, 1965.
6. Naclerio, E. A.: Penetrating wounds of the heart: Experience with 249 patients. Dis. Chest. 46:1, 1964.
7. Borja, A. R., Lansing, A. M., and Ransdell, H. T., Jr.: Immediate operative treatment for stab wounds of the heart. J. Thorac. Cardiovasc. Surg. 59:662, 1970.
8. Sugg, W. L., Rea, W. J., Ecker, R. R., Webb, W. R., Rose, E. F., and Shaw, R. R.: Penetrating wounds of the heart: An analysis of 459 cases. J. Thorac. Cardiovasc. Surg. 56:4, 1968.
9. Beall, A. C., Jr., Ochsner, J. L., Morris, G. C., Cooley, D. A., and DeBakey, M. E.: Penetrating wounds of the heart. J. Trauma 1:195, 1961.
10. Gonzalez, T. A., Vance, M., Helpern, M., and Umberger, C. J.: Legal Medicine Pathology, and Toxicology. 2nd ed. New York, Appleton-Century-Crofts, 1954.
11. Farringer, J. L., Jr., and Carr, D.: Cardiac tamponade. Ann. Surg. 141:437, 1955.
12. Cooley, D. A., Dunn, J. R., Brockman, H. L., and DeBakey, M. E.: Treatment of penetrating wounds of the heart: Experimental and clinical observations. Surgery 37:882, 1955.
13. Reul, G. J., Maddox, K. L., Beall, A. C., and Jordan, J. L., Jr.: Recent advances in the operative management of massive chest trauma. Ann. Thorac. Surg. 16:52, 1973.
14. Elkin, D. C.: Wounds of the heart. Ann. Surg. 120:817, 1944.
15. Griswold, R. A., and Drye, J. C.: Cardiac wounds. Ann. Surg. 138:783, 1954.
16. Bolanowski, P. J. P., Suaminathan, A. P., and Neville, W. E.: Aggressive surgical management of penetrating cardiac injuries. J. Thorac. Cardiovasc. Surg. 66:52, 1973.
17. Hutchinson, J. E., Schmidt, D. M., Cameron, A., and McCord, C. W.: The surgical management of intracardiac defects due to penetrating trauma. J. Thorac. Cardiovasc. Surg. 65:103, 1973.
18. Pate, J. W., and Richardson, R. L., Jr.: Penetrating wounds of cardiac valves. JAMA 207:309, 1969.
19. Hutchinson, J. E., Beach, P. M., Jr., Kaplan, S., and Garvey, J. W.: Management of penetrating cardiac trauma. N.Y. State J. Med. 71:1932, 1971.
20. Ricks, R. K., Powell, J. F., Beall, A. C., and DeBakey, M. E.: Gunshot wounds of the heart: A review of 31 cases. Surgery 57:787, 1965.
21. Carrasquilla, C., Wilson, R. F., Walt, A. J., and Arbulu, A.: Gunshot wounds of the heart. Ann. Thorac. Surg. 13:208, 1972.
22. Parmley, L. F., Manion, W. C., and Mattingly, T. W.: Nonpenetrating traumatic injury to the heart. Circulation, 18:371, 1958.
23. Bright, E. F., and Beck, C. S.: Nonpenetrating wounds of the heart. A clinical experimental study. Am. Heart. J. 10:293, 1935.
24. Kohn, R. M., Harris, R., and Gorham, L. W.: Atrial rupture of the heart: Report of case following atrial infarction and summary of 79 cases collected from the literature. Circulation 10:221, 1954.
25. Ludington, L. G., Boskind, A. S., and Miquel, A.: Rupture of left ventricle from blunt trauma. Review of literature. Ann. Thorac. Surg. 18:195, 1974.
26. Howard, C. P.: Aortic insufficiency due to rupture by strain of a normal aortic valve. Can. Med. Assoc. J. 19:12, 1928.
27. Leonard, J. J., Harvey, W. P., and Hufnagle, C. A.: Rupture of the aortic valve; therapeutic approach. N. Engl. J. Med. 252:208, 1955.
28. Beall, A. C., and Shirkey, A. L.: Successful surgical correction of traumatic aortic valve regurgitation. JAMA 187:507, 1964.
29. Loop, F. D., Hofmeir, G., and Groves, L. K.: Traumatic disruption of aortic valve. Cleve. Clin. Quart. 38:187, 1971.
30. Tchovsky, T. J., Giuliani, E. R., and Ellis, F. H., Jr.: Prosthetic valve replacement for traumatic tricuspid insufficiency. Am. J. Cardiol. 26:196, 1970.

31. Liu, S. M., Sako, Y., and Alexander, C. S.: Traumatic tricuspid insufficiency. Am. J. Cardiol. 26:200, 1970.
32. DeBakey, M. E., Henly, W. S., Cooley, D. A., Morris, G. C., Jr., Crawford, E. S., and Beall, A. C.: Surgical management of dissecting aneurysms of the aorta. J. Thorac. Cardiovasc. Surg. 49:130, 1965.
33. Wheat, M. W., Jr., and Palmer, R. L.: Dissecting aneurysms of the aorta. Curr. Prob. Surg., 1971.
34. Wheat, M. W., Jr., Harris, P. D., Malm, J. R., Kaiser, G., Bowman, F. O., and Palmer, R. F.: Acute dissecting aneurysm of the aorta. Treatment and results in 64 patients. J. Thorac. Cardiovasc. Surg. 58:344, 1969.
35. Daily, P. O., Trueblood, W. H., Stinson, E. B., Wuerflein, R. D., and Shumway, N. E.: Management of acute aortic dissections. Ann. Thorac. Surg. 10:237, 1970.
36. Liotta, D., Hallman, G. L., Milam, J. D., and Cooley, D. A.: Surgical treatment of acute dissecting aneurysm of the ascending aorta. Ann. Thorac. Surg. 12:582, 1971.
37. McFarland, J., Willerson, J. T., Dinsmore, R. E., Austen, W.G., Buckley, M. J., Sanders, C. A., and DeSanctis, R. W.: The medical treatment of dissecting aortic aneurysms. N. Engl. J. Med. 286:115, 1972.
38. DeBakey, M. A., Henly, W. S., Cooley, B. A., Crawford, E. S., and Morris, G. C., Jr.: Surgical treatment of dissecting aneurysm of the aorta. Circulation 24:290, 1961.
39. Gerbode, F., Kerth, W. J., and Hill, J. D.: Surgical management of tumors of the heart. Surgery 61:94, 1967.
40. Bahl, O. P., Oliver, G. C., Ferguson, T. B., Schad, N., Parker, B. M.: Recurrent left atrial myxoma: Report of a case. Circulation 40:673, 1969.
41. Vakil, R. J.: Preinfarction syndrome—management and follow-up. Am. J. Cardiol. 14:55, 1964.
42. Krauss, K. R., Hutter, A. M., Jr., and DeSanctis, R. W.: Acute coronary insufficiency. Circulation 45–46(Suppl. I):66, 1972.
43. Levy, H.: The natural history of changing patterns of angina pectoris. Arch. Intern. Med. 44:1123, 1956.
44. Thomas, C. S., Jr., Alford, W. C., Jr., Burrus, G. R., and Stoney, W. S.: Aorta-to-coronary artery bypass grafting. Ann. Thorac. Surg. 16:201, 1973.
45. Wilson, W. S.: Aortocoronary bypass—State of the art 1974. Cardiovasc. Dis. Bull. Texas Heart Inst. 1:270, 1974.
46. Prinzmetal, M., Ekmekci, A., Kennamer, R., Kwoczynshi, J. K., Shubin, H., and Toyoshima, H.: Variant form of angina pectoris. JAMA 174:1794, 1960.
47. Prinzmetal, M., Kennamer, R., Merlis, R., Wada, T., and Bor, N.: Angina pectoris: I. A variant form of angina pectoris. Am. J. Med. 27:375, 1959.
48. Pifarre, R., Spinazzola, A., Nemickas, R., Scanlon, P. J., and Tobin, J. R.: Emergency aortocoronary bypass for acute myocardial infarction. Arch. Surg. 103:525, 1971.
49. Smullens, S. N., Wiener, L., Kasparian, H., et al.: Evaluation and surgical management of acute evolving myocardial infarction. J. Thorac. Cardiovasc. Surg. 64:495, 1972.
50. Fischl, S. J., Herman, M. V., and Gorlin, R.: The intermediate coronary syndrome—clinical, angiographic, and therapeutic aspects. N. Engl. J. Med. 288:1193, 1973.
51. Cheavechai, C., Effler, D. B., Loop, F. D., et al.: Emergency myocardial revascularization. Am. J. Cardiol. 32:907, 1973.
52. Cohn, L. H., Gorlin, R., Herman, M. V., et al.: Aortocoronary bypass for acute coronary occlusion. J. Thorac. Cardiovasc. Surg. 64:503, 1972.
53. Dawson, J. T., Hall, R. J., Hallman, G. L., et al.: Mortality of coronary artery bypass after previous myocardial infarction. Am. J. Cardiol. 31:128, 1973.

54. Kaiser, G. C., Barner, H. B., Williams, V. L., et al.: Aortocoronary bypass grafting. Arch. Surg. 105:319, 1972.
55. Reul, G. J., Morris, G. C., Howell, J. F., et al.: Current concepts in coronary artery surgery. Ann. Thorac. Surg. 14:243, 1972.
56. Weiner, L., Kasparian, H., Brest, A., and Templeton, J.: Surgical management of acute evolving myocardial infarction. A metabolic and angiographic profile. Am. J. Cardiol. 29:296, 1973. (Abstr.)
57. Cohen, M. V., Cohn, P. D., Herman, M. C., and Gorlin, R.: Diagnosis and prognosis of main left coronary artery obstruction. Circulation 45–46(Suppl. I):57, 1972.
58. Oldham, H. N., Jr., Kong, Y., Bartell, A. G., Morris, J. J., Jr., Behar, V. S., Peter, R. H., Young, G., Jr., and Sabiston, D. C., Jr.: Risk factors in coronary artery bypass surgery. Arch. Surg. 105:918, 1972.
59. Zeft, H. J., Manley, J. C., Huston, J. H., Tector, A. C., and Johnson, W. D.: Direct coronary surgery in patients with left main coronary artery stenosis. Circulation 45–46(Suppl. II): 50, 1972 (Abstr.).
60. Pell, S., and Alonzo, C. A.: Immediate mortality and five year survival of employed men with a first myocardial infarction. N. Engl. J. Med. 270:915, 1964.
61. Schlicter, J., Hellerstein, H. K., and Katz, L. N.: Aneurysm of the heart. Correlative study of 102 proved cases. Medicine 33:43, 1954.
62. Najafi, H., Hunter, J. H., Dye, W. S., Javid, H., Ardakani, R. C., and Julian, O. C.: Emergency left ventricular aneurysmectomy for dying patients. J. Thorac. Cardiovasc. Surg. 10:419, 1969.
63. Ritter, E. R.: Intractable ventricular tachycardia due to ventricular aneurysm with surgical cure. Ann. Intern. Med. 71:1155, 1969.
64. Maloy, W. C., Arrants, J. E., Sowell, B. F., and Hendrix, G. H.: Left ventricular aneurysm of uncertain etiology with recurrent ventricular arrhythmias. N. Engl. J. Med. 255:262, 1971.
65. Meister, S. G., and Helfant, R. H.: Rapid bedside differentiation of ruptured interventricular septum from acute mitral insufficiency. N. Engl. J. Med. 287:1024, 1972.
66. Giuliani, E. R., Danielson, G. K., Pluth, J. R., Odyneic, N. A., and Wallace, R. B.: Postinfarction ventricular septal rupture. Surgical considerations and results. Circulation 49:455, 1974.
67. Austen, W. G., Sanders, C. A., Aberill, J. H., and Friedlich, A. L.: Ruptured papillary muscle: Report of a case with successful mitral valve replacement. Circulation 32:597, 1965.
68. Mundth, E. D., Buckley, M. J., Leinbach, R. C., Gold, H. K., Daggett, W. M., and Austen, W. G.: Surgical intervention for the complications of acute myocardial ischemia. Ann. Surg. 178:379, 1973.
69. Sealy, W. C., Wallace, A. J., Ramming, K. R., Gallagher, J. J., and Swenson, R. H.: An improved operation for the definitive treatment of the Wolff-Parkinson-White Syndrome. Ann. Thorac. Surg. 17:107, 1974.
70. Sealy, W. C., and Wallace, A. G.: The surgical treatment of the Wolff-Parkinson-White Syndrome. Ann. Thorac. Surg. 17:107, 1974.
71. Lloyd, R., Okada, R., Stagg, J., Anderson, R., Brock, H., and Marcus, F.: The treatment of recurrent ventricular tachycardia with bilateral cervicothoracic sympathetic-ganglionectomy: Report of two cases. Circulation 50:382, 1974.
72. Rashkind, W., Waldhausen, J., Miller, W., and Friedman, S.: Palliative treatment in tricuspid atresia. Combined balloon artioseptostomy and surgical alteration of pulmonary blood flow. J. Thorac. Cardiovas. Surg. 57:812, 1969.
73. Bonchek, L. I., and Starr, A.: Total correction of transposition of the great arteries in infancy as initial surgical management. Ann. Thorac. Surg. 14:376, 1972.

INDEX

Page numbers in *italics* refer to illustration; page numbers followed by t, to tables.